Metabolism and Action of Anti-cancer Drugs

Metabolism and Action of Anti-cancer Drugs

Edited by
Garth Powis
Mayo Clinic, Rochester, MN

and **Russell A. Prough**
University of Louisville, KY

Taylor & Francis
London, New York and Philadelphia
1987

UK Taylor & Francis Ltd, 4 John St., London WC1N 2ET

USA Taylor & Francis Inc., 242 Cherry St., Philadelphia, PA 19106–1906

British Library Cataloguing in Publication Data

Metabolism and action of anti-cancer drugs.
1. Cancer—Chemotherapy 2. Antineoplastic agents
I. Powis, Garth II. Prough, Russell A.
615′.7 RC271.C5

ISBN 0-85066-369-5

Library of Congress Cataloging-in-Publication Data

Metabolism and action of anti-cancer drugs.

Includes bibliographies and index.
1. Antineoplastic agents—Metabolism.
2. Antineoplastic agents—Physiological effect.
I. Powis, Garth. II. Prough, Russell A. [DNLM:
1. Antineoplastic Agents—metabolism. 2. Antineoplastic Agents—pharmacodynamics. QV 269 M587]
RC271.C5M47 1987 616.99′4061 86.23179
ISBN 0-85066-369-5

Typeset by Mathematical Composition Setters Ltd, Salisbury, UK
Printed and bound by Taylor & Francis (Printers) Ltd, Rankine Rd, Basingstoke, Hants.

Contents

Prologue

The use of cytotoxic chemicals in the treatment of neoplastic diseases has become a standard practice for the clinical oncologist. The discovery of most of these agents came more by trial-and-error than by rational design and only recently have the metabolism and underlying biochemical mechanisms of action become clear for some of these agents. Success in the application of these agents in cancer treatment spurs our continued interest in these drugs. It is hoped that the various chapters of this book will provide new insights into our understanding of the metabolism and action of these drugs. It is assumed that increased understanding of these two facets of the nature of these drugs might provide better treatment regimens for cancer in the human population.

In planning the book, the Editors sought major researchers involved in the study of the metabolism of cancer chemotherapeutic agents to provide a new look at these agents and their use. Each chapter gives a short history of the agent, together with a brief account of their clinical uses and a detailed review of these agents' metabolism and chemical reactions. The central issues of how metabolism relates to biological activity are stressed in each presentation. Finally, future directions for work on the mechanism of action of the agents and application of this information to cancer therapy are considered.

The first three chapters are concerned with the metabolism and action of alkylating agents. These include the oxazaphosphorines, including the widely used agent cyclophosphamide; 2-chloroethylnitrosoureas, of which there are a number of clinically used examples; and the lone therapeutic alkylhydrazine, procarbazine. Representatives of these classes of drugs have been studied for over two decades and there is a large amount of information available on their chemical reactivities and metabolism. Only now can we begin to understand the complex interrelation between the metabolism, transport and the biological effects of these drugs.

The next two chapters deal with the metabolism of antimetabolites. Folic acid antagonists are among the oldest of the commonly used anti-cancer agents, although their complex metabolism has only recently been appreciated. Purine and pyrimidine antimetabolites are a class of anti-cancer agents whose activity is dependent on metabolic activation. The major pathways of metabolism of purine and pyrimidine antimetabolites are well established, although the modes of action of the agents may be highly complex. Recent attempts have been made to improve the selectivity of the purine and pyrimidine antimetabolites by careful biochemical modulation of the therapeutic activity of individual agents in drug combination. It remains to be seen whether this rational approach will yield improved benefit to patients over the classical empirical approach to combination therapy.

The platinum coordination compounds are a relatively new class of anti-cancer agents. They are not metabolized in the true biochemical sense, but undergo extensive ligand displacement reactions with biological nucleophiles. These reactions probably are responsible for much of their biological activity. The next section of the book includes two chapters which deal with the metabolism of the antibiotic anti-tumour agents, bleomycin and the anthracyclines. Recent evidence suggests that metabolism may be important for the toxicity of bleomycin to normal tissues, although its relationship to anti-tumour activity is not clear. The anthracycline antibiotics undergo numerous metabolic conversions including the intriguing ability to form organic free radicals. Whether free radical formation can explain the biological activity of the anthracyclines, as has been suggested by many workers, remains to be established.

In a separate chapter, the anti-steroidal agents are shown to be a widely used class of anti-cancer agents that undergo their own special type of metabolic conversion and the possible relationship between their metabolism and biological activity is considered. Cancer chemotherapy is a continually evolving area and the last chapter of the book considers the metabolism of some new and different agents that are currently in clinical development. Although they demonstrate unique activities, their application will require continued testing and study to understand their use as anti-cancer drugs.

We trust that this book will provide an up-to-date account of the mode of action of these agents. It is hoped that the chapters will stimulate refinement of cancer treatment by providing a well documented reference text related to the metabolism and action of the commonly used anti-cancer drugs. It has not been the goal of the authors to document exhaustively all of the work in the field during the preparation of these chapters, but to provide a focus on the mechanism of action of the drugs and to point to how the compounds might be optimally utilized in the treatment of human malignancies.

G. Powis
R. A. Prough
August 1986

Contributors

Matthew M. Ames
Department of Oncology,
Mayo Clinic,
200 First Street, S. W.,
Rochester, MN 55905

Richard F. Borch
Department of Pharmacology,
University of Rochester,
Rochester, NY 14642

Andrew E. Filderman
Department of Medicine,
Yale University School of Medicine
333 Cedar Street,
New Haven, CT 06510

V. Craig Jordan
Department of Human Oncology,
University of Wisconsin Clinical Cancer Center,
600 Highland Avenue,
Madison, WI 53792

Barton A. Kamen
Department of Pediatrics,
Southwestern Medical School,
The University of Texas Health Science Center at Dallas,
5323 Harry Hines Boulevard,
Dallas, TX 75235

John S. Lazo
Department of Pharmacology,
Yale University School of Medicine,
333 Cedar Street,
New Haven, CT 06510

Daniel S. Martin
St. Anthony's Hospital, 89/15,
Woodhaven Boulevard,
Woodhaven, NY 11421

Garth Powis
Department of Pharmacology,
Mayo Clinic,
200 First Street, S.W.,
Rochester, MN 55905

Russell A. Prough
Department of Biochemistry
University of Louisville School of Medicine,
Louisville, KY 40292

Donald J. Reed
Department of Biochemistry and Biophysics,
Oregon State University
Corvallis, OR 97331

Simon P. Robinson
Department of Human Oncology,
University of Wisconsin Clinical Cancer Center,
600 Highland Avenue,
Madison, WI 53792

Said M. Sebti
Department of Pharmacology
Yale University School of Medicine,
333 Cedar Street,
New Haven, CT 06510

Norman E. Sladek
Department of Pharmacology,
3-260 Millard Hall,
University of Minnesota,
Minneapolis, MN 55455

Donald J. Tweedie
Department of Biochemistry
University of Louisville School of Medicine,
Louisville, KY 40292

Abbreviations

ACNU	1-(2-chloroethyl)-3-(4-amino-2-methylpyrimidine-5-yl)methyl-1-nitrosourea
ACTH	adrenocorticotrophic hormone
AD32	*N*-trifluoroacetyl doxorubicin 14-valerate
AICAR	5-aminoimidazole-4-carboxamide ribotide
ALD	*N*-isopropyl-*p*-formylbenzamide (benzaldehyde)
ALL	acute lymphoblastic leukaemia
6-AN	6-aminonicotinamide
APRTase	adenine phosphoribosyltransferase
Ara-C	cytosine arabinoside
A-TDA	2-ethylamino-1,3,4-thiadiazole
AUC	area under the serum concentration curve
Azo	*N*-isopropyl-α-(2-methylazo)-*p*-toluamide (azo procarbazine)
Azoxy I	*N*-isopropyl-α-(2-methyl-*NNO*-azoxy)-*p*-toluamide
Azoxy II	*N*-isopropyl-α-(2-methyl-*ONN*-azoxy)-*p*-toluamide
AZQ	diaziquone (aziridinylbenzoquinone or NSC 182986)
BCNU	1,3-bis(2-chloroethyl)-1-nitrosourea
BLM	bleomycin
BSO	buthionine sulphoximine
BUN	blood urea nitrogen
CCNU	1-(2-chloroethyl)-3-cyclohexyl-1-nitrosourea
CENUs	2-chloroethylnitrosoureas
Cisplatin	*cis*-diamminedichloroplatinum (II) or Peyrone's chloride
CNS	central nervous system
CPS II	carbamoyl phosphate synthase (cytosolic)
CR	clearance ratio
CSF	cerebrospinal fluid
CV	Covalent binding
DDTC	diethyldithiocarbamate
DHFR	dihydrofolate reductase
DHO	dihydroorotate oxidase or dehydrogenase
DMPO	dimethyl-1-pyrroline-1-oxide
dR-1-P	deoxyribose-1-phosphate

E^1	reduction potential
ENU	1-ethyl-1-nitrosourea
EPP	ethylphenyl(2-formylethyl)phosphinate, aldehyde dehydrogenase inhibitor
ESR	elecron spin resonance
F-ara-AMP	fludarabine phosphate (9-β-D-arabinofuranosyl-2-fluoroadenine 5′-monophosphate)
FdUDP	5-fluoro-2′-deoxyuridine 5′-diphosphate
FdUMP	5-fluoro-2′-deoxyuridine 5′-monophosphate
FdUTP	5-fluoro-2′-deoxyuridine 5′-triphosphate
Fe(II)	ferrous iron
Fe(III)	ferric iron
FUDP	5-fluorouridine diphosphate
FUdR	5-fluoro-2′-deoxyuridine
FUMP	5-fluorouridine monophosphate
FUR	5-fluorouridine
FUra	5-fluorouracil
FUTP	5-fluorouridine triphosphate
GANU	1-(2-chloroethyl)-3-(β-D-glucopyranosyl)-1-nitrosourea
GAR	glycinamide ribonucleotide
GTN	gestational trophoblastic neoplasms
HDMTX	high dose methotrexate
HECNU	1-(2-chloroethyl)-1-nitroso-3-(2-hydroxyethyl)urea
HGPRTase	hypoxanthine guanosine phosphoribosyltransferase
7OHMTX	7-hydroxymethotrexate
HPLC	High performance liquid chromatography
Hydrazone	*N*-isopropyl-*p*-formylbenzamide methylhydrazone
IMP	iosine 5′-monophosphate or inosinic acid
LD_{10}	dose in mice to produce 10% lethality
LH	luteinizing hormone
LHRH	luteinizing hormone releasing hormone
LV	leucovorin or 5-formyltetrahydrofolate (citrovorum factor)
MAO	monoamine oxidase
MeCCNU	1-(2-chloroethyl)-3-(*trans*-4-methylcyclohexyl)-1-nitrosourea or methylCCNU
MELD-10	mouse equivalent LD_{10} in dog
Melphalan	cyclophosphamide
5,10-MeTHF	N_5,N_{10}-methylene tetrahydrofolate
MHE	*N*-2-methyl-9-hydroxyellipticine
MMPR	6-methylmercaptopurine ribonucleoside
MMPR-P	6-methylmercaptopurine ribonucleoside 5′-phosphate
MOPP	Combination therapy consisting of Mechlorethamine (nitrogen mustard), Oncovin (vincristine), procarbazine, and prednisolone

6-MP	6-mercaptopurine
MRA-CN	3′-deamino-3′-(3″-cyano-4″-morpholinyl)doxorubicin
MTD	maximal tolerated dose
MTX	methotrexate
MTX-PG	methotrexate polyglutamates
OMP	orotidine-5′-phosphate
OPRTase	orotate phosphoribosyltransferase
Orimeten	*p*-aminoglutethimide
P-450	cytochrome P-450
PAH	polycyclic aromatic hydrocarbons
PALA	*N*-(phosphonacetyl)-L-aspartate
PB	phenobarbital
PCNU	1-(2-chloroethyl)-3-(2,6-dioxo-3-piperidyl)-1-nitrosourea
PCV	combination therapy consisting of procarbazine, CCNU, and vincristine
PMR	proton magnetic resonance
PRPP	5-phosphoribosylpyrophosphate
PRTase	phosphoribosyltransferase
Q	quinone
$Q^{\cdot}$	semiquinone
QH_2	hydroquinone
SCEs	sister-chromatid exchanges
SKF 525A	diethylaminoethyl 2,2-diphenylvalerate hydrochloride
SL-CNU	1-(2-chloroethyl)-3-(1-oxyl-2,2,6,6-tetramethylpiperidinyl)-1-nitrosourea
TAC (acid)	*N*-isopropylterephthalamic acid
TS	thymidylate synthetase
6-TG	6-thioguanine
6-thio-IMP	6-thioinosate, MPRP, or 6-thio-IMP
6-thioGMP	6-thioguanylate
TXMP	6-thioxanthylate
UdR	deoxyuridine
UR	uridine

1. 2-Chloroethylnitrosoureas

Donald J. Reed

Historical background

The Cancer Chemotherapy National Service Center screening program provided the initial interest and resources for the development of *N*-nitrosoureas as anti-tumour drugs. 1-Methyl-3-nitro-1-nitrosoguanidine was found to increase the life-span of mice implanted intraperitoneally with leukaemia L1210 cells. Investigators at the Southern Research Institute observed that 1-methyl-1-nitrosourea was an even more effective agent against L1210 cells (Johnston *et al.*, 1963). They subsequently initiated a programme which has resulted in the synthesis and testing of hundreds of *N*-nitrosoureas. The congeners of major importance are those containing a 2-chloroethyl moiety on the nitrogen atom attached to the nitroso group. Three drugs emerged and underwent intense testing: 1,3-bis(2-chloroethyl)-1-nitrosourea (BCNU); 1-(2-chloroethyl)-3-cyclohexyl-1-nitrosourea (CCNU); and 1-(2-chloroethyl)-3-(*trans*-4-methylcyclohexyl)-1-nitrosourea (methyl CCNU). Because of the ability of these lipophilic drugs to cross the blood–brain barrier and to be effective against solid tumours (including brain tumours), as well as leukaemias, great interest developed in their clinical efficacy. A large body of literature exists from over 20 years of study of these and of other nitrosoureas. The National Cancer Institute considers nitrosoureas to be one of the most important classes of anti-tumour agents developed by the Cancer Chemotherapy Program (Carter *et al.*, 1972). The structures of many of the 2-chloroethylnitrosoureas (CENUs) are shown in Table 1.

Clinical uses

Recent clinical uses of the CENUs that have been reported in the literature and described in Table 2 include combination therapy such as PCV (Procarbazine, CCNU and vincristine) via intracarotid administration for brain tumours (Brufman *et al.*, 1984) and BCNU, cisplatin and VM-26 (Stewart *et al.*, 1984). A major study has been completed on the treatment of malignant gliomas with

Table 1. Nitrosoureas and certain of their metabolites.

Code	Compound	R− = NH−C(=O)−N(NO)−CH_2−CH_2−Cl
BCNU NSC 409962	1,3-Bis(2-chloroethyl)-1-nitrosourea	R−CH_2−CH_2−Cl
CCNU NSC 79037	1-(2-Chloroethyl)-3-cyclohexyl-1-nitrosourea	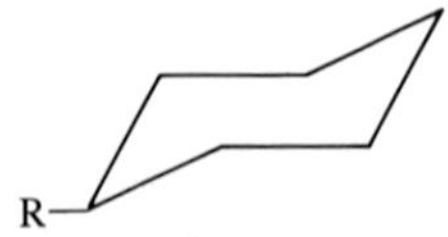
trans-2-hydroxy CCNU NSC 253947	1-(2-Chloroethyl)-3-*trans*-2-hydroxycyclohexyl)-1-nitrosourea	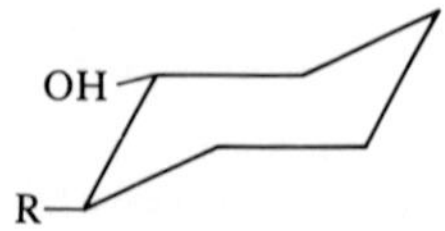
Me CCNU NSC 95441	1-(2-Chloroethyl)-3-(*trans*-4-methylcyclohexyl)-1-nitrosourea	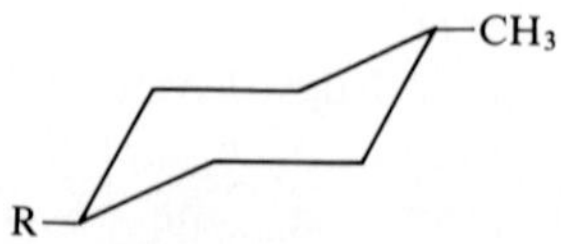
Chlorozotocin NSC 178248	1-(2-Chloroethyl)-3-(D-2-glucopyranosyl)-1-nitrosourea	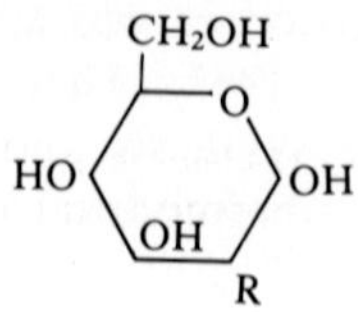
cis-Acid NSC 153174	1-(2-Chloroethyl)-3-(4-*cis*-carboxycyclohexyl)-1-nitrosourea	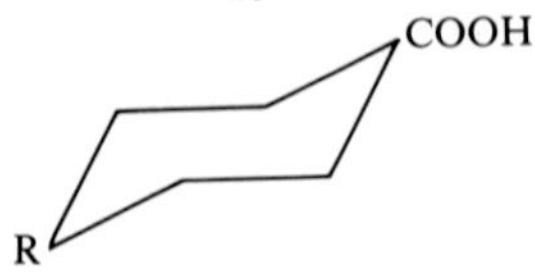
MCNU	1-(2-Chloroethyl)-3-(methyl-α-D-glucopyranose-6-yl)-1-nitrosourea	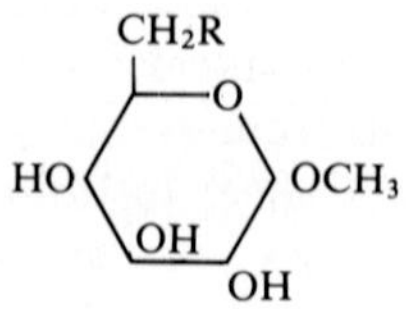
TA-077	1-(2-Chloroethyl)-3-isobutyl-3-(β-maltosyl)-1-nitrosourea	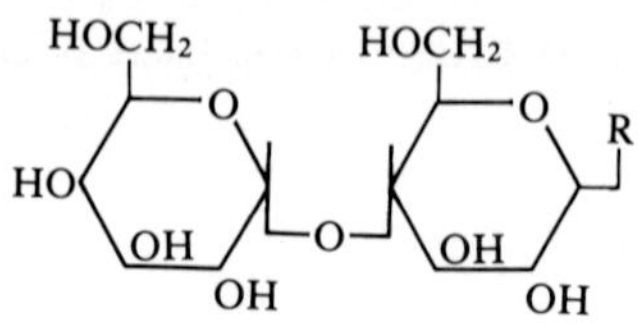
GANU NSC D 254157	1-(2-Chloroethyl)-3-(β-D-glucopyranosyl)-1-nitrosourea	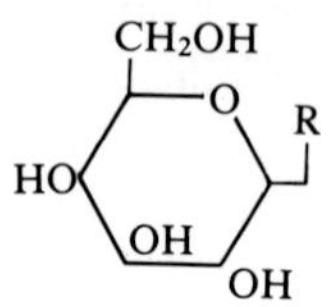

Table 1. (Continued)

Code	Compound	R— = NH—C(=O)—N(NO)—CH_2—CH_2—Cl
ACNU	1-(2-Chloroethyl)-3-(4-amino-2-methylpyrimidine-5-yl) methyl-1-nitrosourea	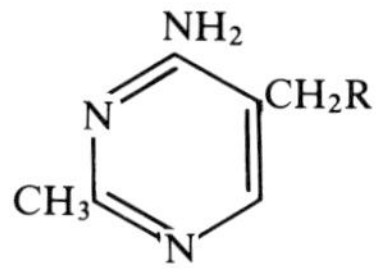
HECNU NSC 294895	1-(2-Chloroethyl)-3-(2-hydroxy-ethyl-1-nitrosourea	R—CH_2—CH_2OH
CNCC 1.C.1.G.1325	*N*,*N'*-Bis [*N*-(2-chloroethyl)-*N*-nitrosocarbonyl] cystamine	S—CH_2—CH_2—R | S—CH_2—CH_2—R
RPCNU 1.C.1.G.1163	1-(2-Chloroethyl)-3-(2,3,4-triacetyl-1-ribopyranosyl)-1-nitrosourea	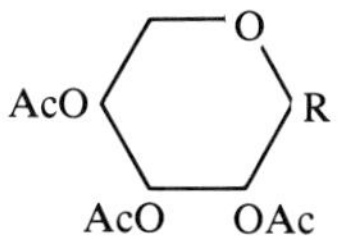
RFCNU 1.C.1.G.1105	1-(2-Chloroethyl)-3-[2,3-isopropylidene 5-(nitro-4-benzoyl)-1-ribofuranosyl]-1-nitrosourea	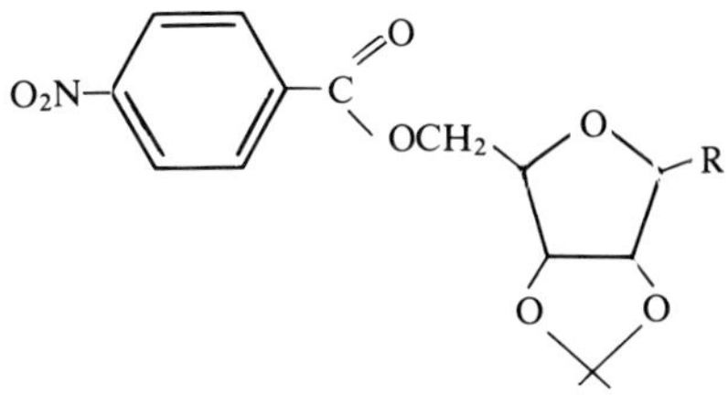

Code	Compound	R = Bisnitrosourea
BCyNU NSC-80590	1,3-Bis(cyclohexyl)-1-nitrosourea	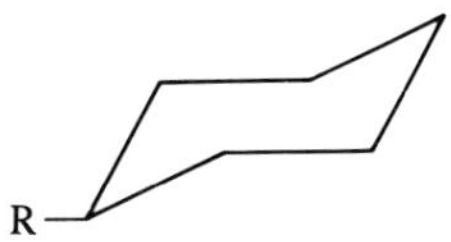
trans-4-Hydroxy BCyNU NSC-305715	1,3-Bis(*trans*-4-hydroxycyclo-hexyl)-1-nitrosourea	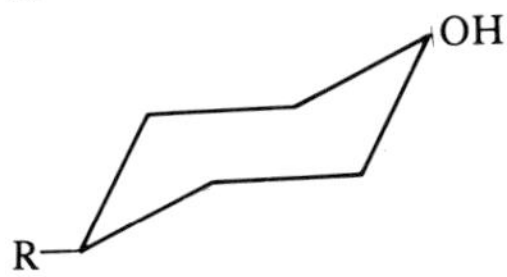
cis-4-Carboxyl BCyNU NSC-305716	1,3-Bis(*cis*-4-carboxylcyclo-hexyl)-1-nitrosourea	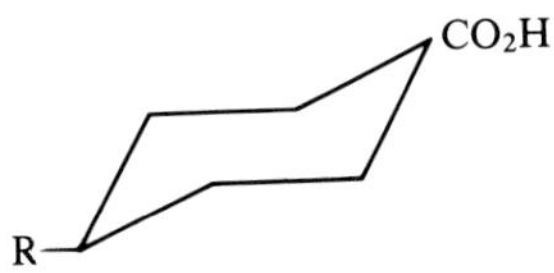

Table 2. Some recent clinical trials.

Treatment	Type of tumour	Patient number	Number of patients responding	Mean duration	Mean survival	Reference
Procarbazine + CCNU + vincristine (PCV)	Brain	12	3—	9.3 months Responders Non-responders	 11.7 months 3.6 months	Brufman *et al.* (1984)
	Metastatic brain	1	Partial response—lymphoma of the brain			
5-Fluorouracil and CCNU followed by hydroxyurea, misonidazole (5500 rads)	Brain stem gliomas	28 Children	Disease free	32 weeks 44 weeks		Levin *et al.* (1984)
BCNU- intra-arterial (internal carotid artery) with absorbent resin cartridge in ipsilateral jugular drainage	Cerebral gliomas	4	Calculated pharmacokinetic advantage (brain:body exposure ratio) was between 21 and 55:1 when the combined treatment was used			Oldfield *et al.* (1985)
BCNU Intraarterial one month after postoperative radiotherapy repeated every 8–10 weeks	Malignant gliomas	10	Higher anti-tumour activity as compared to intravenous BCNU therapy			Safdari (1985)
Three courses		4				
Two courses		6				
BCNU cisplatin VM-26 combination via intracarotid administration	Intracranial Primary or metastatic tumours	37 13				Stewart *et al.* (1984)

ACNU every 4–6 weeks intravenous 2–3 courses	Advanced colorectal cancer	46	One complete remission three partial remissions	Fiebig *et al.* (1984)
	(distant metastases)	37		
	(Unresectable primary tumour)	6		
	Colon	24		
	Rectal	19		
	(prior anticancer drug treatment)	34		
	(nitrosourea pretreatment)	11		
BCNU and PALA	Advanced large bowel carcinoma (advanced metastatic colorectal carcinoma)	30	1 partial response for 3 month's duration.	Rubin *et al.* (1984)
	(no prior chemotherapy)	15		
	(one or more cytotoxic agents)	15		
PCNU	Small cell carcinoma	19	One patient had a minor response. No major.	Chapman *et al.* (1984)
			Median time to tumour progression (weeks): BCNU / PVV	
BCNU or combination of procarbazine, CCNU and vincristine (PCV) administered after radiotherapy with hydroxyurea.	Malignant gliomas (glioblastoma multiforme)	76	BCNU 32, 40*; PVV 31, 70*	Levin *et al.* (1985a)
	(Other analplastic Gliomas)	72	BCNU 77; PVV 123	

*25th percentile times to progression.

PCV which has administered after radiotherapy accompanied by hydroxyurea treatment (Levin *et al.*, 1985a). Trials have been underway with BCNU monochemotherapy by intra-arterial administration after post-operative radiotherapy for malignant gliomas (Safdari *et al.*, 1985). Higher doses of BCNU have been possible in the treatment of cerebral gliomas by internal carotid artery administration in combination with an adsorbent resin cartridge placed in the ipsilateral jugular drainage (Oldfield *et al.*, 1985). In this manner, malignant gliomas have been treated with intensive BCNU monochemotherapy and autologous marrow transplantation with 36 patients (Phillips *et al.*, 1986). Twelve of the 27 patients with progressive disease responded; two remain disease-free 84 and 60 months after BCNU treatment. Three patients of nine in the adjuvant therapy group (nine without progression) remain progression-free at 70, 48, and 27 months after BCNU therapy. These results are considered encouraging as they surpass the results with conventional therapy (Oldfield *et al.*, 1985). Children with brain stem gliomas have been treated with 5-fluorouracil and CCNU followed by hydroxyurea, misonidazole and irradiation (Levin *et al.*, 1984).

Structural features

Many CENUs have been synthesized and the variety of congeners is indicated in Table 1. Prominent infrared absorption bands in the carbonyl-stretching region (1620–1750 cm^{-1}) characterize the nitrosoureas. Nitrosation of urea functions was found to cause consistently a shift toward higher wavenumbers in the carbonyl region (Johnston *et al.*, 1963). Nitroso isomer identification has been established by proton magnetic resonance (PMR) spectroscopy by demonstrating a spectral symmetry of the $ClCH_2CH_2N(NO)$ group (A_2B_2 system) (Johnston *et al.*, 1966; Machinami *et al.*, 1975). Mass spectral fragmentation patterns have been shown to be very useful in establishing nitroso isomer identification (May *et al.*, 1975, 1979). Ultraviolet (UV) absorbance at about 230 nm provides a means of detection and quantitation of nitrosoureas. Quantitation by HPLC at nanomole levels is made possible with sensitive UV flow detectors (May *et al.*, 1975, 1979). An elegant analytical method based on stable isotope dilution analysis and mass spectrometry has been described for BCNU (Weinkam *et al.*, 1978).

Decomposition of 2-chloroethylnitrosoureas in aqueous solution is spontaneous and dependent on pH, buffer and temperature. Typical decomposition rates afford a range of half-lives from 46 min for chlorozotocin (Montgomery, 1976) to 70 min for methyl CCNU (Reed *et al.*, 1975). Isocyanate formation during nitrosourea degradation was established in early studies (Garrett *et al.*, 1965). Alkylating species were observed indirectly with the nitrobenzylpyridine assay method (Wheeler and Chumley, 1967). Vinyl carbonium ions were suggested as the alkylating species from BCNU (Montgomery *et al.*, 1967). However, Reed and co-workers (1975) examined in detail the decomposition of CCNU and methyl CCNU at pH 7·4 in phosphate buffer and found the major alkylating species to be capable of 2-chloroethylation. 2-Chloroethanol is a major decomposition product with small amounts of acetaldehyde, vinyl chloride and ethylene. At the same time, Colvin *et al.* (1974) concluded that BCNU decomposition produced primarily a chloroethylcarbonium ion intermediate as the alkylating species. Dependence on pH was later noted for the difference in degradation products, with low pH producing acetaldehyde, whereas neutral pH produces greatly enhanced quantities of 2-chloroethanol (Montgomery *et al.*, 1975).

Recent studies illustrate the complexity of the degradation events of the 2-chloroethylnitrosoureas. Lown and Chauhan (1981) described the synthesis of three 2-(alkylimino)-3-nitrosooxazolidines that correspond to degradation intermediates of BCNU, CCNU and methyl CCNU. These intermediates are proposed to be formed via a minor pathway of degradation, yet may account in part for the 2-hydroxyethylated nucleoside products reported by other workers. The appropriateness of chloride ion as a leaving group for 2-chloroethylnitrosoureas has been discussed in terms of an effective chemical compromise in reactivity. Chloride leaving group ability is low enough to not favour competing pathways of nitrosourea degradation involving oxadiazoline, imino-*N*-nitrosooxazolidinones, or hybrid migrations which can limit 2-chloroethyl alkylations. Yet after chloroethylation, labilization of the chloride and production of inter-strand cross-links can occur. It appears that the probability of cross-linking events is maximized with chloroethylation compared to other haloethylation (Kohn, 1977). Interestingly, FCCNU, which contains a decafluorocyclohexyl ring, rapidly converts to the corresponding 1-(1*H*-decafluorocyclohexyl)-3-nitrosoimidazolidin-2-one by chloride being a leaving group (Foster *et al.*, 1980). CCNU did not form a detectable quantity of the imidazolidine derivative, which suggests that a decafluorocyclohexyl moiety enhances the nucleophilicity of the N-3 nitrogen atom to facilitate the cyclization and the loss of chloride ion (Foster *et al.*, 1980).

Brundrett (1980) has found evidence for the intermediacy of 4,5-dihydro-1,2,3-oxadiazole in BCNU decomposition. Formation of ethylene glycol as a degradation product of BCNU was noted. He concluded that its formation is best explained by an oxadiazole intermediate. Again this intermediate is thought to play only a minor role in the decomposition of BCNU at physiological pH and to have little or no anti-tumour activity (Brundrett, 1980).

Efforts to utilize 2-chloroethylnitrosoureas for the treatment of solid tumours have led to the development of CENUs that could undergo preferential bioreductive activation in hypoxic tumours. Two of these agents are 3,3′-bis-[*N*-(2-chloroethyl)-*N*-nitrosocarbamoyl]propyl disulphide (Lown *et al.*, 1980) and a mixture of dinitrosated derivatives of *N*,*N*′-bis-[*N*-(2-chloroethyl)-*N*-carbamoyl]cystamine (CNCC-(D)) which contains a mixture of three dinitrosated isomers (CNCC-(C), (S), and (M)) (Imbach *et al.*, 1981).

N-Me cis-CCNU, which is a nitrosourea that is incapable of the facile decomposition that characterizes the clinically useful nitrosoureas, has latent activity against an experimental solid tumour (Johnston *et al.*, 1984 a). Prior studies had suggested activation via enzymatic demethylation of fully substituted congeners as the basis for the latent activity. An important property of N-Me cis-CCNU is solubility in cold phosphate buffer with a half-life at pH 7·4 of 4·2 h (Johnston *et al.*, 1984 a).

Other new analogues of CENUs that are water-soluble such as 1-(2-chloroethyl)-1-nitroso-3-(2-hydroxyethyl)urea (HECNU) are more effective anti-tumour agents in most model systems than are the clinically used compounds such as BCNU or chlorozotocin, according to preclinical studies. In this regard, HECNU was less toxic and less carcinogenic, and these differences were supported by its carbamoylating and alkylating potential, and glutathione reductase inhibition that did not parallel either its anti-tumour effectiveness or its chronic toxicity or carcinogenic potential (Eisenbrand, 1984). Thus HECNU and other CENUs with higher anti-tumour activity in preclinical trials also display a higher potential for DNA–DNA inter-strand cross-link *in vivo* (Eisenbrand, 1984). More recently, several CENU analogues of 2′-deoxyuridine and 2′-deoxy-5-fluorouridine have been synthesized and tested for anti-tumour activity (Lin *et al.*, 1986). 3′-CTNU was found to be three times more potent than BCNU in the inhibition of L1210 leukaemia cells in culture. Possibly of greater interest, pyrimidine deoxyribonucleosides such as thymidine, 2′-deoxyuridine and 2′-deoxycytidine specifically prevent the inhibitory effects of the thymidine CENU, 3′-CTNU which produced "cures" in animal tests (Lin *et al.*, 1986) and 3′-CdUNU and 3′-CFdUNU which produced 90% and 60% "cures" (survival > 60 days), respectively, when administered to mice bearing L1210 cells (Lin *et al.*, 1986).

Weinkam and Dolan (1983) have compared the physical, chemical and kinetic parameters of five different CENUs in terms of the toxic effects on the growth of cultured P388 cells. They conclude that since the CENUs tested have the same activity at the cellular level, the difference in activity *in vivo* may be explained by differences in biodistribution (Weinkam and Dolan, 1983).

Because alterations of the "carrier" moiety of CENUs affect both their physical and chemical properties, a major effort has been expended on nitrosourea derivatives containing a glucose carrier. TA-077 (1-(2-chloroethyl)-3-isobutyl-3-(β-maltosyl)-1-nitrosourea) is disubstituted at the N-3 position and upon activation does not produce an isocyanate moiety for carbamoylation. Evidence of toxicity of TA-077 in BDF_1 mice indicates that it is a suitable drug for consecutive administration, in part because of the lack of toxicity associated with carbamoylation reactions (Fujimoto and Ogawa, 1985).

Interesting new additions to the CENUs are the spin-labelled nitrosourea, 1-(2-chloroethyl)-3-(1-oxyl-2,2,6,6-tetramethylpiperidinyl)-1-nitrosourea (SL-CNU), and several of its analogues (Sosnovsky and Li, 1985). At equal molar doses, or at doses of equal toxicity level, SLCNU was found to be more active than CCNU.

The anti-cancer activity of several *N*-(2-fluoroethyl)-*N*-nitrosoureas has been determined, and a dihydroxycyclohexyl derivative was found to be the most effective (Johnston *et al.*, 1984 b).

A main feature of the CENUs is that the chemistry of the nitrosoureas is complex and new degradation products and metabolites continue to be identified. New pathways illustrate the steps that may occur in the formation of these degradation and metabolic products. Some products are very reactive intermediates that appear to be essential for the biological effects of the nitrosoureas by mechanisms that remain poorly understood.

Animal metabolism

The therapeutic efficacies of the CENUs appear to involve their spontaneous chemical decomposition to yield electrophilic species that alkylate cellular macromolecules. The isocyanates may either carbamoylate macromolecules or undergo intramolecular carbamoylation to form cyclic urethanes. Alternative pathways of decomposition account for the diversity of products which are highly dependent upon the structure of individual CENUs.

The short half-lives of the nitrosoureas in buffer at physiological pH and *in vivo* as plasma half-lives led to an initial assumption that these drugs would have little opportunity to undergo metabolism *in vivo* (for a review see Reed, 1981). Not only was this assumption erroneous, but it is now generally accepted that the biological activity of CCNU is expressed through its metabolites; these are formed by an extremely rapid monohydroxylation of the cyclohexyl ring by cytochrome P-450 dependent-enzymes. Evidence is accumulating to suggest that *in vivo* denitrosation is important to the pharmacodynamics of certain nitrosoureas.

Cytochrome P-450 mono-oxygenase dependent hydroxylation

During the past 15 years cytochrome P-450-dependent enzymes have been established as the major enzymes responsible for the biotransformation of lipophilic drugs. Lipophilic nitrosoureas, including CCNU and methyl CCNU, undergo cytochrome P-450-dependent mono-oxygenation at cyclohexyl ring carbon atoms. Methyl CCNU is also hydroxylated in the 2-chloroethyl side-chain. Cytochrome P-450 present in rat liver microsomes prepared from liver of phenobarbital-induced rats catalyses rapid mono-oxygenation of CCNU to yield five hydroxy CCNU metabolites (May *et al.*, 1974, 1975; Reed, 1981; Reed and May, 1975, 1977; Hilton and Walker, 1975). Within 2 min after intravenous administration of CCNU to rats, a majority of the CCNU in the liver is metabolized and hydroxy CCNU metabolites are detectable in all organs examined (Reed and May, 1977). Methyl CCNU displays a slower rate of mono-oxygenation than CCNU and has a more complex metabolic pattern than CCNU (May *et al.*, 1979). The presence of a *trans*-4-methyl group decreases the rate of mono-oxygenation of methyl CCNU 25% compared to CCNU (May *et al.*, 1979). The methyl group is hydroxylated to some extent and a small amount of *trans*-4-hydroxy-*cis*-4-methyl CCNU formation occurs, possibly via a free-radical intermediate which facilitates some methyl group "flip" (Potter and Reed, 1980).

Efforts have been made towards metabolism-directed design of new nitrosourea congeners. An attempt was made to direct the metabolic formation of specific hydroxy CCNU metabolites with specific deuterium labelling of the cyclohexyl ring (Farmer *et al.*, 1978). Whereas a metabolic shift is achieved, the fraction of the metabolite desired, *trans*-2-hydroxy CCNU, remains too small compared to total metabolite formation for a noticeable change in therapeutic effect.

More recently, fluorinated congeners of CCNU were synthesized and tested, in the hope that such congeners would be more effective anti-tumour agents than CCNU due to possible blocking of ring hydroxylation and changes in physicochemical characteristics (Foster *et al.*, 1980). The 3-(1*H*-decafluorocyclohexyl) analogue of CCNU (FCCNU) was found to be more toxic and possess less anti-tumour activity than CCNU. This congener favours chemical decomposition via a 3-nitroso imidazolidin-2-one intermediate. A mixture of this intermediate and a 1-(nonafluorocyclohexyl) derivative appears to be responsible for the observed toxicity of FCCNU (Foster *et al.*, 1980).

Nitrosourea denitrosation

The lack of anti-tumour activity of methylurea as well as other ureas demonstrates the requirement for the *N*-nitroso moiety (Skipper *et al.*, 1961). Chemically, the nitroso moiety of methyl CCNU can be quantitatively removed with the formation of methyl CCNU by hydrogenation in ethanol in the presence of 5% rhodium in charcoal at 25°C and 1 atmos. (May *et al.*, 1979). Biologically, BCNU undergoes denitrosation, which is catalysed by liver microsomes in the presence of NADPH (Hill *et al.*, 1975). Recent evidence has demonstrated that nitric oxide is formed as a product of denitrosation under anaerobic conditions (Potter and Reed, 1981). Cytochrome P-450 can form a nitroso complex during denitrosation of CCNU with an absorption maximum at 445 nm (Reed and May, 1977). Certain nitrosoureas can undergo denitrosation *in vivo* with loss of anti-tumour activity, especially after induction of the liver endoplasmic reticulum with phenobarbital. Phenobarbital pretreatment of rats bearing intracerebral 9L tumours eliminates the anti-tumour activity of BCNU and decreases the efficacy of PCNU (1-(2-chloroethyl)-3-(2,6-dioxo-3-piperidyl)-1-nitrosourea) and CCNU (Levin *et al.*, 1979). Decreased systemic toxicity to the host rats is observed, which agrees with a microsomal-catalysed rate of BCNU disappearance that doubles by phenobarbital pretreatment (Levin *et al.*, 1979).

Denitrosation is a factor which may have importance in the design and efficacy of new nitrosourea drugs. Every nitrosourea examined so far can undergo anaerobic denitrosation catalysed by liver microsomes in the presence of NADPH (Potter and Reed, 1981). The rates of denitrosation reveal a sufficient variation between the nitrosoureas tested to indicate that a low denitrosation rate may modify the therapeutic index of a congener.

ACNU metabolism

The degradation and metabolism of ACNU *in vitro* includes the spontaneous formation in phosphate buffer, pH 7·4, of an intramolecular cyclized product, 3,4-dihydro-7-methylpyrimido-[4,5-*d*] pyrimidin-2(1*H*)-one, with simultaneous liberation of the alkylating moiety. Rat liver enzyme preparations metabolized ACNU to three metabolites. The nature of the metabolites and enzymes indicates that at least two enzymatic steps are involved which cause an oxidative dechlorination to 1-[(4-amino-2-methyl-5-pyrimidinyl)methyl]-5-hydroxy-3-nitroso-2-imidazolidinone by a microsomal mixed-function oxidase and a denitrosation process to yield 1-[(4-amino-2-methyl-5-pyrimidinyl) methyl]-3-(2-chloroethyl)urea. The denitrosated product of the oxidative dechlorination was the remaining metabolite (Nishigaki *et al.*, 1985 a).

The major urinary metabolites of ACNU have been identified following intravenous administration of [^{14}C]ACNU into rats (Nishigaki *et al.*, 1985 b). An imidazolidinone compound, 1-[(4-amino-2-methyl-5-pyrimidinyl) methyl]-5-hydroxy-2-imidazolidinone, was the main metabolite with one of the other major metabolites being a nitrosated compound of the main metabolite, i.e., 1-[(4-amino-2-methyl-5-pyrimidinyl)methyl]-5-hydroxy-3-nitroso-2-imidazolidinone. Also observed was the denitrosated parent urea and a cyclized pyrimidopyrimidine (Nishigaki *et al.*, 1985 b).

In a study of the central nervous system (CNS) toxicity and cerebrospinal fluid (CSF) pharmacokinetics of intraventricularly administered ACNU in beagles, it was concluded that the disappearance of ACNU from CSF was due to hydrolytic decomposition with a half-time for CSF elimination of 18 min (Levin *et al.*, 1985 b). Treatment of meningeal neoplasia may be limited since CSF elimination of ACNU is rapid compared to its equilibration time from ventricle to spinal–cerebral convexity–subarachnoid space (Levin *et al.*, 1985 b).

CNCC metabolism

CNCC metabolism in rats displays a first-pass metabolism to yield four main metabolites (Godeneche *et al.*, 1985). These metabolites arise from the bioreduction of the disulphide bridge of CNCC followed by S-methylation and oxidation to sulphinyl and sulphonyl derivatives. *In vitro* studies (Godeneche *et al.*, 1986) have shown that a cytosolic thioreductase, a microsomal and cytosolic *S*-methyltransferase and a microsomal oxidase catalyse very rapid enzymatic reactions, which explains the non-detectable reduction products. An equally rapid metabolic sequence appears to cause a loss of the nitroso groups. All metabolic intermediates that retain both the nitroso group and the 2-chloroethyl moiety are potentially active anti-tumour agents.

Human metabolism

Clinical pharmacology of the CENUs has been reviewed (Levin, 1981). Unfortunately, the clinical relevance of analogues other than BCNU has not been assessed in terms of their pharmacokinetics and very little human metabolic data has been reported.

Human brain tumours have been examined for the pharmacokinetics of positron-labelled BCNU with positron emission tomography, and the results compared to those of normal brain (Diksic *et al.*, 1984). Distribution of radioactivity in brain and plasma indicates a different rate of BCNU decomposition in the tumour than in normal brain, and the clearance of total radioactivity from the tumour is significantly slower than from the contralateral brain and plasma (Diksic *et al.*, 1984).

Relationship between metabolism and biological activity

Many nitrosoureas are remarkable in their ability to achieve complete cures of various tumours in test animals. Except for one factor, these drugs undoubtedly would be equally impressive in achieving cures of many neoplasms in humans. This factor, toxicity to normal cells as well as malignant cells, is extremely severe with the nitrosoureas. A wide range of toxicities is exhibited when nitrosoureas are administered to either test animals or humans. These include bone marrow suppression (myelosuppression or myelotoxicity), alopecia (loss of hair), interference with spermatogenesis, and of particular importance to patients, nausea and vomiting. Since rapidly proliferating cells or tissue have growth characteristics similar to tumour cells, they are the most susceptible to these cytotoxic effects. Alteration of genetic material is expressed not only by cytotoxicity, but also by the ability of the nitrosoureas to be mutagenic and somewhat carcinogenic. These effects have been reviewed (Ludlum, 1977). Cytotoxicity is so severe with the 2-chloroethylnitrosoureas that cancer cell kill plays a greater role than transformation of normal cells to malignancy and tumour formation.

Non-enzymic degradation of 2-chloroethylnitrosoureas, which may be protein-mediated under certain conditions (Weinkam *et al.*, 1980), is responsible for the generation of a common but penultimate alkylating intermediate, 2-chloroethyldiazene hydroxide. This hypothetical intermediate (also known as a diazo-hydroxide) is very unstable and yet appears to have an important role in the selective alkylation events of DNA. This role has been discussed in detail for the corresponding diazene hydroxides derived from degradation of methyl and ethylnitrosourea (Jensen and Reed, 1978; Jensen, 1978). Formation of either 2-chloroethanol or 1-bromo-2-chloroethane in the presence of bromide ion during CCNU degradation is strong evidence for an intermediate capable of 2-chloroethylation of biological molecules (Reed *et al.*, 1975). Evidence against a classical S_N1 reaction mechanism for BCNU alkylation has been reported by Brundrett *et al.* (1976) from studies with deuterated BCNU. They proposed that a reaction which has a 2-chloroethylcarbonium ion intermediate would yield products predominantly from rearranged 1-chloroethylcarbonium ion and cyclic chloronium ions. The major product, 2-chloroethanol, was mostly unrearranged (90%) (Brundrett *et al.*, 1976). Since S_N2 reactions of the diazene hydroxide are of low activation energy, little selectivity is proposed for the concerted loss of N_2 and alkylation of either sulphur, oxygen or nitrogen atoms (Brundrett *et al.*, 1976). Differences in oxygen atom alkylation by ethyl- and methylnitrosoureas would suggest that alkylation site affinity for the diazene hydroxide cannot be ruled out entirely (Jensen, 1978).

Ludlum and co-workers have studied extensively alkylation modifications of DNA and RNA bases by nitrosoureas. Properties of these derivatives are reviewed (Ludlum and Tong, 1981). The modified bases have been categorized into two classes: those derived from a single substitution at a nucleophilic site and those involving a two-step modification. The haloethyl, hydroxyethyl, and aminoethyl modified bases are placed in the first group (Ludlum and Tong, 1981). The formation of diguanylethane represents a DNA cross-linking event which probably is intra-strand in nature but inter-strand cross-linking cannot be ruled out at this time (Tong and Ludlum, 1981). Some of the unique cytotoxic properties of the nitrosoureas may relate to inter-strand DNA cross-linking processes which were first observed with purified DNA by physical studies by Kohn (1977) and Lown and co-workers (1978). We are still unable to describe these events chemically and therefore we cannot fully assess their impact on loss of cellular function, including cellular repair processes. Studies on DNA cross-linking have been reviewed (Kohn *et al.*, 1981). Efforts to quantitate alkylation of DNA in intact cells and bone marrow have led workers to conclude that differences in DNA alkylation may relate to difference of bone marrow toxicity of nitrosoureas (Green *et al.*, 1981). These workers conclude that decreased myelotoxicity of an individual nitrosourea compared to other nitrosoureas may relate more to localization of DNA modification within chromatin than alteration of rate and extent of DNA repair. In this regard, Tew (1981) has observed that within the nuclear matrix there exist transcriptionally active regions to chromatin that are preferentially modified by nitrosoureas. This rather speculative hypothesis of nitrosourea cytotoxicity is greatly limited by our meagre knowledge of the structure of chromatin and the molecular events necessary for nuclear DNA function.

Carbamoylation

Carbamoylation events can occur after nitrosourea degradation to yield an organic isocyanate and a diazene hydroxide. As mentioned previously, the organic moiety of the isocyanate may contain a functional group such as a hydroxyl group leading to a possible intramolecular carbamoylation reaction to form a cyclic urethane. Extensive *in vitro* intramolecular carbamoylation is known to occur with chlorozotocin (Johnston *et al.*, 1975) but whether exclusive intramolecular carbamoylation takes precedence *in vivo* over intermolecular carbamoylation is not known. The extent of intermolecular carbamoylation *in vitro* has been assayed by the carbamoylation of [^{14}C]lysine and quantitation of products by chromatography (Wheeler *et al.*, 1974). This assay has been utilized extensively on the basis that the isocyanate would attack in a random manner any amino, hydroxyl or thiol functional group. Thus, classification of nitrosoureas based on their comparative carbamoylation of lysine *in vitro* has been utilized extensively to rank them on their *in vivo* or intracellular carbamoylating ability. It is now apparent that such a comparison is not an adequate estimate of protein modification because many organic isocyanates are excellent pseudosubstrates which are capable of irreversible inactivation of a specific enzyme at its catalytic site.

Originally, Brown and Wold (1973 a,b) found that butyl isocyanate and octyl isocyanate were active-site-directed inactivators of elastase and chymotrypsin, respectively. Babson *et al.* (1977) observed that active-site-specific inactivation of chymotrypsin occurred by cyclohexyl isocyanate released during degradation of CCNU. A 70-fold excess of lysine over chymotrypsin concentration is necessary to detect any effect on the stoichiometric inactivation of chymotrypsin (Babson *et al.*, 1977). Subsequently, Frischer and Ahmad (1977) observed that only glutathione reductase out of 19 erythrocyte enzymes assayed is inactivated *in vivo* during chemotheraphy of patients with BCNU. Further studies by Babson and Reed (1978) have shown that inactivation of glutathione reductase occurs only when the enzyme is in a reduced state (i.e., NADPH reduction) and two thiol groups are present at the active site. The inactivation of catalytic activity appears to occur as a thiocarbamate adduct forms between the isocyanate and possibly the distal thiol group at the active site (Babson and Reed, 1978).

The importance of these observations is that certain enzymes and proteins have either a catalytic or functional site at a region of hydrophobicity that is capable of high-affinity binding of organic isocyanate with R groups of proper size and character. Thus a very high probability exists for a successful collision between a particular isocyanate and protein functional group. Active-site-directed interactions of this type take precedence over undirected reactions between other functional groups lacking the associated hydrophobic region for initial binding of the R group of the isocyanate. Such pockets or crevices in proteins have a very important role in the overall specificity and affinity of enzymes and other proteins (i.e., receptor proteins) for substrates and/or pseudosubstrates. The ability of cyclohexylisocyanate to prevent stoichiometrically the polymerization of brain tubulin is another example of highly specific irreversible binding of isocyanate to a protein (Brodie *et al.*, 1980).

Alkylation versus carbamoylation effects

Much of the effort on development of new nitrosoureas has been directed towards decreasing the dose-limiting bone marrow suppression. Chlorozotocin is an example of a drug which was designed to maintain therapeutic efficacy while attempting to minimize host toxicity (Anderson *et al.*, 1975). The next section of this chapter will provide some views as to why chlorozotocin does not achieve this goal to the extent desired.

A comparison of chemical structure of carbamoylating groups suggests that for the 2-chloroethylnitrosoureas, bifunctional alkylation is essential for anti-glioma activity and that myelosuppression is at least partly correlated with carbamoylation (Ali-Osman *et al.*, 1985). However, structural entities in the carbamoylating isocyanate, rather than a quantitative degree of carbamoylation, may be important in the degree of potential myelotoxicity (Ali-Osman *et al.*, 1985).

Thiols potentiate the inter-strand cross-linking of DNA by CNCC-(C) as well as other CCNUs, which is explained by nucleophilic attack at the carbonyl group and subsequent stereoelectronically controlled decomposition of the tetrahedral intermediate (Lown *et al.*, 1985). The reduced cytotoxic potential of CNCC-(S) has been described as an interaction between GSH and the drug, thereby protecting other more critical nucleophilic targets within the nucleus (Lown *et al.*, 1985). It has been suggested that the decreased cytotoxic potential of CNCC-(S) is in agreement with a prolongation in the half-life of production of alkylating carbonium species and the lack of capacity to cross-link macromolecules (Farhi *et al.*, 1984).

Four plasma metabolites of CNCC have been synthesized and evaluated for their anti-tumour activity. The metabolities are *N'*-(2-chloroethyl)-*N*-[2-(methylsulphinyl)ethyl]- and *N'*-(2-chloroethyl)-*N*-[2-(methylsulphonyl) ethyl]-*N*- or *N'*-nitrosoureas (Madelmont *et al.*, 1985). Two of the four metabolites exhibited a greater anti-tumour activity than CNCC.

Specificity in ACNU and CCNU binding to the nucleosomal DNA of murine bone marrow and L1210 cells is in contrast to chlorozotocin and GANU binding preferentially to the linker DNA of bone marrow, but not tumour, cell chromatin (Dean *et al.*, 1985). Differences in DNA linker length does not appear to be the basis for these quantitative differences in the tissue-specific toxicity of these 2-chloroethylnitrosureas which contain sugar moieties (Dean *et al.*, 1985).

An in-depth investigation of resistance to DNA cross-linking agents in 9L cell lines with different sensitivities to CENUs has revealed that cellular resistance to CENUs is highly specific (Bodell *et al.*, 1985 a). DNA repair processes may mediate cellular resistance to CENUs, since the mechanism of resistance does not allow cross-resistance with other DNA cross-linking agents. Thus other cross-linking agents will not be cross-resistant unless they form alkylation products that are affected by repair processes which mediate resistance to CENUs (Bodell *et al.*, 1985 a).

Repair of DNA inter-strand cross-link precursors, which is mediated by O^6-alkylguanine-DNA alkyltransferase activity, may be an important determinant of MeCCNU cytotoxicity. Evidence for this correlation comes from measurement of the extent of tumour regression and the level of O^6-methylguanine-DNA methyltransferase activity in tumour extracts of six different human rhabdomyosarcoma lines grown in immune-deprived female CBA/CaJ mice after treatment with MeCCNU (Brent *et al.*, 1985). The level of this repair enzyme may be a clinically useful prediction of sensitivity of human tumour cells to the CENUs (Brent *et al.*, 1985).

The induction of sister-chromatid exchanges (SCEs) in 9L rat brain tumour cells is 143-fold greater with ACNU than with 1-ethyl-1-nitrosourea (ENU) (Bodell *et al.*, 1985 b). Since on an equimolar basis ^{14}C labelling for [^{14}C]ACNU was about 3·2-fold higher than for [^{14}C]ENU, after correction for this difference the induction difference may be about 45-fold. The increased induction of SCEs caused by ACNU is thought to be a result of the formation of DNA inter-strand cross-links (Bodell *et al.*, 1985 b). Potentiation of BCNU-induced cytotoxicity in 9L cells by pretreatment with 6-thioguanine may result from increased formation of DNA cross-links derived from the formation of S^6-(2-chloroethyl)-6-thioguanine in cellular DNA (Bodell *et al.*, 1985 c).

The levels of induction of SCEs and the cytotoxicity of ENU, MNU, ACNU and BCNU have been compared (Bodell *et al.*, 1985 d). The CENUs are 200-fold more cytotoxic and induce SCEs with 45-fold greater efficiency than ECU and MNU, which are not capable of cross-linking. It is suggested that cross-linking is probably the most important molecular event that leads to cell death and induction by SCEs.

A relationship may exist between the repair of O^6-substituted guanine derivatives and cellular resistance to CENUs in human tumour cells. Resistance of 9L-2, HU-188, and HU-253-2 cells to SCE induction and cytotoxicity by CENUs correlates to their increased capacity to remove O^6-(2-chloroethyl)guanine in DNA. O^6-Methylguanine-DNA methyltransferase removes a chloroethylation product that forms DNA cross-links (Brent, 1984; Robins *et al.*, 1983). Resistant cell lines have a higher cellular level of O^6-methylguanine-DNA methyl transferase, increased repair of

O^6-methylguanine, and 50% fewer DNA inter-strand cross-links formed than do sensitive cells treated with the same concentration of CENU (Bodell *et al.*, 1985 d).

A major difference between 2-chloroethyl-(methylsulphonyl)methane sulphonate (ClEtSoSo) and the CENUs is that the CENUs, during chemical degradation, yield 2-hydroxyethyl intermediates and 7-hydroxyethyl hydroxylation products, whereas ClEtSoSo causes only chloroethylated products such as 7-chloroethylguanine (Gibson *et al.*, 1986). Such a difference is thought to be important in the overall biological effects of these agents. In this regard, three chloroethylating anti-tumour agents have been compared for their DNA sequence selectivities of guanine-N^7 alkylation. Cis-2-OH CCNU, ClEtSoSo, and mitozolomide alkylation of pBR322 DNA, followed by use of the Maxam and Gilbert sequencing technique to determine the alkylation of runs of three or more guanines in the DNA showed differences in the degree of alkylation of specific guanine bases (Hartley *et al.*, 1986). ClEtSoSo alkylated all guanines to the same extent, while cis-2-OH CCNU preferentially alkylated the middle guanines as did mitozolomide, but not as intensely as cis-2-OH CCNU. Both 7-chloroethylation and 7-hydroxyethylation were similarly enhanced by the presence of adjacent guanines when cis-2-OH CCNU was the alkylator. The results imply that the alkylating intermediates, 2-chloroethyldiazohydroxide and 2-hydroxyethyldiazohydroxide react preferentially with the middle guanines because of the enhanced electronegativity created by the presence of neighbouring guanines. The cationic character of these diazo intermediates is thought to be greater than with the other two alkylating agents.

It is suggested that CCNU has carbamoylating activity that is associated with inhibition of RNA processing and with the degree of chemopotentiation achieved with MISO (Hill *et al.*, 1984 a). Also, such chemopotentiation by misonidazole (MISO) does not appear to occur equally in all cell subpopulations derived from solid KHT sarcomas, and therefore some specificity of enhanced cell killing exists (Hill *et al.*, 1984 b). No loss in tumour cell sensitization was found with fractionation of CCNU treatment during chemopotentiation *in vivo* with KHT sarcoma, with and without MISO (Hill and Siemann, 1984). The combination of MISO with repeated low-dose treatment of CCNU results in a therapeutic gain (Hill and Siemann, 1984). The variable response to BCNU of human glioma cells, sorted according to DNA content, suggests a problem imposed by heterogeneity with regard to chemosensitivity even within a single tumour (Kobayashi *et al.*, 1984).

Cross-linking mediated by X-rays has been proposed as the mechanism through which cell kill is increased by combination with BCNU that also induces DNA inter-strand cross-linking (Tofilon *et al.*, 1984).

A comparison of the alkylation of bone marrow DNA by chlorozotocin and CCNU indicates a quantitative equivalent level of DNA alkylation (Byrne *et al.*, 1984). However, the bone marrow sparing effects of chlorozotocin may exist because in contrast to CCNU, chlorozotocin predominantly alkylates the transcriptionally inactive regions of chromatin. The lethal damage of CENU's alkylation in human bone marrow may be principally expressed in transcriptionally active regions of chromatin (Byrne *et al.*, 1984).

The differential bone marrow toxicity exhibited by CENUs does not appear to be a carbamoylation-mediated difference in the rate and extent of DNA–DNA inter-strand cross-link removal (Bedford and Eisenbrand, 1984). In the repair of DNA damage in the bone marrow of rats, the kinetics of cross-link removal was identical for chlorozotocin and BCNU (Bedford and Eisenbrand, 1984). These results are in agreement with studies on effects of carbamoylation on cell survival and DNA repair in normal human embryo cells (IMR-90). Carbamoylation may inhibit nucleotide excision repair that is not involved in the repair process of O^6-methylguanine-DNA methyltransferase (Sariban *et al.*, 1984).

Evidence for *in vivo* carbamoylation of proteins by nitrosoureas includes not only organ and tissue distribution of radiolabel following administration of nitrosoureas radiolabelled in the isocyanate precursor moiety, but also the nature of the urinary metabolites. Kohlhepp *et al.* (1981) observed that major urinary metabolites of CCNU have molecular weights of 629, 413, 329 and 243 and they represent 5%, 20%, 20% and 5%, respectively of total excreted ^{14}C following administration of ^{14}C ring-labelled CCNU. They concluded that the higher molecular weight metabolites are conjugates of peptides derived from active site-directed inactivation of specific enzymes. Lysine does not contribute significantly to the composition of the urinary metabolites. Major amino acids present in the peptides were cysteine, serine, glutamic acid, alanine, glycine and aspartic acid (Kohlhepp *et al.*, 1981).

One must conclude that selective alkylation and carbamoylation events that modify macromolecules are both important in correlation of structure–activity relationships and that *in vitro* assays are unable to measure the selectivity of such specific macromolecular modifications *in vivo*.

Organ toxicity

Nephrotoxicity

Renal toxicity has been observed in patients after chemotherapy with MeCCNU (Weiss *et al.*, 1983). Such toxicity is characterized as being cumulative dose dependent (>1400 mg/m^2), delayed in onset (>12 months), and often fatal (Kramer *et al.*, 1986). Other CENUs cause renal failure, including CCNU (Weiss and Poster, 1982; Ellis *et al.*, 1985) and chlorozotocin (Moriconi *et al.*, 1985).

A model for CENU nephrotoxicity is based on a single, sublethal dose of MeCCNU or chlorozotocin to the Fischer 344 (F344) rat that produces chronic and progressive changes in renal function (Kramer *et al.*, 1986). At equimolar doses chlorozotocin is a much more potent nephrotoxicant even though it causes much less carbamoylation of cellular macromolecules. Karyomegaly by MeCCNU and chlorozotocin was taken as evidence that both CENUs may have their toxic effects by virtue of extensive alkylation of renal DNA (Kramer *et al.*, 1986).

Lung toxicity

Lung damage caused by BCNU is characterized by fibrosing alveolitis and interstitial pneumonitis that can lead to pulmonary fibrosis, restrictive pulmonary failure, and death (Smith and Boyd, 1984 a; Muggia *et al.*, 1983; Weiss *et al.*, 1981). Initial injury may occur in endothelial cells, causing changes in pulmonary and serum angiotensin converting enzyme activity (Smith and Boyd, 1984 a). Preferential destruction of lung glutathione reductase by BCNU precedes the development of severe lung injury (Smith and Boyd, 1984 b).

BCNU has been shown to accentuate acute lung damage in mice with pre-existing lung damage that was produced by the administration of butylated hydroxytoluene (Kehrer and Klein-Szanto, 1985). A single dose of BCNU alone had a minimal toxic effect on lung tissue, whereas high doses of BCNU administered one day after butylated hydroxytoluene were related to the ability of BCNU to inhibit pulmonary glutathione reductase activity and the increased DNA synthesis after butylated hydroxytoluene (Kehrer and Klein-Szanto, 1985).

The future

Because current anti-tumour agents are toxic to both malignant and non-maligant cells, a major chemotherapeutic goal is to make available selective therapy regimens having limited potential to injure normal cells. Rapidly proliferating cells are major targets, and selectivity continues to be a major problem. However, some cells lack such a high mitotic index and yet are highly susceptible to injury, e.g., endothelial cells found in endothelium (Lazo, 1986). CENU toxicity to endothelial cells and pulmonary fibrosis needs further investigation. Such studies could utilize very effectively the availability of CENUs with varying alkylating and carbamoylating capabilities to establish which reactive moiety is important in dose-limiting toxicity of these drugs.

The ability of the nitrosoureas to cross the blood–brain barrier, while many anti-tumour drugs fail to do so, has resulted in much interest in the lipophilic character of the nitrosoureas. Based on cancer quantitative structure–activity relationship (QSAR), some guidelines for the design of new nitrosoureas have been advanced. After an extensive study of a QSAR for 90 nitrosoureas against L1210 leukaemia in mice, it was concluded that the lipophilic character of the nitrosoureas is the most important parameter determining their anti-tumour activity (Hansch *et al.*, 1980). *P*-values were measured for 43 nitrosoureas and efforts to make nitrosourea congeners somewhat more hydrophilic became a central point in the study. Justified concern was expressed about the limitation of functional groups such as COOH, which are almost completely ionized at physiological pH, pH 7·4, to confer greater hydrophilicity when un-ionized functional groups showed a better correlation. Making the R group more polar yet un-ionized with a disaccharide was suggested (Hansch *et al.*, 1980). Interestingly, at about the same time, this approach was being tested with three nitrosoureas containing either a β-maltosyl, β-lactosyl, or β-cellobiosyl R group (Suami *et al.*, 1979). Testing of these congeners against various types of tumours is continuing.

Increasing evidence supports the concept that carbamoylation capability remains an important factor in the design of new nitrosourea congeners. DNA alkylation events have a greater chance for cell killing when the rate of DNA repair is decreased. Day *et al.* (1980) have identified a group of eight (among 39) human tumour cell strains that are deficient in DNA repair ability. This deficiency is being studied in regard to susceptibility to DNA cross-links caused by CNU, BCNU, and CCNU (Day *et al.*, 1980; Erickson *et al.*, 1980). Eisenbrand *et al.* (1976) have designed and synthesized a congener series of 1,1′-polymethylene bis-3-(2-chloroethyl)-3-nitrosoureas as transport forms of polymethylene diisocyanates. These compounds may cause some interesting cross-linking reactions primarily with proteins. Studies with these and other new nitrosoureas have led Eisenbrand and co-workers (1981) to conclude that the non-alkylating part of the 2-chloroethylnitrosourea is important for the biological effects of these drugs.

Certain nitrosoureas have been shown to cause a prolonged *in vivo* depression of cytochrome P-450 content and cytochrome P-450-dependent enzyme activities of liver microsomes when measured *in vitro* (Reed and May, 1978; Litterst, 1981). A single non-lethal dose of CCNU *in vivo* decreased liver cytochrome P-450 content and drug metabolism of rat liver microsomes by 40–70% for up to six weeks. This unique suppression is without parallel by any other drug and cannot be explained, except for possible persistent alkylation and/or carbamoylation effects by the degradation intermediates of the nitrosoureas. This effect could well be the basis for a new congener series that could modulate the activity of these and other drugs which are substrates for the cytochrome P-450 enzymes.

Conclusions

Nitrosourea cytotoxicity remains a very complex effect with unique characteristics. Much more needs to be understood at the molecular level to provide even rudimentary explanation of the chemical modifications caused by the alkylations and carbamylating events of the nitrosoureas. If potent toxicity of the nitrosoureas could be ameliorated without sacrificing tumour cell cytotoxicity, the clinical impact of these drugs would be enormous. Design and testing of new congeners on a rational basis should continue to be a worthwhile activity in the years ahead.

Acknowledgements

The author wishes to acknowledge support by Grant CH109 from the American Cancer Society.

References

The following books are the proceedings of recent international symposia on the nitrosoureas: *Nitrosoureas: Current Status and New Developments*, edited by A. W. Prestayko, S. T. Crooke, L. H. Baker, S. K. Carter and P. S. Schein (New York: Academic Press, 1981, 416 pp.) and *Nitrosoureas in Cancer Treatment*, edited by B. Serrou, P. S. Schein and J.-L. Imbach (New York: Elsevier, 1981, 310 pp.).

Ali-Osman, F., Giblin, J., Berger, M., Murphy, M. J., Jr. and Rosenblum, M. L., 1985, Chemical structure of carbamoylating groups and their relationship to bone marrow toxicity and antiglioma activity of bifunctionally alkylating and carbamoylating nitrosoureas. *Cancer Res.*, **45**, 4185–4191.

Anderson, T., McMenamin, M. G. and Schein, P. S., 1975, Chlorozotocin, 2[3-(2-chloroethyl)-3-nitrosoureido]-*D*-glucopyranose, an antitumor agent with modified bone marrow toxicity. *Cancer Res.*, **35**, 761–765.

Babson, J. R. and Reed, D. J., 1978, Inactivation of glutathione reductase by 2-chloroethyl nitrosourea-derived isocyanates. *Biochem. Biophys. Res. Commun.*, **83**, 754–762.

Babson, J. R., Reed, D. J. and Sinkey, M. A., 1977, Active site specific inactivation of chymotrypsin by cyclohexyl isocyanate formed during degradation of the carcinostatic 1-(2-chloroethyl)-3-cyclohexyl-1-nitrosourea. *Biochemistry*, **16**, 1584–1589.

Bedford, P. and Eisenbrand, G., 1984, DNA damage and repair in the bone marrow of rats treated with four chloroethylnitrosoureas. *Cancer Res.*, **44**, 514–518.

Bodell, W. J., Gerosa, M., Aida, T., Berger, M. S. and Rosenblum, M. L., 1985 a, Investigation of resistance to DNA cross-linking agents in 9L cell lines with different sensitivities to chloroethylnitrosoureas. *Cancer Res.*, **45**, 3460–3464.

Bodell, W. J., Aida, T. and Rasmussen, J., 1985 b, Comparison of sister-chromatid exchange induction caused by nitrosoureas that alkylate or alkylate and crosslink DNA. *Mutat. Res.*, **149**, 95–100.

Bodell, W. J., Morgan, W. F., Rasmussen, J., Williams, M. E. and Deen, D. F., 1985 c, Potentiation of 1,3-bis(2-chloroethyl)-1-nitrosourea (BCNU)-induced cytotoxicity in 9L cells by pretreatment with 6-thioguanine. *Biochem. Pharmacol.*, **34**, 515–520.

Bodell, W. J., Toshimitsu, A., Berger, M. S. and Rosenblum, M. L., 1985 d, Repair of O^6-(2-chloroethyl)guanine mediates the biological effects of chloroethylnitrosoureas. *Environ. Health Persp.*, **62**, 119–126.

Brent, T. P., 1984, Suppression of cross-link formation in chloroethylnitrosourea-treated DNA by an activity in extracts of human leukemic lymphoblasts. *Cancer Res.*, **44**, 1887–1892.

Brent, T. P., Houghton, P. J. and Houghton, J. A., 1985, O^6-Alkylguanine-DNA alkyltransferase activity correlates with the therapeutic response of human rhabdomyosarcoma xenografts to 1-(2-chloroethyl)-3-(trans-4-methylcyclohexyl)-1-nitrosourea. *Proc. Natl. Acad. Sci. USA*, **82**, 2985–2989.

Brodie, A. E., Babson, J. R. and Reed, D. J., 1980, Inhibition of tubulin polymerization by nitrosourea-derived isocyanates. *Biochem. Pharmacol.*, **29**, 652–654.

Brown, W. E. and Wold, F., 1973 a, Alkyl isocyanates as active-site-specific reagents for serine proteases. Reaction properties. *Biochemistry*, **12**, 828–834.

Brown, W. E. and Wold, F., 1973 b, Alkyl isocyanates as active-site-specific reagents for serine proteases. Identification of the active-site serine as the site of reaction. *Biochemistry*, **12**, 835–840.

Brufman, G., Halpern, J., Sulkes, A., Catane, R. and Biran, S., 1984, Procarbazine, CCNU and vincristine (PCV) combination chemotherapy for brain tumors. *Oncology*, **41**, 239–241.

Brundrett, R. B., 1980, Chemistry of nitrosoureas. Intermediacy of 4,5-dihydro-1,2,3-oxadiazole in 1,3-bis(2-chloroethyl)-1-nitrosourea decomposition. *J. Med. Chem.*, **23**, 1245–1247.

Brundrett, R. D., Cowens, J. W., Colvin, M. and Jardine, I., 1976, Chemistry of nitrosoureas. Decomposition of deuterated 1,3-bis(2-chlorothyl)-1-nitrosourea. *J. Med. Chem.*, **19**, 958–961.

Byrne, P., Tew, K., Jemionek, J., MacVittie, T., Erickson, L. and Schein, P., 1984, Cellular and molecular mechanisms of the bone marrow sparing effects of the glucose chloroethylnitrosourea chlorozotocin. *Blood*, **63**, 759–767.

Carter, S. K., Schabel, F. M., Jr., Broder, L. S. and Johnson, T. P., 1972, 1,3-bis (2-chloroethyl)-1-nitrosourea (BCNU) and other nitrosoureas in cancer treatment: A review. *Adv. Cancer Res.*, **16**, 273–332.

Chapman, B. A., Natale, R. B., Young, C. W. and Wittes, R. E., 1984, Phase II trial of 1-(2-chloroethyl)-3-(2,6-dioxo-3-piperidyl)-1-nitrosourea in small cell cancer of the lung. *Am. J. Clin. Oncol.*, **7**, 413–414.

Colvin, M., Cowens, J. W., Brundrett, R. B., Kramer B. S. and Ludlum, D. B., 1974, Decomposition of BCNU [1,3-*bis*(2-chloroethyl)-1-nitrosourea] in aqueous solution. *Biochem. Biophys. Res. Commun.*, **60**, 515–520.

Day, R. S., III, Ziolkowski, C. H. J., Scudiero, D. A., Meyer, S. A., Lubiniecki, A. S., Girardi, A. J., Galloway, S. M. and Bynum, G. D., 1980, Defective repair of alkylated DNA by human tumour and SV40-transformed human cell strains. *Nature*, **288**, 724–727.

Dean, S. W., Tew, K. D., Clark, A. E. and Schein, P. S., 1985, DNA repeat length in chromatin from murine bone marrow and L1210 leukaemia cells. *Br. J. Cancer*, **52**, 377–382.

Diksic, M., Sako, K., Feindel, W., Kato, A., Yamamoto, Y. L., Farrokhzad, S. and Thompson, C., 1984, Pharmacokinetics of positron-labeled 1,3-bis(2-chloroethyl)nitrosourea in human brain tumors using positron emission tomography. *Cancer Res.*, **44**, 3120–3124.

Eisenbrand, G., 1984, Anticancer nitrosoureas: investigations on antineoplastic, toxic and neoplastic activities. *IARC Sci. Publ.*, **57**, 695–708.

Eisenbrand, G., Fiebig, H. H. and Zeller, W. J., 1976, Some new congeners of the anticancer agent 1,3-bis(2-chloroethyl)-1-nitrosourea (BCNU). Synthesis of bifunctional analogs and water soluble derivatives and preliminary evaluation of their chemotherapeutic potential. *Z. Krebsforsch*, **86**, 279–286.

Eisenbrand, G., Habs, M., Zeller, W. J., Fiebig, H., Berger, M., Zelesmy, O. and Schmahl, D., 1981, New nitrosoureas—therapeutic and long-term toxic effects of selected compounds in comparison to established drugs, in *Nitrosoureas in Cancer Treatment*, edited by B. Serrou, P. S. Schein and J. L. Imbach (New York: Elsevier), pp. 175–191.

Ellis, M. E., Weiss, R. B. and Kuperminc, M., 1985, Nephrotoxicity of lomustine: A case report and literature review. *Cancer Chemother. Pharmacol.*, **15**, 174–175.

Erickson, L. C., Laurent, G., Sharkey N. A. and Kohn, K. W., 1980, DNA cross-linking and monoadduct repair in nitrosourea-treated human tumour cells. *Nature*, **288**, 727–729.

Farhi, J. J., Bennoun, M., Tapiero, H., Wang, A. L. and Tew, K. D., 1984, Biochemical and cytotoxic properties of the isomeric forms of N,N′-bis[N-2-chloroethyl)-N-nitrosocarbamoyl] cystamine. *Biochem. Pharmacol.*, **33**, 2575–2580.

Farmer, P. B., Foster, A. B., Jarman, M., Oddy, M. R. and Reed, D. J., 1978, Synthesis, metabolism, and antitumor activity of deuterated analogues of 1-(2-chloroethyl)-3-cyclohexyl-1-nitrosoureas. *J. Med. Chem.*, **21**, 514–520.

Fiebig, H. H., Wellens, W., Peukert, M., Henss, H., Arnold, H., Westerhausen, M. and Liohr, G. W., 1984, Phase II Study of the water-soluble nitrosourea compound ACNU in advanced colorectal carcinomas. *Onkologie*, **7**, 370–377.

Foster, A. B., Jarman, M., Coe, P. L., Sleigh, P. and Tatlow, J. C., 1980, Fluorinated analogues of 1(2-chloroethyl)-3-cyclohexyl-1-nitrosourea: An attempt to control metabolism. *J. Med. Chem.*, **23**, 1226–1229.

Frischer H. and Ahmad, T., 1977, Severe generalized glutathione reductase deficiency after antitumor chemotherapy with BCNU [1,3-bis(chloroethyl)-1-nitrosourea]. *J. Lab. Clin. Med.*, **89**, 1080–1089.

Fujimoto, S. and Ogawa, M., 1985, Toxicological study on a new nitrosourea derivative, 1-(2-chloroethyl)-3-isobutyl-3-(beta-maltosyl)-1-nitrosourea. *Jap. J. Cancer Res.*, **76**, 651–656.

Garrett, E. R., Goto, S. and Stubbins, J. F., 1965, Kinetics of solvolyses of various *N*-alkyl-*N*-nitrosoureas in neutral and alkaline solutions. *J. Pharm. Sci.*, **54**, 119–123.

Gibson, N. W., Hartley, J. A., Strong, J. M. and Kohn, K. W., 1986, 2-Chloroethyl (methylsulfonyl)methanesulfonate (NSC-338947), a more selective DNA alkylating agent than the chloroethylnitrosoureas. *Cancer Res.*, **46**, 553–557.

Godeneche, D., Madelmont, J. C., Moreau, M. F., Duprat, J., Chabrad, J. L., Plagne, R. and Meyniel G., 1985, Metabolic disposition of 2-chloroethyl nitrosocarbamoylcystamine in rats. *Drug Metab. Dispos.*, **13**, 220–226.

Godeneche, D., Madelmont, J. C., Moreau, M. F., Duprat, J., Plagne, R. and Meyniel G., 1986, Metabolism of 2-chloroethyl nitrosocarbamoylcystamine by rat liver subcellular fractions. *Drug Metab. Dispos.*, **14**, 112–117.

Green, D., Ahlgreen, J. D. and Schein, P. S., 1981, A molecular basis for differences in nitrosourea bone marrow toxicity, in *Nitrosoureas in Cancer Treatment*, edited by B. Serrou, P. S. Schein and J. L. Imbach (New York: Elsevier). pp. 49–59.

Hansch, C., Leo, A., Schmidt, C., Jow, P. Y. C. and Montgomery, J. A., 1980, Antitumor structure-activity relationships. Nitrosoureas vs. L-1210 leukemia. *J. Med. Chem.*, **23**, 1095–1101.

Hartley, J. A., Gibson, N. W., Kohn, K. W. and Mattes, W. B., 1986, DNA sequence selectivity of guanine-N7 alkylation by three antitumor chloroethylating agents. *Cancer Res.*, **46**, 1943–1947.

Hill, S. A. and Siemann, D. W., 1984, Chemopotentiation *in vivo*: no loss of sensitization with fractionation. *Br. J. Cancer*, **50**, 509–517.

Hill, D. L., Kirk, M. C. and Struck, M. F., 1975, *Cancer Res.*, **35**, 296.

Hill, S. A., Bauer, K. D., Keng, P. C. and Siemann, D. W., 1984 a. The effect in the KHT sarcoma of CCNU and MISO on cell cycle progression evaluated by flow-cytometry. *Int. J. Radiat. Oncol. Biol. Phys.*, **10**, 1619–1622.

Hill, S. A., Keng, P. C. and Siemann, D. W., 1984 b, Survival in subpopulations of cells derived from solid KHT sarcomas by centrifugal elutriation following treatment with CCNU and MISO. *Int. J. Radiat. Oncol. Biol. Phys.*, **10**, 1615–1618.

Hilton J. and Walker, M. D., 1975, Hydroxylation of 1(2-chloroethyl)-3-cyclohexyl-1-nitrosourea. *Biochem. Pharmacol.*, **24**, 2153–2158.

Imbach, J. L., Martinez, J., Oiry, J., Bourut, Ch., Chenu, E., Maral, R. and Mathe, G., 1981, New nitrosoureas derivatives and related compounds, in *Nitrosoureas in Cancer Treatment*, edited by B. Serrou, P. S. Schein and J. L. Imbach (New York: Elsevieer), pp. 123–137.

Jensen, D. E., 1978, Reaction of DNA with alkylating agents. Differential alkylation of poly[dA-dT] by methylnitrosourea and ethylnitrosourea. *Biochemistry*, **17**, 5108—5113.

Jensen D. E. and Reed, D. J., 1978, Reaction of DNA with alkylating agents. Quantitation of alkylation by ethylnitrosourea of oxygen and nitrogen sites on poly [dA-dT] including phosphotriester formation. *Biochemistry*, **17**, 5098–5107.

Johnston, T. P., McCaleb, G. S. and Montgomery, J. A., 1963, The synthesis of antineoplastic agents. XXXII. N-Nitrosoureas. I. *J. Med. Chem.*, **6**, 669–681.

Johnston, T. P., McCaleb, G. S., Opliger, P. S. and Montgomery, J. A., 1966, The synthesis of potential anticancer agents. XXXVI. N-nitrosourceas. II. Haloalkyl derivatives. *J. Med. Chem.*, **9**, 892–911.

Johnston, T. P., McCaleb, G. S. and Montgomery, J. A., 1975, Synthesis of chlorozotocin, the 2-chloroethyl analog of the anticancer antibiotic streptozocin. *J. Med. Chem.*, **18**, 104–106.

Johnston, T. P., McCaleb, G. S., Rose, W. C, and Montgomery, J. A., 1984 a, *Cis*-4-[[[(2-Chloroethyl)nitrosoamino]carbonyl]methylamino] cyclohexanecarboxylic acid, a nitrosourea with latent activity against an experimental solid tumor. *J. Med. Chem.*, **27**, 97–99.

Johnston, T. P., Kussner, C. L., Carter, R. L., Frye, J. L., Lomax, N. R., Plowman, J. and Narayanan, V. L., 1984b, Studies on synthesis and anticancer activity of selected N-(2-fluoroethyl)-N-nitrosoureas. *J. Med. Chem.*, **27**, 1422–1426.

Kehrer, J. P. and Klein-Szanto, A. J., 1985, Enhanced acute lung damage in mice following administration of 1,3-bis(2-chloroethyl)-1-nitrosourea. *Cancer Res.*, **45**, 5707–5713.

Kobayashi, S., Hoshino, T., Dougherty, D. V. and Rosenblum, M. L., 1984, Variable response to 1,3-bis(2-chloroethyl)-1-nitrosourea of human glioma cells sorted according to DNA content. *J. Neurooncol.*, **2**, 5–11.

Kohlhepp, S. J., May, H. E. and Reed, D. J., 1981, Urinary metabolites of 1-(2-chloroethyl)-3-cyclohexyl-1-nitroso urea and 1-(2-chloroethyl)-3-(*trans*-4-methylcyclohexyl)-1-nitrosourea. *Drug Metab. Dispos.*, **9**, 135–141.

Kohn, K. W., 1977, Interstrand cross-linking of DNA by 1,3-bis(2-chloroethyl)-1-nitrosourea and other 1-(2-haloethyl)-1-nitrosoureas. *Cancer Res.*, **37**, 1450–1454.

Kohn, K. W., Erickson, L. C. and Laurent, G., 1981, DNA alkylation, crosslinking and repair. In *Nitrosoureas in Cancer Treatment*, edited by B. Serrou, P. S. Schein and J. L. Imbach (New York: Elsevier), pp. 33–48.

Kramer, R. A., Boyd, M. R. and Dees, J. H., 1986, Comparative nephrotoxicity of 1-(2-chloroethyl)-3-(trans-4-methylcyclohexyl)-1-nitrosourea (MeCCNU) and chlorozotocin: functional–structural correlations in the Fischer 344 rat. *Toxicol. App. Pharmacol.*, **82**, 540–550.

Lazo, J. S., 1986, Endothelial injury caused by antineoplastic agents. *Biochem. Pharmacol.*, **35**, 1919–1923.

Levin, V. A., 1981, Clinical pharmacology of the nitrosoureas. In *Nitrosoureas:*

Current Status and New Developments, edited by C. A. W. Prestayko, S. T. Crooke, L. H. Baker, S. K. Carter and P. S. Schein (New York: Academic Press), pp. 171–180.

Levin, V. A., Stearns, J., Byrd, A., Finn, A. and Weinkam, R. J., 1979, The effect of phenobarbital pretreatment on the antitumor activity of 1,3-bis(2-chloroethyl)-1-nitrosourea (BCNU), 1-(2-chloroethyl)-3-cyclohexyl-1-nitrosourea (CCNU) and 1-(2-chloroethyl)-3-(2,6-dioxo-3-piperidyl)-1-nitrosourea (PCNU), and on the plasma pharmacokinetics and biotransformation of BCNU. *J. Pharmacol. Exp. Ther.*, **208**, 1–6.

Levin, V. A., Edwards, M. S., Wara, W. M., Allen, J., Ortega, J. and Vestnys, P., 1984, 5-Fluorouracil and 1-(2-chloroethyl)-3-cyclohexyl-1-nitrosourea (CCNU) followed by hydroxyurea, misonidazole, and irradiation for brain stem gliomas: a pilot study of the Brain Tumor Research Center and the Childrens Cancer Group. *Neurosurgery*, **14**, 679–681.

Levin, V. A., Wara, W. M., Davis, R. L., Vestnys, P., Resser, K. J., Yatsko, K., Nutik, S., Gutin, P. H. and Wilson, C. B., 1985 a, Phase III comparison of BCNU and the combination of procarbazine, CCNU, and vincristine administered after radiotherapy with hydroxyurea for malignant gliomas. *J. Neurosurg.*, **63**, 218–223.

Levin, V. A., Byrd, D., Campbell, J., Giannini, D. D., Borcich, J. K. and Davis, R. L., 1985 b, Central nervous system toxicity and cerebrospinal fluid pharmacokinetics of intraventricular 3-[(4-amino-2-methyl-5-pyrimidinyl)ethyl]-1-(2-chloroethyl)-1-nitrosoureas and other nitrosoureas in beagles. *Cancer Res.*, **45**, 3803–3809.

Lin, T. S., Brubaker, W. F., Jr., Wang, Z. H., Park, S. and Prusoff, W. H., 1986, Antineoplastic activity of 3′-(chloroethyl)nitrosourea analogues of 2′-deoxyuridine and 2′-deoxy-5-fluorouridine. *J. Med. Chem.*, **29**, 862–865.

Litterst, C. L., 1981, Prolonged depression of hepatic microsomal drug metabolism and hemoprotein levels following a single dose of 1-(2-chloroethyl)-3-cyclohexyl-1-nitrosourea (CCNU). *Biochem. Pharmacol.*, **30**, 1014–1016.

Lown J. W. and Chauhan, S. M. S., 1981, Synthesis of specifically ^{15}N- and ^{13}C-labeled antitumor (2-haloethyl)nitrosoureas. The study of their conformations in solution by nitrogen-15 and carbon-13 nuclear magnetic resonance and evidence for stereoelectronic control in their aqueous decomposition. *J. Med. Chem.*, **24**, 5309–5321.

Lown, J. W., McLaughlin, L. W. and Y-M. Chang., 1978, Mechanism of action of 2-haloethylnitrosoureas on DNA and its relation to their antileukemic properties. *Bioorganic Chem.*, **7**, 97–110.

Lown, J. W., Joshua A. V. and McLaughlin, L. W., 1980, Novel antitumor nitrosoureas and related compounds and their reactions with DNA. *J. Med. Chem.*, **23**, 798–805.

Lown, J. W., Koganty, R. R., Tew, K. D., Oiry, J. and Imbach, J. L., 1985, Mechanism of action of 2-haloethylnitrosoureas on deoxyribonucleic acid. Pathways of aqueous decomposition and pharmacological characteristics of new anticancer disulfide-linked nitrosoureas. *Biochem. Pharmacol.*, **34**, 1015–1024.

Ludlum, D. B., 1977, Alkylating agents and the nitrosoureas, in *Cancer, A Comprehensive Treatise*, edited by F. F. Becker, Vol. 5 (New York: Plenum Press), pp. 285–307.

Ludlum, D. B. and Tong, W. P., 1981, Modification of DNA and RNA bases by the nitrosoureas. In *Nitrosoureas in Cancer Treatment*, edited by B. Serrou, P. S. Schein and J.-L. Imbach (New York: Elsevier), pp. 21–31.

Machinami, T., Nishiyama, S., Kikushi, K. and Suami, T., 1975, Synthesis of (2-chloroethyl)-nitrosourea derivatives of carbohydrate. *Bull. Chem. Soc. Jap.*, **48**, 3763–3764.

Madelmont, J. C., Godeneche, D., Parry, D., Duprat, J., Chabard, J. L., Plagne, R., Mathe, G. and Meyniel, G., 1985, New cysteamine (2-chloroethyl)nitrosoureas. Synthesis and preliminary antitumor results. *J. Med. Chem.*, **28**, 1346–1350.

May, H. E., Boose, R. and Reed, D. J., 1975, Microsomal monooxygenation of the carcinostatic 1-(2-chloroethyl)-3-cyclohexyl-1-nitrosourea. Synthesis and identification of *cis* and *trans* monohydroxylated products. *Biochemistry*, **14**, 4723–4730.

May, H. E., Boose, R. and Reed, D. J., 1975, Microsomal monooxygenation of the carcinostatic 1-(2-chloroethyl)-3-cyclohexyl-l-nitroso urea. Synthesis and identification of *cis* and *trans* monohydroxylated products. *Biochemistry*, **13**, 4723–4730.

May, H. E., Kohlhepp, S. J., Boose, R. B. and Reed, D. J., 1979, Synthesis and identification of products derived from the metabolism of the carcinostatic 1-(2-chloroethyl)-3-(*trans*-4-methylcyclohexyl)-1-nitrosourea by rat liver microsomes. *Cancer Res.*, **39**, 762–772.

Montgomery, J. A., 1976, Chemistry and structure–activity studies of the nitrosoureas. *Cancer Treat. Rep.*, **60**, 651–664.

Montgomery, J. A., James, R., McCaleb, G. S. and Johnston, T. P., 1967, The modes of decomposition of 1,3-bis-(2-chloroethyl)-1-nitrosourea and related compounds. *J. Med. Chem.*, **10**, 668–674.

Montgomery, J. A., James, R., McCaleb, G. S., Kirk, M. C. and Johnston, T. P., 1975, Decomposition of *N*-(2-chloroethyl)-*N*-nitrosoureas in aqueous media. *J. Med. Chem.*, **18**, 568–571.

Moriconi, W. J., Taylor, S., Slavik, M., Belt, R. J., Haas, C. D. and Hoogstraten, B., 1985, Phase I evaluation of chlorozotocin (NSC-178248): Weekly schedule. *Invest. New Drugs*, **3**, 57–62.

Muggia, F. M., Louie, A. C. and Sikic, B. I., 1983, Pulmonary toxicity of antitumor agents. *Cancer Treat. Rev.*, **10**, 221–243.

Nishigaki, T., Nakamura, K. and Tanaka, M., 1985a, *In vitro* metabolism of ACNU. *J. Pharmacobiodyn.*, **8**, 409–416.

Nishigaki, T., Nakamura, K., Kinoshita, T., Kuwano, H. and Tanaka, M., 1985 b, Identification of major urinary metabolites of ACNU, 3-[(4-amino-2-methyl-5-pyrimidinyl)methyl]-1-(2-chloroethyl)-1-nitrosourea hydrochloride in rats. *J. Pharmacobiodyn.*, **8**, 401–408.

Oldfield, E. H., Dedrick, R. L., Yeager, R. L., Clark, W. C., DeVroom, H. L., Chatterji, D. C. and Doppman, J. L., 1985, Reduced systemic drug exposure by combining arterial intra-chemotherapy with hemoperfusion of regional venous drainage. *J. Neurosurg.*, **63**, 726–732.

Phillips, G. L., Wolff, S. N., Fay, J. W., Herzig, R. H., Lazarus, H. M., Schold, C. and Herzig, G. P., 1986, Intensive 1,3-bis (2-chloroethyl)-1-nitrosourea (BCNU) monochemotherapy and autologous marrow transplantation for malignant glioma. *J. Clin. Oncol.*, **4**, 639–645.

Potter, D. W. and Reed, D. J., 1980, Loss of methylcyclohexyl stereospecificity during cytochrome P-450-dependent monooxygenation, in *Microsomes, Drug Oxidations, and Chemical Carcinogenesis*, edited by M. J. Coon *et al.*, Vol. 2 (New York: Academic Press), pp. 371–374.

Potter, D. W. and Reed, D. J., 1981, Denitrosation of carcinostatic nitrosoureas by NADPH dependent microsomal catalysis to yield nitric oxide under anaerobic conditions. *Pharmacologist*, **23**, 168.

Reed, D. J., 1981, Metabolism of nitrosoureas, in *Nitrosoureas: Current Status and New Developments*, edited by A. W. Prestayko, S. T. Crooke, L. H. Baker, S. K. Carter, and P. S. Schein (New York: Academic Press), pp 57–67.

Reed, D. J. and May, H. E., 1975, Alkylation and carbamoylation intermediates from the carcinostatic 1-(2-chloroethyl)-3-cyclohexyl-1-nitrosourea (CCNU). *Life Sci.*, **16**, 1263–1270.

Reed, D. J. and May, H. E., 1977, Formation of alkylation and carbamylation intermediates and cytochrome P-450 catalyzed monooxygenation of the 2-chloroethylnitrosoureas CCNU and methyl CCNU, in *Microsomes and Drug Oxidations*, edited by V. Ullrich, I. Roots, A. Hildebrandt, R. W. Estabrook, and A. H. Conney (New York: Pergamon), pp. 680–687.

Reed, D. J. and May, H. E., 1978, Cytochrome P-450 interactions with the 2-chloroethylnitrosoureas and procarbazine. *Biochimie*, **60**, 989–995.

Reed, D. J., May, H. E., Boose, R. B., Gregory, K. M. and Beilstein, M. A., 1975, 2-Chloroethanol formation as evidence for a 2-chloroethyl alkylating intermediate during chemical degradation of 1(2-chloroethyl)-3-cyclohexyl-1-nitrosourea and 1-(2-chloroethyl)-3-(*trans*-4-methylcyclohexyl)-1-nitrosourea. *Cancer Res.*, **35**, 568–576.

Robins, P., Harris, A. L., Goldsmith, I. and Lindahl, T., 1983, Cross-linking of DNA induced by chloroethyl nitrosourea is prevented by O^6-methyl guanine-DNA methyl transferase. *Nucl. Acid Res.*, **11**, 7743–7758.

Rubin, J., Schutt, A. J., O'Connell, M. J., Gertz, M. A., Moertel, C. B., 1984, A phase II study of the combination, 1,3-bis(2-chloroethyl)-1-nitrosourea (BCNU) and N-(phosphonacetyl)-L-aspartate (PALA), in patients with advanced large bowel cancer. *Am. J. Clin. Oncol.*, **7**, 523–525.

Safdari, H., Mompeon, B., Dubois, J. B. and Gros, C., 1985, Intraarterial 1,3-bis(2-chloroethyl)-1-nitrosourea chemotherapy for the treatment of malignant gliomas of the brain: a preliminary report. *Surg. Neurol.*, **24**, 490–497.

Sariban, E., Erickson, L. C. and Kohn, K. W., 1984, Effects of carbamoylation on cell survival and DNA repair in normal human embryo cells (IMR-90) treated with various 1-(2-chloroethyl)-1-nitrosoureas. *Cancer Res.*, **44**, 1352–1357.

Skipper, H. E., Schabel, F. M., Jr., Trader, M. W. and Thomson, J. R., 1961, Experimental evaluation of potential anticancer agents. VI. Anatomical distribution of leukemic cells and failure of chemotherapy. *Cancer Res.*, **21**, 1154–1164.

Smith, A. C. and Boyd, M. R., 1984 a, Effects of bis-chloronitrosourea (BCNU) on pulmonary and serum angiotensin converting enzyme activity in rats. *Biochem. Pharmacol.*, **32**, 3719–3722.

Smith, A. C. and Boyd, M. R., 1984 b, Preferential effects of 1,3-bis-(2-chloroethyl)-1-nitrosourea (BCNU) on pulmonary glutathione reductase and glutathione/glutathione disulfide ratios: possible implications for lung toxicity. *J. Pharmacol. Exp. Ther.*, **229**, 658–663.

Sosnovsky, G. and Li, S. W., 1985, In the search for new anticancer drugs. XII. Synthesis and biological evaluation of spin labeled nitrosoureas. *Life Sci.*, **36**, 1479–1483.

Stewart, D. J., Grahovac, Z., Benoit, B., Addison, D., Richard, M. T., Dennery, J., Hugenholtz, H., Russell, N., Peterson, E. and Maroun, J. A., 1984, Intracarotid chemotherapy with a combination of 1,3-bis(2-chloroethyl)-1-nitrosourea (BCNU), cis-diaminedichloroplatinum (cisplatin), and 4′-O-demethyl-1-O(4,6-O-2-thenylidene-beta-D-glucopyranosyl) epipodophyllotoxin (VM-26) in the treatment of primary and metastatic brain tumors. *Neurosurgery*, **15**, 828–833.

Suami, T., Machinami, T. and Hisamatsu, T., 1979, Synthesis and activities of antitumor agents. *J. Med. Chem.*, **22**, 247–250.

Tew, K. D., 1981, A molecular rationale for nitrosourea induced cytotoxicity. In *Nitrosoureas in Cancer Treatment*, edited by B. Serrou, P. S. Schein and J.-L. Imbach, (New York: Elsevier), pp. 61–77.

Tofilon, P. J., Williams, M. E. and Deen, D. F., 1984, The effects of X rays on BCNU-induced DNA crosslinking. *Radiat. Res.*, **99**, 165–174.

Tong, W. P. and Ludlum, D. B., 1981, Formation of the cross-linked base, diguanylethane, in DNA treated with *N,N'*-bis(2-chloroethyl)-N-nitrosourea. *Cancer Res.*, **41**, 380–382.

Weinkam, R. J., Wen, J. H. C., Furst, D. E. and Levin, V. A., 1978, Analysis for 1,3-bis(2-chloroethyl)-1-nitrosourea by chemical ionization mass spectrometry. *Clin. Chem.*, **24**, 45–49.

Weinkam, R. J., Liu, T-Y. J. and Lin, H-S., 1980, Protein mediated chemical reactions of chloroethylnitrosoureas. *Chem.-Biol. Interactions*, **31**, 167–177.

Weinkam, R. J. and Dolan, M. E., 1983, An analysis of 1-(2-chloroethyl)-1-nitrosourea activity at the cellular level. *J. Med. Chem.*, **26**, 1656–1659.

Weiss, R. B. and Poster, D. S., 1982, The renal toxicity of cancer chemotherapeutic agents. *Cancer Treat. Rev.*, **9**, 37–56.

Weiss, R. B., Poster, D. S. and Penta, J. S., 1981, The nitrosoureas and pulmonary toxicity. *Cancer Treat. Rev.*, **8**, 111–125.

Weiss, R. B., Posada, J. G., Jr., Kramer, R. A. and Boyd, M. R., 1983, Nephrotoxicity of semustine. *Cancer Treat. Rep.*, **67**, 1105–1112.

Wheeler, G. P. and Chumley, S., 1967, Alkylating activity of 1,3-bis(2-chloroethyl)-1-nitrosourea and related compounds. *J. Med. Chem.*, **10**, 259–261.

Wheeler, G. P., Bowden, B. J., Grimsley, J. A. and Lloyd, H. H., 1974, Interrelationships of some chemical, physicochemical, and biological activities of several 1-(2-haloethyl)-1-nitrosoureas. *Cancer Res.*, **34**, 194–200.

2. Procarbazine

Russell A. Prough and Donald J. Tweedie

Introduction

A large number of organic chemicals, including procarbazine [*N*-isopropyl-α-(2-methylhydrazino)-*p*-toluamide, Matulane, natulan, ibenzmethyzin, Ro4-6467, NSC-77213], were synthesized during the early 1960s as potential inhibitors of the enzyme monoamine oxidase (Zeller *et al.*, 1963). Subsequently, several of the alkylhydrazine derivatives prepared were tested for anti-cancer activity (Bollag, 1963, 1964; Bollag and Grunberg, 1963). 1-Methyl-2-benzylhydrazine, the parent compound of procarbazine, displayed anti-cancer activity, but was noted to be very hepatotoxic. Procarbazine was then selected as a less toxic, but equally efficacious antineoplastic derivative. Procarbazine (Figure 1) was first used successfully in clinical trials two decades ago (Martz *et al.*, 1963) and it has subsequently been adopted for treatment of a number of neoplastic diseases. In particular the most successful use of procarbazine has been in the treatment of Hodgkin's disease, primarily in combination therapy with other antineoplastic compounds, namely, nitrogen mustard, vincristine and prednisone (DeVita *et al.*, 1970).

Procarbazine has been shown to act as a methylating agent (Kreis, 1970) and it is this property which has been assumed to lead to its cytotoxic activity. To date, a number of reviews have been published relating to the history, pharmacology and mode of action of procarbazine as an anti-cancer agent (Oliverio, 1973; Reed, 1975; Reed and May, 1978; Weinkam and Shiba, 1982). Reed (1975) surveyed much of the literature regarding the anti-cancer activity of the compound in rodents and discussed its presumed mode of action as it was understood at that time. In particular, the review contains an extensive survey of the experiments in which the methylhydrazine derivatives were successfully used against a number of tumours in rodents. The present chapter will focus on recent developments and will describe the routes of metabolism of procarbazine and the nature of its metabolic activation to chemically reactive methylating species.

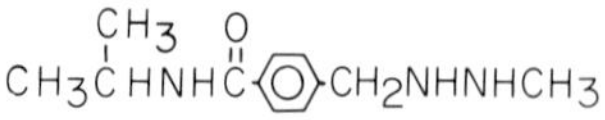

Figure 1. Procarbazine.

Clinical use

Martz *et al.* (1963) reported the first successful clinical trials with procarbazine involving patients with malignant lymphoma. Subsequent studies of Bonadonna *et al.* (1969) and Miller (1970) presented more detailed information regarding the use of procarbazine as an anti-cancer agent. Of patients with Hodgkin's disease who were refractory to other therapeutic regimens, 46–57% responded to treatment with procarbazine. DeVita *et al.* (1969, 1970) provided evidence that combination therapy with nitrogen mustard, vincristine, procarbazine and prednisone was effective against Hodgkin's disease. Of the patients administered the combination therapy, 81% achieved complete remission, with a 29–42 month median duration of remission following completion of treatment. The use of the MOPP combination therapy consisting of Mechlorethamine (nitrogen mustard), Oncovin (vincristine), procarbazine and prednisone has become a standard treatment for this disease.

Interestingly, procarbazine displays anti-cancer activity with solid tumours in animals, e.g., the advanced mast cell P815 in CD_2F_1 mice, Dunning leukaemia in Fischer rats (Oliverio *et al.*, 1964), advanced LPC-1 plasma cell tumours in Balb/c mice (Abraham *et al.*, 1967), and spontaneous mammary tumours in C3H mice (Gelzer and Loustalot, 1967). However, clinical studies of patients with solid tumours suggested that procarbazine was without pronounced effect in humans (Martz *et al.*, 1963). Consequently, procarbazine is used less frequently in the treatment of neoplastic diseases other than Hodgkin's disease. However, the drug has been used with some success against non-Hodgkin's lymphoma, malignant melanoma, bronchogenic carcinoma, and brain tumours in children (Dorr and Fritz, 1980).

Structural features

Procarbazine (*N*-isopropyl-α-(2-methylhydrazino)-*p*-toluamide hydrochloride) is a symmetrically substituted hydrazine derivative whose physical form is a white crystalline powder. It is soluble in aqueous solutions and is rapidly oxidized in the presence of oxygen and redox-active metals to yield the azo derivative and hydrogen peroxide (Reed, 1975). Figure 2 shows some of the biological and chemical products of procarbazine and their trivial names used in this chapter. The two adjacent heteroatom nitrogens provide a unique set of chemistry which is apparently responsible for the biological reactivity of the

$CH_3{-}N{=}N{-}CH_2{-}R$

Azo procarbazine
N-Isopropyl-α-(2-methylazo)-*p*-toluamide

$CH_3{-}NH{-}N{=}CH{-}R$

Hydrazone
N-Isopropyl-*p*-formylbenzamide methylhydrazone

$CH_3{-}N{=}\overset{\overset{\displaystyle O}{|}}{N}{-}CH_2{-}R$

Azoxy I
N-Isopropyl-α-(2-methyl-*NNO*-azoxy)-*p*-toluamide

$CH_3{-}\overset{\overset{\displaystyle O}{|}}{N}{=}N{-}CH_2{-}R$

Azoxy II
N-Isopropyl-α-(2-methyl-*ONN*-azoxy)-*p*-toluamide

$H{-}CO{-}R$

Benzaldehyde
N-Isopropyl-*p*-formylbenzamide

$HO{-}CO{-}R$

Acid
N-Isopropylterephthalamic acid

where $R = -C_6H_4{-}CO{-}NH{-}CH(CH_3)_2$

Figure 2. The structure of the derivatives of procarbazine.

molecule (Smith, 1966). For example, the *N*-isopropylamide function at the *para*-position of the benzyl group apparently causes the hydrazine moiety to be less easily oxidized to form either the hydrazone or azo derivatives (D. L. Dunn and R. A. Prough, unpublished results). This is important for the preparation and storage of the compound, as the parent analogue, 1-methyl-2-benzylhydrazine, is far more easily oxidized than procarbazine. Electron-withdrawing groups at the *para*-position of the ring ($-CN$, $-CONHCH(CH_3)_2$) decrease the ease of oxidation of the hydrazine, while electron-donating groups (–OH,–NH_2) increase the ease of chemical oxidation. This decrease in reactivity with metal-catalysed oxidation reactions may be an important factor for prolonging the shelf-life of the compound and in decreasing its toxicity relative to 1-methyl-2-benzylhydrazine.

We have noted in liquid preparations of procarbazine obtained from several area hospitals in Dallas, Texas and Louisville, Kentucky, that there are appreciable amounts of the azo and hydrazone derivatives of procarbazine (J. E. Erikson and R. A. Prough, unpublished results). As procarbazine is an air-sensitive compound and the hydrazone derivative is most likely toxic, care must be taken in the formulation and storage of the compound. Upon oxidation with inorganic oxidants such as HgO, $K_3Fe(CN)_6$ and Fe^{3+}, procarbazine is converted to its azo and hydrazone products as shown in Figure 3 (Dunn *et al.*, 1979). Normally, the azo derivative (*N*-isopropyl-α-(2-methylazo)-*p*-toluamide) is formed in higher yields in the presence of chemical oxidants, but is slowly converted to its hydrazone tautomer (*N*-isopropyl-*p*-formylbenzamide methylhydrazone). This tautomerization reaction is potentiated at lower pH values. At pH 1, the hydrazone is hydrolysed to form methylhydrazine and *N*-isopropyl-*p*-formylbenzamide (Dunn *et al.*, 1979). However, in aprotic solvents, the azo derivative is relatively stable compared to the monoazo compounds formed during the oxidation of alkyl- or arylhydrazines (Smith, 1966).

The azoxy derivatives (*N*-isopropyl-α-(2-methyl-*NNO*-azoxy)-*p*-toluamide (azoxy I) and *N*-isopropyl-α-(methyl-*ONN*-azoxy)-*p*-toluamide (azoxy II) can be formed by oxidation of the azo derivative with peracid oxidants such as *m*-chloroperbenzoic acid. These metabolites are relatively stable in organic solvents. The azoxy II derivative is however unstable in aqueous phase. This isomer would be expected to undergo facile oxidation of the benzylic carbon by inorganic metals (K. G. Taylor, personal communication). HPLC and GC–MS procedures have been described for separation of the chemical and biological products of procarbazine (Dunn *et al.*, 1979; Weinkam and Shiba, 1978).

A final note regarding structure can be drawn from early studies of the effect of various hydrazine derivatives on cell cytotoxicity. Bollag (1963, 1964)

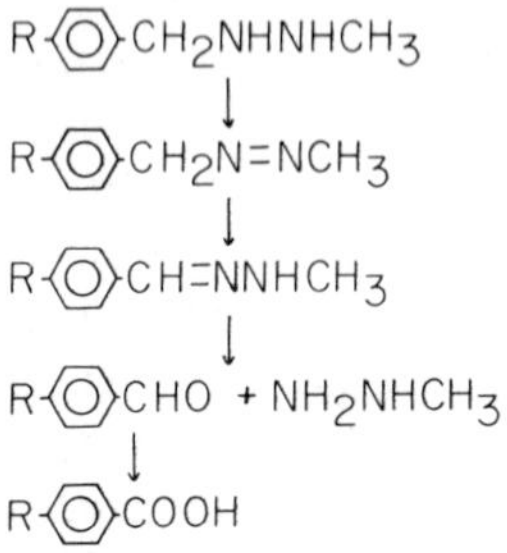

Figure 3. The pathway for chemical degradation of procarbazine. R = $-C_6H_4-CONHCH(CH_3)_2$.

demonstrated that the biological activity was absolutely dependent on the methyl group of the molecule. In the intervening years, no definitive data have emerged to satisfactorily link the metabolism of procarbazine with its biological activity.

Animal metabolism

Chemical reactivity

Procarbazine is oxidized in aqueous solutions containing oxygen and metal ions, such as ferric ion, to yield azoprocarbazine and its hydrazone tautomer as shown in Figure 3 (Oliverio *et al.*, 1964; Weinkam and Shiba, 1978). The other product formed is hydrogen peroxide. Early studies on the mode of action of the drug led to postulates that it was the hydrogen peroxide which served as the DNA-damaging species (Berneis *et al.*, 1963). However, Gale *et al.* (1967) demonstrated, using cultured Ehrlich ascites tumour cells, that the amount of hydrogen peroxide formed was not sufficient to account for the DNA damage seen. Under the same conditions, the drug did cause inhibition of DNA and RNA synthesis with L5178Y ascites cells (Sartorelli and Tsunamura, 1966).

Although the rates of chemical degradation (Figure 3) are slow, many of the breakdown products are also formed by biological systems both *in vivo* and *in vitro* during the metabolism of procarbazine (Prough, 1985). In general, the rate of formation of the azo, hydrazone and benzaldehyde derivatives by chemical processes is less than 5% of that seen with enzyme-catalysed reactions.

Studies *in vivo*

Studies to evaluate the kinetics of excretion and distribution of ^{14}C-labelled procarbazine demonstrated that the half-life of the radioactive label in the systemic circulation was 7 min in humans, 12 min in dogs and 24 min in rats (Raaflaub and Schwartz, 1965). The radioactivity accumulated mainly in the liver, kidney, intestine and skin of rats and mice administered doses of the drug i.p. (Schwartz *et al.*, 1967). Excretion and expiration of radioactivity occurs mainly over the first 24 h (Baggiolini *et al.*, 1965; Schwartz, 1966; Schwartz *et al.*, 1967). A comparison of the excretion of [^{14}C]procarbazine, labelled either on the carbonyl carbon or on the *N*-methyl carbon, showed that 74% of the [*carbonyl*-^{14}C]procarbazine was excreted in the urine over 4 days, whereas only 36% of the [*N-methyl*-^{14}C]procarbazine was isolated from the urine in that time (Schwartz *et al.*, 1967). This discrepancy could mostly be accounted for by expiration of $^{14}CO_2$. Peak expiration of $^{14}CO_2$ occurred as early as 30–60 min after i.p. administration. In man, 20% of the dose of [^{14}C]procarbazine was measured as expired $^{14}CO_2$ in 6 h (Gescher and Raymont, 1981; Schwartz *et al.*, 1967). Over the four days of the study, 4–12% of the administered radioactivity was excreted in the faeces, while 8–12% was retained in the tissues.

Azoprocarbazine has long been recognized as the primary circulating metabolite of procarbazine (Raaflaub and Schwartz, 1965; Kuttab *et al.*, 1982). In addition, an estimated 67–70% of the administered dose is excreted in the urine within the first 24 h (Schwartz *et al.*, 1967). The major urinary metabolite was shown to be *N*-isopropylterephthalamic acid (Oliverio *et al.*, 1964). Less than 5% of the dose is excreted as unchanged drug. Oliverio *et al.* (1964) also reported the presence of an unspecified glucuronide conjugate from mouse urine, although they could not find a similar conjugate in dog urine.

It has been suggested that CO_2 is released from methylhydrazine as a chemical degradation product of the hydrazone derivative of procarbazine (Dewald *et al.*, 1969; Raaflaub and Schwartz, 1965). However further studies by Baggiolini and Dewald (Baggiolini *et al.*, 1965; Dewald *et al.*, 1969) comparing the metabolism of methylhydrazine to that of procarbazine, both in the rat *in vivo* and in the isolated rat liver, showed that there were significant differences in the rates of CO_2 production from these two compounds, suggesting that methylhydrazine was not an intermediate in the conversion of procarbazine to CO_2. These differences were substantiated by observations of differential effects with the mono-oxygenase inhibitor SKF 525A and the cytochrome P-450 inducers phenobarbital and methylcholanthrene.

Methane (Dost and Reed, 1967; Schwartz *et al.*, 1969), formaldehyde and methylamine (Schwartz, 1966) have also been proposed as products of procarbazine metabolism *in vivo*. However, methylamine has not subsequently been found and Schwartz was unable to isolate the benzylamine derivative which would be produced by an N–N bond splitting reaction (Schwartz, 1966). Early metabolic pathways for procarbazine metabolism were based on the route of chemical breakdown (Figure 3) (Oliverio *et al.*, 1964; Raaflaub and Schwartz, 1965). Subsequent measurements *in vitro* demonstrated that the azo derivative was relatively stable and that little isomerization to the hydrazone occurred under physiological conditions (Baggiolini *et al.*, 1969) or during enzymatic oxidation of procarbazine (Moloney and Prough, 1983; Weinkam and Shiba, 1978).

HPLC isolation and mass spectral analysis of products of procarbazine metabolism both *in vivo* (Garsen *et al.*, 1980; Rucki *et al.*, 1980; Weinkam and Shiba, 1978) and *in vitro* (Dunn *et al.*, 1979; Weinkam and Shiba, 1978) demonstrated alternative pathways of metabolic activation of procarbazine. Two additional metabolites have been detected in the plasma of rats after i.p. administration of procarbazine and in incubation mixtures which contained postmitochondrial supernatant fractions or microsomes. These appeared to result from the *N*-oxidation of the azo derivative to yield the two azoxyprocarbazine isomers, azoxy I (*N*-isopropyl-α-(2-methyl-*NNO*-azoxy)-*p*-toluamide) and azoxy II [*N*-isopropyl-α-(2-methyl-*ONN*-azoxy)-*p*-toluamide). Further metabolism of the azoxy isomers by *C*-hydroxylation *in vitro* was suggested based on the metabolic activation pathway proposed for 1,2-dimethylhydrazine by Druckrey (1970) in which methylazoxymethanol was shown to be formed (Fiala, 1977). It was proposed that degradation of the *C*-hydroxy-azoxy metabolites would yield the benzaldehyde derivative and possibly diazomethane or formaldehyde (Weinkam and Shiba, 1978). The diazomethane can then decompose to form a methyl carbonium ion which can either alkylate cellular nucleophiles or undergo solvolysis to form methanol. Carbon dioxide may be released from oxidation of either methanol or formaldehyde *in vivo*. Also, the benzaldehyde derivative can be converted *in vivo* to the terephthalamic acid derivative by oxidation in the presence of aldehyde dehydrogenase. In reaction mixtures containing washed microsomes (where there is little aldehyde dehydrogenase), the benzaldehyde derivative is the ultimate metabolite (Weinkam and Shiba, 1978; Tweedie, Spearman and Prough, unpublished results).

A comparison of the rates of CO_2 formed in the isolated, perfused rat liver and *in vivo* demonstrated that the efflux rates of CO_2 from the isolated liver, corresponded to 75–80% of the mean CO_2 expired following administration of procarbazine *in vivo* (Baggiolini *et al.*, 1965). These authors therefore concluded that the liver was the primary site of procarbazine metabolism. Schwartz (1966) also demonstrated that the cytochrome P-450 inhibitor SKF 525A could inhibit the metabolism of procarbazine *in vivo*, supporting a significant role for hepatic oxidative enzymes.

The possibility that procarbazine is rapidly cleared by a cytochrome P-450 dependent process was further substantiated by the observed prolongation of barbitone-induced sleeping time by procarbazine (Eade *et al.*, 1972; Lee and Lucier, 1976). Although procarbazine is itself an hypnotic, non-hypnotic doses were shown to prolong sleeping times by 6–7-fold (Lee and Lucier, 1976). Procarbazine was also shown to inhibit the metabolism of a number of substrates of P-450 (Eade *et al.*, 1972; Lee and Lucier, 1976; Reed, 1976). This effect could be decreased by pretreatment with phenobarbital, an inducer of cytochrome P-450, and could be attenuated by SKF 525A, a known inhibitor of cytochrome P-450 *in vivo* and *in vitro* (Lee and Lucier, 1976).

Studies *in vitro*

Wittkop *et al.* (1969) demonstrated that a demethylase activity for procarbazine existed in the microsomal fraction of the liver. Several lines of evidence indicated that the demethylase activity was dependent on cytochrome P-450. For example, procarbazine demethylase activity could be induced by phenobarbital or methylcholanthrene treatment *in vivo* and inhibited by addition of CO, steapsin or cholate *in vitro*. Addition of procarbazine to suspensions of liver microsomes yielded a Type II substrate interaction spectrum with the microsomal cytochrome P-450. Although other alkylhydrazines were converted to their parent alkanes by microsomal cytochrome P-450, procarbazine was poorly converted to methane. This suggested that procarbazine was not a good substrate for the alkylhydrazine oxidase described by Prough *et al.* (1969).

The conversion of procarbazine to the azo derivative was shown to be mediated by liver microsomal cytochrome P-450 by its dependence on NADPH, O_2 and cytochrome P-450 reductase, as well as by the effects of various inhibitors and inducers (Dunn *et al.*, 1979; Prough *et al.*, 1977; Wittkop *et al.*, 1969). A colorimetric and an HPLC assay were devised to accurately measure the rates of metabolism of procarbazine to azoprocarbazine (Dunn *et al.*, 1979). The rate of conversion was approximately 10–18 nmol product/min/mg protein; a value similar to the best drug substrates of cytochrome P-450. These results confirmed the contentions of others that the liver is the main site of metabolism of procarbazine and that its disposition may be one of first-pass kinetics.

The metabolism of procarbazine to azoprocarbazine by an NADPH-independent mechanism was discovered using isolated rat hepatocytes (Coomes and Prough, 1983). Dilution of the cytosolic pool of NADPH by sonication of the hepatocytes did not greatly reduce the rate of procarbazine oxidation, whereas the rates of biphenyl hydroxylation, a cytochrome P-450 mediated reaction, were markedly decreased. This oxidase activity was localized in the mitochondrial fraction of the cells, could be inhibited by the monoamine oxidase (MAO) inhibitor *N*, *N*-dimethylpropargylamine, and was not linked to mitochondrial electron transport. The activity also co-purified with benzylamine oxidase activity. The product of procarbazine metabolism by MAO was the azo derivative, but azoprocarbazine was shown not to be a substrate of MAO (Prough *et al.*, 1983).

Based on the specific activity of both the NADPH-dependent (cytochrome P-450) and NADPH-independent (MAO) reactions, it was estimated that in the non-induced rat hepatocyte, MAO is responsible for at least 40% of the total procarbazine oxidation to azoprocarbazine, while in the PB-induced hepatocyte this value decreased to 25% (Coomes and Prough, 1983). The relative contributions of these two enzyme systems in the metabolism of procarbazine in rat liver and lung have been studied (Erikson and Prough, 1986 a). Monoamine oxidase oxidized the N–N bond of all classes of hydrazines, while cytochrome P-450 only preferentially metabolized the N–N bond of 1,2-disubstituted hydrazines, including procarbazine. Other hydrazines, such as monoalkylhydrazines, appeared to be oxidized across the N–C bond. There did not appear to be any specificity towards the two isozymes of monoamine oxidase (MAO-A or MAO-B) in the metabolism of procarbazine or of hydrazines in general. Unlike other hydrazine compounds (Patek and Hellerman, 1974), procarbazine does not inactivate MAO, but serves as a competitive substrate against benzylamine or kynurenine oxidase activity.

Prough and Ziegler (1977) were able to distinguish two enzyme activities involved in the microsomal metabolism of a number of *N*-methylamines, i.e. an *N*-oxygenase activity (due to FAD-containing mono-oxygenase) and a demethylase activity (due to cytochrome P-450). Subsequent studies with a number of hydrazine derivatives demonstrated that although the microsomal FAD-containing mono-oxygenase (amine oxidase) was capable of metabolizing a number of these compounds at rates comparable to that obtained with *N*, *N*-dimethylamine (a preferred substrate of this enzyme), procarbazine was not a good substrate (Prough *et al.*, 1981).

Multiple forms of cytochrome P-450 have been implicated in both the oxidation of procarbazine to azoprocarbazine (Dunn *et al.*, 1979; Wiebkin and Prough, 1980) and in the subsequent *N*-oxygenation of azoprocarbazine (Prough *et al.*, 1984). This is manifested by the induction of stereoselective *N*-oxygenation reactions by phenobarbital and polycyclic aromatic hydrocarbons (PAH). For example, microsomes from PAH-treated rats preferentially *N*-oxidized the nitrogen closest to the methyl group (Dunn *et al.*, 1979; Wiebkin and Prough, 1980) with a 20 : 1 product ratio. In addition, microsomes from untreated or phenobarbital-pretreated rats had identical product ratios of the two isomeric azoxy metabolites, but treatment with phenobarbital increased the total rate of azoxy synthesis 3–5-fold. The azoxy II derivative was formed in a 4 :1 ratio to azoxy I (azoxy with N–O bond closest to benzyl group). Based on these results, a subsequent set of experiments was performed with purified cytochromes P-450 and with antibodies directed toward various purified forms of cytochrome P-450. Of the eight isozymes studied (Guengerich *et al.*, 1982), most of the activity (> 80%) involved in the *N*-oxidation of azoprocarbazine was mediated by a minor form, P-450_{PB-C} and a major form, P-$450_{\beta NF-B}$ (P-450c). A small portion of the activity was also noted with the major form, P-450_{PB-B} (P-450b). The product ratios of the two azoxy isomers formed with either purified isozymes or their respective microsome sources were similar. Experiments using specific inhibitory antibodies supported these contentions.

Preliminary experiments on the metabolism of the azoxy metabolites suggested that cytochrome P-450 might further metabolize these compounds. Weinkam and Shiba (1978) also demonstrated that in ether extracts of incubation mixtures containing procarbazine and rat liver microsomes or post-mitochondrial supernatant, an unknown compound could be observed based on a mass spectrum with a parent ion at *m*/*e* 252. This structure corresponds to that of a putative *C*-hydroxy-azoxy metabolite. However, we have observed that the azoxy II derivative (azoxy with N–O bond closest to the methyl group) decomposes chemically at appreciable rates in aqueous solutions to an intermediate which apparently leads to covalent binding to protein (Moloney *et al.*, 1985). The other product of this chemical decomposition reaction is the benzaldehyde derivative, *N*-isopropyl-*p*-formylbenzamide. The azoxy II isomer possesses a readily oxidizable C–H methylene bond and apparently decomposes to produce a protein-binding species, probably a methyl carbonium ion (Moloney *et al.*, 1985; K. G. Taylor, personal communication).

This reaction can be accelerated in the presence of purified cytosolic protein(s) which also produce the benzaldehyde derivative as the major metabolite and an uncharacterized alkylating species (D. J. Tweedie and R. A. Prough, unpublished observation). Studies currently in progress suggest the presence of two forms of the enzyme which metabolize azoxy compounds; this work will be the subject of future publications. In the presence of the cytosolic NADH-dependent aldehyde dehydrogenase, the benzaldehyde derivative is rapidly converted to the organic acid, *N*-isopropylterephthalamic acid (TAC). This reaction, no doubt, accounts for the formation of TAC as the major urinary metabolite observed by others (Oliverio *et al.*, 1964; Weinkam and Shiba, 1978).

The other product formed *in vivo* and *in vitro* from procarbazine is the respired product, methane. Some confusion has existed as to the route of formation of methane from procarbazine. It must be pointed out that this product is unique for procarbazine, as 1,2-dimethylhydrazine, another 1,2-substituted hydrazine does not yield methane as a product either *in vivo* (Dost *et al.*, 1966) or *in vitro* (Prough, 1983). In addition, only alkylhydrazines were shown to yield these alkane products. The pathway leading to methane formation from procarbazine has recently been elucidated *in vitro* by Moloney and Prough (1983). Previous suggestions that methane was produced via methylhydrazine formation from the hydrazone tautomer of azoprocarbazine were dispelled on the basis of kinetic and inhibitor studies. The V_{max} and apparent K_m values for methane formation from the hydrazone derivative and from methylhydrazine itself demonstrated that the hydrazone derivative had a lower apparent K_m and a higher V_{max} value than did methylhydrazine. This clearly indicates that the hydrazone is a better substrate for methane production than methylhydrazine. The inhibition studies employed methimazole and ethylhydrazine. While methimazole could inhibit methane formation from procarbazine and azoprocarbazine, it stimulated methane formation from methylhydrazine. Ethylhydrazine strongly inhibited methane formation from monomethylhydrazine and hydrazone, but had less of an effect on methane formation from procarbazine or azoprocarbazine. Thus, formation of the hydrazone or monomethylhydrazine would not appear to contribute significantly to methane production *in vivo* or *in vitro*.

Moloney and Prough (1983) also demonstrated a lag in the production of methane from procarbazine which would be consistent with the formation of methane from a metabolite of procarbazine, namely, azoprocarbazine (Baggiolini *et al.*, 1969; Dewald *et al.*, 1969; Dost and Reed, 1967). Methane is not produced from the azoxy isomers (Moloney and Prough, 1983) and although methane can be produced in the hydrazone pathway, the isomerization of azo to hydrazone is not fast enough to account for this reaction. In addition, little hydrazone is formed during the biological *N*-oxidation reaction (Moloney and Prough, 1983). Based on the chemical literature (Smith, 1966), one must assume that the methane formed from azoprocarbazine is derived from some putative diazene or a *C*-hydroxyazo intermediate which decomposes to yield a methyl free radical (Moloney *et al.*, 1985). In addition, Sinha (1984) has demonstrated that radicals are formed during the metabolism of procarbazine. The decomposition products of the diazene intermediate (i.e., the methyl free radicals) apparently can either bind to cellular macromolecules or can abstract a proton, e.g. from reduced glutathione or protein thiols, to yield methane (Moloney and Prough, 1983; Moloney *et al.*, 1985; Spearman *et al.*, 1985).

Human metabolism

The information available in the literature would support the contention that humans metabolize procarbazine, azoprocarbazine, and the azoxy isomers in a manner similar to that seen in rats (Oliverio *et al.*, 1964; Raaflaub and Schwartz, 1965; Shiba and Weinkam, 1983). The early metabolic work of Schwartz and others (Oliverio *et al.*, 1964; Raaflaub and Schwartz, 1965; Schwartz *et al.*, 1967) demonstrated the presence of *N*-isopropylterephthalamic acid as a major urinary metabolite and $^{14}CO_2$ as a respired product in both rodents and humans. These findings have been confirmed in later studies which also demonstrated the formation of the azoxy metabolites of procarbazine (Shiba and Weinkam, 1983). Wolff *et al.* (1985) have reported that human liver microsomes metabolize azoprocarbazine to azoxyprocarbazine metabolites and we have observed that human liver microsomes and mitochondria metabolize procarbazine to azoprocarbazine, presumably involving cytochrome P-450 and monoamine oxidase (M. W. Coomes and R. A. Prough, unpublished results). Work is in progress to deduce the characteristics of the cytosolic enzymes in rodents and humans which metabolize the azoxy metabolites.

Relationship between metabolism and biological activity

Procarbazine possesses considerable potential as a carcinogenic and toxic chemical. Marked side-effects are seen in human patients during drug therapy (DeVita *et al.*, 1970) which can lead to loss of function of the immune system, depression of bone marrow and decreases in sperm viability. A recent study by Lewis (1984) demonstrated a procarbazine-associated irritation of the lung tissue of humans. A number of effects on the central nervous system have been reported as well, including depression, confusion, decreased reflexes and other neuropathies (Reed, 1985; Weinkam and Shiba, 1982). As the drug is a good substrate for monoamine oxidase and readily crosses the blood–brain barrier, it may exert certain of its pharmacological side-effects by interfering with the metabolism of biogenic amines. Finally, procarbazine has been shown to be teratogenic (Chaube and Murphy, 1969), mutagenic (Pueyo, 1979), and carcinogenic (Kelly *et al.*, 1969; Sieber *et al.*, 1978).

The proposed pathways of procarbazine metabolism, based on the literature, are summarized in Figure 4. The reactive intermediates shown may contribute to the toxic and carcinogenic action of the drug. The formation of the first oxidative metabolite of procarbazine, the azo derivative, has been well documented. This appears to have little chemical reactivity (Prough, 1985). Tautomerization of the azo derivative to its hydrazone form is a very minor pathway and no evidence exists demonstrating the conversion of the hydrazone to azoxy metabolites. However, azoprocarbazine, the hydrazone tautomer and methylhydrazine all can be metabolized by cytochrome P-450 to yield methane as a product. Based on the studies by Moloney and Prough (1983), it would seem unlikely that the methane formed during the metabolism of procarbazine *in vivo* involves the intermediacy of the hydrazone derivative or methylhydrazine. If impure preparations of procarbazine are administered, the hydrazone or methylhydrazine present could lead to methane formation. Moloney *et al.* (1985) have demonstrated a correlation between methane formation and covalent binding of the methyl group on azoprocarbazine to microsomal protein without involvement of the azoxy metabolites. This may provide a rationale for more than one potential mechanism of reactivity of procarbazine metabolites, besides the azoxy pathway described below. Similar conclusions were made regarding the spermatogenic toxicity (Yost *et al.*, 1985) and anti-cancer activity of procarbazine metabolites (G. Yost, private communication).

Further *N*-oxidation of azoprocarbazine leads to formation of the two isomeric azoxy metabolites. The presence of a *C*-hydroxylated metabolite of the azoxy II intermediate was proposed based on mass spectral data presented by Weinkam and Shiba (1978) and by analogy to the metabolism of 1,2-dimethylhydrazine (Fiala, 1977). As the azoxy II isomer possesses a readily oxidizable C–H bond, it is presumed that this metabolite may be the *C*-hydroxylated derivative of azoxy II. The presence of this metabolite has not been further documented by other groups.

In addition, we have observed that the azoxy II (azoxy with N–O bond closest to the methyl group) decomposes at appreciable rates in aqueous solutions to an intermediate which apparently leads to covalent binding, probably through a methyl carbonium ion (Moloney *et al.*, 1985; K. G. Taylor, personal communication). The amount of covalent binding of the terminal methyl group of azoxy II procarbazine to microsomal protein (chemical decomposition) was 30% as large as that seen from azoprocarbazine in the presence of

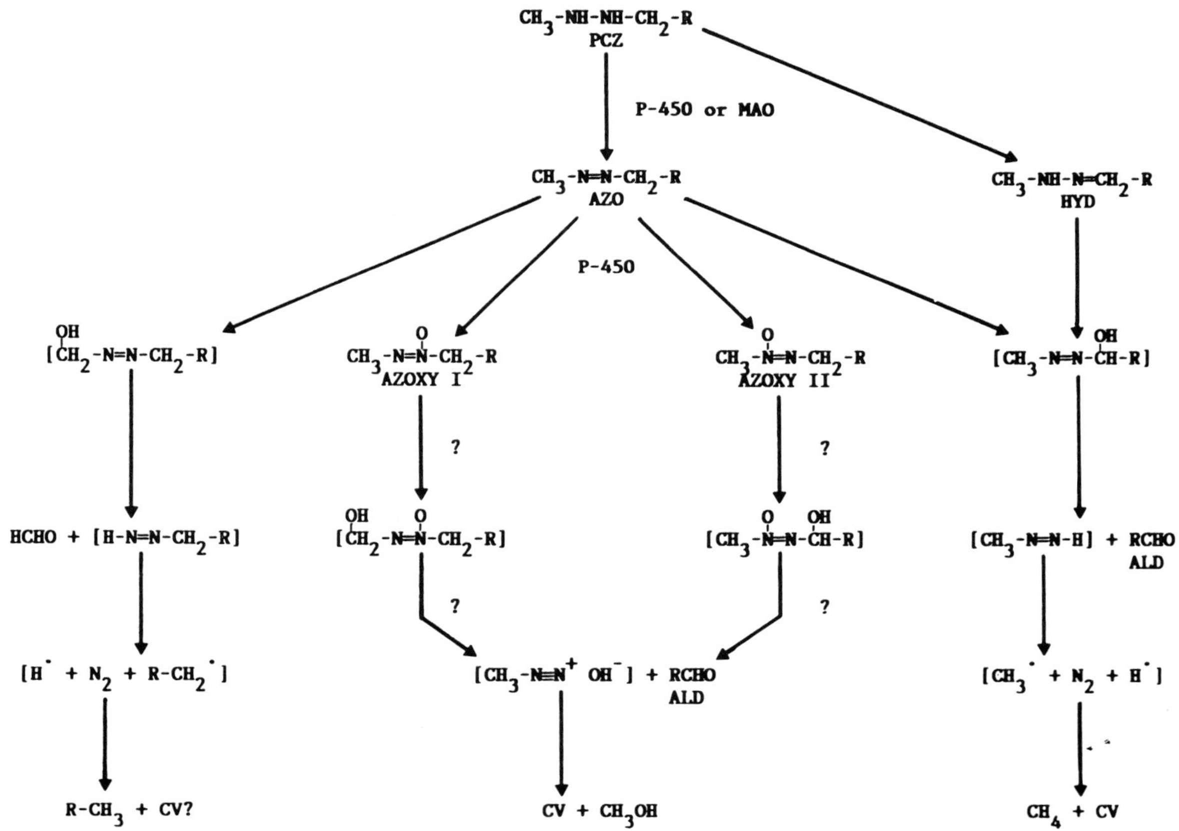

Figure 4. The metabolic pathway of procarbazine activation. CV, Covalent binding. $R = -C_6H_4\text{-}CONHCH(CH_3)_2$.

NADPH (enzymic decomposition). Therefore, a portion of the covalent binding of azo- or azoxyprocarbazine to liver microsomal protein and presumably other cellular nucleophiles could be due to a chemical decomposition reaction of azoxy II. We have also demonstrated that the azoxy II can be metabolized by a cytosolic protein to form the benzaldehyde derivative. This pathway could also lead to biologically-generated, chemically-reactive intermediates, since the background rates of azoxy II disappearance in aqueous solutions are less than one half of the protein-associated rate. This situation is similar to that shown by Grab and Zedeck (1977) for methylazoxymethanol conversion to reactive methylating agents in the presence of several alcohol dehydrogenases.

Recently, Erikson, Ducore and Prough have studied the DNA-damaging potential of procarbazine and its metabolites in L1210 tumour cells in culture (Erikson *et al.*, 1986 b). The azoxy derivatives are the most potent agents in causing single-strand breaks and alkali-labile sites in DNA. In addition, the cytosolic enzyme(s) capable of metabolizing the azoxy derivatives have been shown to be present in L1210 cells. Future studies will evaluate the role of the(se) enzyme(s) in tumour cell cytotoxicity and DNA damage. Based on these reports from the literature, the pathways of biological oxidation of the benzylic or methyl carbon of the azoxy isomers to form *C*-hydroxyazoxy intermediates may also be of importance in the mode of action of procarbazine as a cytotoxic or carcinogenic agent. However, our studies on the metabolic activation of the azoxy metabolites are not complete at this time.

Thus, three potential mechanisms for the mode of action of procarbazine can be visualized, i.e. a diazene metabolite from azoprocarbazine, direct chemical reactivity of azoxy II, and the reactivity of a *C*-hydroxyazoxy metabolite of the azoxy derivatives. However, insufficient evidence is present to unambiguously state which mode of action of the drug contributes to its cytotoxic or carcinogenic activity. Indeed, it is possible that future experiments will demonstrate a different mechanism for the cytotoxic and carcinogenic activities.

Future directions

Procarbazine appears to be unique as an anti-tumour agent. Only one chemical form of the drug has been shown to be useful for treatment and the drug has a selectivity in a limited number of tumours in humans. Therefore it is possible that little can be done to enhance the use of the drug beyond the experimental approaches provided in the past. However, the *in vitro* studies by our group describing the enzymology of the metabolism of procarbazine and the *in vivo* studies of Shiba and Weinkam (1982, 1983) clearly demonstrate that the formation of azoprocarbazine and the azoxy procarbazines can be easily modulated by induction of the enzymes involved in their metabolic activation. For example, a regiospecific metabolism of azoprocarbazine to give the two isomeric azoxy compounds can be obtained by treatment of rodents with either phenobarbital or 5,6-benzoflavone (Wiebkin and Prough, 1980). Likewise, Shiba and Weinkam (1982, 1983) have shown that phenobarbital treatment of tumour-bearing mice before administration of procarbazine causes a 20–40% increased lifetime. It is possible that with an understanding of the enzymes which activate azo and azoxyprocarbazine, a more selective treatment regimen might be established. This possibility justifies more focused studies on the metabolism and mechanism of action of procarbazine.

References

Abraham, D., Carbone, P. P., and Venditti, J. M., 1967, Evaluation of chemical agents against the plasma cell tumor LPC-1 in mice. *Biochem. Pharmacol.*, **16**, 665–673.

Baggiolini, M., Bickel, M. H. and Messiha, F. S., 1965, Demethylation *in vivo* of Natulan, a tumour-inhibiting methylhydrazine derivative. *Experientia* (*Basel*), **21**, 334–336.

Baggiolini, M., Dewald, B. and Aebi, H., 1969, Oxidation of *p*-(N^1-methylhydrazinomethyl)-*N*-isopropyl benzamide (procarbazine) to the methylazo derivative and oxidative cleavage of the N^2–C bond in the isolated perfused rat liver. *Biochem. Pharmacol.*, **18**, 2187–2196.

Berneis, K., Kofler, M., Bollag, W., Kaiser, A., and Langemann, A., 1963, The degradation of deoxyribonucleic acid by new tumor inhibiting compounds: the intermediate formation of hydrogen peroxide. *Experientia* (*Basel*), **19**, 132–133.

Bollag, W., 1963, The tumor-inhibitory effects of the methylhydrazine derivative Ro 4-6467/1 (NSC-77213). *Cancer Chemother. Rep.*, **33**, 1–4.

Bollag, W., 1964, Investigations with methylhydrazine derivatives. In *Chemotherapy of Cancer*, edited by P. A. Plattner (Amsterdam: Elsevier), pp. 191–197

Bollag, W. and Grunberg, E., 1963, Tumour inhibitory effects of a new class of cytotoxic agents: Methylhydrazine derivatives. *Experientia* (*Basel*), **19**, 130–131.

Bonadonna, G., Monfardini, S. and Oldini, C., 1969, Comparative effects of vinblastine and procarbazine in advanced Hodgkin's disease. *Eur. J. Cancer*, **5**, 393–402.

Chaube, S. and Murphy, M. L., 1969, Fetal malformations produced in rats by *N*-isopropyl-α-(2-methylhydrazino)-*p*-toluamide hydrochloride (procarbazine). *Teratology*, **2**, 23–31.

Coomes, M. W. and Prough, R. A., 1983, The mitochondrial metabolism of 1,2-disubstituted hydrazines, procarbazine and 1,2-dimethylhydrazine. *Drug Metab. Dispos.*, **11**, 550–555.

DeVita, V. T., Serpick, A. A., and Carbone, P. P., 1969, Combination chemotherapy of advanced Hodgkin's disease (HD): the NCI program, a progress report. *Proc. Am. Ass. Cancer Res.*, **10**, p. 19.

DeVita, V. T., Serpick, A. A., and Carbone, P. P., 1970, Combination chemotherapy in the treatment of advanced Hodgkin's disease. *Ann. Int. Med.*, **73**, 881–895.

Dewald, B., Baggiolini, M. and Aebi, H., 1969, *N*-Demethylation of *p*-(N^1-methylhydrazinomethyl)-*N*-isopropyl benzamide (procarbazine), a cytostatically active methylhydrazine derivative, in the intact rat and in the isolated perfused rat liver. *Biochem. Pharmacol.*, **18**, 2179–2186.

Dorr, R. T. and Fritz, W. L., 1980, Procarbazine, In *Cancer Chemotherapy Handbook* (New York: Elsevier), pp. 593–601.

Dost, F. N. and Reed, D. J., 1967, Methane formation *in vivo* from, *N*-isopropyl-α-(2-methylhydrazino)-*p*-toluamide hydrochloride, a tumor-inhibiting methylhydrazine derivative. *Biochem. Pharmacol.*, **16**, 1741–1746.

Dost, F. N., Reed, D. J. and Wang, C. H., 1966, The metabolic fate of monomethylhydrazine and unsymmetrical dimethylhydrazine. *Biochem. Pharmacol.*, **15**, 1325–1332.

Dunn, D. L., Lubet, R. A. and Prough, R. A., 1979, Oxidative metabolism of *N*-isopropyl-α-(2-methylhydrazino)-*p*-toluamide hydrochloride (procarbazine) by rat liver microsomes. *Cancer Res.*, **39**, 4555–4563.

Druckrey, H., 1970, Production of colonic carcinomas by 1,2-dimethylhydrazines and azo alkanes. In *Carcinoma of the Colon and Antecedent Epithelium*, edited by W. J. Burdette (Springfield, IL: C. C. Thomas), pp. 267–279.

Eade, N. R., MacLeod, S. M., and Renton, K. W., 1972, Inhibition of hepatic microsomal drug metabolism by the hydrazines RO 4-4602, MK 486, and procarbazine hydrochloride. *Can. J. Physiol. Pharmacol.*, **50**, 721–724.

Erikson, J. E. and Prough, R. A., 1986 a, Oxidative metabolism of some hydrazine derivatives by rat liver and lung tissue fractions. *J. Biochem. Toxicol.*, **1**, 41–52.

Erikson, J. E., Ducore, J. M., and Prough, R. A., 1986 b, Potential of procarbazine (*N*-isopropyl-α-(2-methylhydrazino)-*p*-toluamide) and its metabolites to damage DNA in L1210 cells. *The Pharmacologist*, **28**, p. 444.

Fiala, E. S., 1977, Investigations into the metabolism and mode of action of the colon carcinogens 1,2-dimethylhydrazine and azoxymethane. *Cancer*, **40**, 2436–2445.

Gale, G. R., Simpson, J. G., and Smith, A. B., 1967, Studies of the mode of action of *N*-isopropyl-α-(2-methylhydrazino)-*p*-toluamide. *Cancer Res.*, **27**, 1186–1191.

Gelzer, J. and Loustalot, P., 1967, Biological and chemotherapeutic studies on primary mammary tumors in C3H and C3HO mice. *Int. J. Cancer*, **2**, 179–187.

Gescher, A. and Raymont, C., 1981, Studies of the metabolism of *N*-methyl containing anti-tumour agents. $^{14}CO_2$ breath analysis after administration of ^{14}C-labelled *N*-methyl drugs, formaldehyde and formate in mice. *Biochem. Pharmacol.*, **30**, 1245–1252.

Gorsen, R. M., Weiss, A. J. and Manthei, R. W., 1980, Analysis of procarbazine and metabolites by gas chromatography-mass spectrometry. *J. Chromatog.*, **221**, 309–318.

Grab, D. J. and Zedeck, M. S., 1977, Organ-specific effects of the carcinogen methylazoxymethanol related to metabolism by nicotinamide adenine dinucleotide-dependent dehydrogenases. *Cancer Res.*, **37**, 4182–4189.

Guengerich, F. P., Dannan, G. A., Wright, S. T., Martin, M. V., and Kaminsky, L. S., 1982, Purification and characterization of liver microsomal cytochromes P-450: electrophoretic, spectral, catalytic, and immunochemical properties and inducibility of eight isozymes isolated from rats treated with phenobarbital and β-naphthoflavone. *Biochemistry.*, **21**, 6019–6030.

Kelly, M. G., O'Gara, R. W., Yancey, S. T. Gadekar, K., Botkin, C. and Oliverio, V. T., 1969, Comparative carcinogenicity of *N*-isopropyl-α-(2-methylhydrazino)-*p*-toluamide HCl (procarbazine hydrochloride), its degradation products, other hydrazines, and isonicotinic acid hydrazide. *J. Natl. Cancer Inst.*, **42**, 337–344.

Kreis, W, 1970, Metabolism of an antineoplastic methylhydrazine derivative in a P815 mouse neoplasm. *Cancer Res.*, **30**, 82–89.

Kuttab, S. H., Tanglertpaibul, S. and Vouros, P., 1982, Studies on the metabolism of procarbazine by mass spectrometry. *Biomed Mass Spectrom.*, **9**, 78–84.

Lee, I. P. and Lucier, G. W., 1976, The potentiation of barbiturate-induced narcosis by procarbazine. *J. Pharmacol. Exp. Ther.*, **196**, 586–593.

Lewis, L. D., 1984, Procarbazine associated alveolitis. *Thorax*, **39**, 206–207.

Martz, G., D'Alessandri, A., Keel, H. J., and Bollag, W., 1963, Preliminary clinical results with a new anti-tumor agent Ro 4-6467 (NSC-77213). *Cancer Chemother. Rep.*, **33**, 5–14.

Miller, E., 1970, Development of procarbazine. In *Procarbazine (Matulane: NSC-77213): Development and Application*, edited by S. K. Carter (Bethesda: Cancer Therapy Evaluation Branch, National Cancer Institute), pp. 3–8.

Moloney, S. J. and Prough, R. A., 1983, Studies on the pathway of methane formation from procarbazine, a 2-methylbenzylhydrazine derivative, by rat liver microsomes. *Arch. Biochem. Biophys.*, **221**, 577–584.

Moloney, S. J., Wiebkin, P., Cummings, S. W. and Prough, R. A., 1985, Metabolic activation of the terminal *N*-methyl group of *N*-isopropyl-α-(2-methylhydrazino)-*p*-toluamide hydrochloride (procarbazine). *Carcinogenesis*, **6**, 397–401.

Oliverio, V. T., 1973, Derivatives of triazenes and hydrazines. In *Cancer Medicine*, edited by J. F. Holland and E. Frei (Philadelphia: Lea and Febiger), pp. 806–817.

Oliverio, V. T., Denham, C., DeVita, V. T, and Kelly, M. G., 1964, Some pharmacologic properties of a new antitumor agent, *N*-isopropyl-α-(2-methylhydrazino)-*p*-toluamide hydrochloride (NSC-77213). *Cancer Chemother. Rep.*, **42**, 1–7.

Patek, D. R. and Hellerman, L., 1974, Mitochondrial monoamine oxidase. Mechanism of inhibition by phenylhydrazine and by aralkylhydrazines. Roles of enzymatic oxidation. *J. Biol. Chem.*, **249**, 2373–2380.

Prough, R. A., 1973, The *N*-oxidation of alkylhydrazines catalyzed by the microsomal mixed-function amine oxidase. *Arch. Biochem. Biophys.*, **158**, 442–444.

Prough, R. A., 1985, The biological *N*-oxidation of hydrazines and azo-compounds. In *Biological Oxidation of Nitrogen in Organic Molecules*, edited by J. W. Gorrod and L. A. Damani (Chichester: Ellis Horwood), ch. 29, pp. 267–277.

Prough, R. A., and Ziegler, D. M., 1977, The relative participation of liver microsomal amine oxidase and cytochrome P-450 in *N*-demethylation reactions. *Arch. Biochem. Biophys.*, **180**, 363–373.

Prough, R. A. Wittkop, J. A. and Reed, D. J., 1969, Evidence for the hepatic metabolism of some monoalkylhydrazines. *Arch. Biochem. Biophys.*, **131**, 369–373.

Prough, R. A., Coomes, M. L. and Dunn, D. L., 1977, The microsomal metabolism of carcinogenic and/or therapeutic hydrazines. In *Microsomes and Drug Oxidations*, edited by V. Ullrich, I. Roots, A. Hildebrandt, R. W. Estabrook and A. H. Conney (Oxford: Pergamon Press), pp. 500–507.

Prough, R. A., Freeman, P. C. and Hines, R. N., 1981, The oxidation of hydrazine derivatives catalyzed by the purified liver microsomal FAD-containing monooxygenase. *J. Biol. Chem.*, **256**, 4178–4184.

Prough, R. A., Brown, M. I., Amrhein, C. A. and Marnett, L. J., 1983, Metabolism of azo and hydrazine derivatives to reactive intermediates. In *Extrahepatic Drug Metabolism and Chemical Carcinogenesis*, edited by J. Rydstrom, J. Montelius, and M. Bengtsson (Amsterdam: Elsevier), pp. 489–498.

Prough, R. A., Brown, M. I., Dannan, G. A. and Guengerich, F. P., 1984, Major isozymes of rat liver microsomal cytochrome P-450 involved in the *N*-oxidation of *N*-isopropyl-α-(2-methylazo)-*p*-toluamide, the azo derivative of procarbazine. *Cancer Res.*, **44**, 543–548.

Pueyo, C; 1979, Natulan induces forward mutations to L-arabinose-resistance in *Salmonella typhimurium*. *Mutat. Res.*, **67**, 189–192.

Raaflaub, J. and Schwartz, D. E., 1965, Uber den Metabolismus eines cytostatisch wirksamen Methylhydrazin-Derivats (Natulan). *Experientia (Basel)*, **21**, 44–45.

Reed, D. J., 1975, Procarbazine. In *Handbook of Experimental Pharmacology*,

Antineoplastic and Immunosuppressive Agents, edited by A. C. Sartorelli and D. G. Johns (New York: Springer Verlag), Vol. 38/2, Ch. 70, pp. 747–765.

Reed, D. J., 1976, Effects *in vivo* of lymphoma ascites tumors and procarbazine, alone and in combination, upon hepatic drug-metabolizing enzymes of mice. *Biochem. Pharmacol.*, **25**, 153–156.

Reed, D. J. and May, H. E., 1978, Cytochrome P-450 interactions with 2-chloroethylnitrosoureas and procarbazine. *Biochimie*, **60**, 989–995.

Rucki, R. J., Ross, A. and Moros, S. A., 1980, Application of an electrochemical detector to the determination of procarbazine hydrochloride by high-performance liquid chromatography. *J. Chromatog.*, **190**, 359–365.

Sartorelli, A. C. and Tsunamura, S., 1966, Studies on the biochemical mode of action of a cytotoxic methylhydrazine derivative, *N*-isopropyl-α-(2-methylhydrazino)-*p*-toluamide. *Mol. Pharmacol.*, **2**, 275–283.

Schwartz, D. E., 1966, Comparative metabolic studies with natulan, methylhydrazine and methylamine in rats. *Experientia* (*Basel*), **22**, 212–213.

Schwartz, D. E., Bollag, W. and Obrecht, P., 1967, Distribution and excretion studies of procarbazine in animals and man. *Arzneimittel-Forsch.*, **17**, 1389–1393.

Schwartz, D. E., Brubaker, G. B. and Vecchi, M., 1969, Metabolic formation of methane from *N*-methyl-substituted hydrazine compounds and carcinostatic activity. *J. Labelled Compounds*, **111**, 487–488.

Shiba, D. A. and Weinkam, R. J., 1982, Quantitative analysis of procarbazine, procarbazine metabolites and chemical degradation products with application to pharmacokinetic studies. *J. Chromatog.*, **229**, 397–407.

Shiba, D. A. and Weinkam, R. J., 1983, The *in vivo* cytoxic activity of procarbazine and procarbazine metabolites against L1210 ascites leukemia cells in CDF_1 mice and the effects of pretreatment with procarbazine, phenobarbital, diphenylhydantoin, and methylprednisolone upon *in vivo* procarbazine activity. *Cancer Chemother. Pharmacol.*, **11**, 124–129.

Sieber, S. M., Correa, P., Dalgard, D. W., and Adamson, R. H., 1978, Carcinogenic and other adverse effects of procarbazine in nonhuman primates. *Cancer Res.*, **38**, 2125–2134.

Sinha, B. K., 1984, Metabolic activation of procarbazine. Evidence for carbon-centred free radical intermediates. *Biochem. Pharmacol.*, **33**, 2777–2781.

Smith, P. A. S., 1966, *The Chemistry of Open-chain Organic Nitrogen Compounds* (New York: W. A. Benjamin), Vol. 2, pp. 119–209.

Spearman, M. E., Franck, T. G., Moloney, S. J. and Prough, R. A., 1985, Influence of cytosolic factors on hydrazine and hydrazide metabolism. In *Biological Oxidation of Nitrogen in Organic Molecules*, edited by J. W. Gorrod and L. A. Damani (Chichester: Ellis Horwood), ch. 30, pp. 290–296.

Weinkam, R. J. and Shiba, D. A., 1978, Metabolic activation of procarbazine. *Life Sci.*, **22**, 937–946.

Weinkam, R. J. and Shiba, D. A., 1982, Nonclassical alkylating agents. Procarbazine. In *Pharmacologic Principles of Cancer Treatment*, edited by B. Chabner (Philadelphia: Saunders), Ch. 15, pp. 340–362.

Wiebkin, P. and Prough, R. A., 1980, Oxidative metabolism of *N*-isopropyl-α-(2-methylazo)-*p*-toluamide (azoprocarbazine) by rodent liver microsomes. *Cancer Res.*, **40**, 3524–3529.

Wittkop, J. A., Prough, R. A. and Reed, D. J., 1969, Oxidative demethylation of *N*-methylhydrazines by rat liver microsomes. *Arch. Biochem. Biophys.*, **134**, 308–315.

Wolff, T., Distlerath, L. M., Worthington, M. T., Groopman, J. D., Hammons, G. J., Kadlubar, F. F., Prough, R. A., Martin, M. V. and Guengerich, F. P., 1985, Substrate specificity of human liver cytochrome P-450 debrisoquine hydroxylase probed using immunochemical inhibition and chemical modeling. *Cancer Res.*, **45**, 2116–2122.

Yost, G. S., Horstman, M. G., El Walily, A. F., Gordon, W. P. and Nelson, S. D., 1985, Procarbazine spermatogenesis toxicity: Deuterium isotope effects point to regioselective metabolism in mice. *Toxicol. Appl. Pharmacol.*, **80**, 316–322.

Zeller, P., Gutmann, H., Hegedus, B., Kaiser, A., Langemann, A., and Muller, M., 1963, Methylhydrazine derivatives, a new class of cytotoxic agents. *Experientia (Basel)*, **19**, 129.

3. Oxazaphosphorines

N. E. Sladek

Introduction

Synthesis of what was to be the first clinically useful 2-chloroethylamido-oxazaphosphorine, namely cyclophosphamide, was reported by Arnold and Bourseaux in 1958. The therapeutic efficacy of this agent in the treatment of certain cancers and for the purpose of immunosuppression is now widely recognized (American Medical Association, 1983; Calabresi and Parks, 1985). Thus various myeloproliferative and lymphoproliferative disorders, solid malignancies and disorders with an autoimmune component all respond, at least in some cases and/or to some extent, to cyclophosphamide therapy. Its immunosuppressive properties have also proven useful in the preparation of patients for bone marrow transplantation (Thomas *et al.*, 1975). Most recently, analogues of "activated" cyclophosphamide (see below) have been used *ex vivo* for the purpose of purging autologous bone marrow of neoplastic cells before transplantation (Sharkis *et al.*, 1980; Lu *et al.*, 1984; Kluin-Nelemans *et al.*, 1984); *ex vivo* purging of allogeneic bone marrow of the cells that give rise to graft-versus-host disease is also being examined (F. R. Kohn and N. E. Sladek, unpublished observations).

From the viewpoint of the medicinal chemist, the design of cyclophosphamide and like compounds was based on an intellectually satisfying rationale. It was already well known that certain rather chemically simple bis-(β-chlorethyl)amines (nitrogen mustards) such as mechlorethamine were highly cytotoxic to various neoplastic cells by virtue of their ability to form highly reactive carbonium ions. Unfortunately, these compounds exhibited only minimal selectivity. It was also known that addition of an electron-withdrawing group to the nitrogen of bis-(β-chloroethyl)amine would decrease the chemical reactivity by decreasing the rate of carbonium ion formation. Finally, it had been reported that a number of malignant epithelial tumours had, relative to normal tissues, high levels of phosphoroamidase activity (Gomori, 1948). Phosphoroamidases catalyse the hydrolysis of nitrogen–phosphorus bonds. Hence, the idea was to conjugate bis-(β-chloroethyl)amine with a suitable electron-withdrawing substituted phsophoryl group, thus producing a "transport" or "latent" form of the drug, i.e., a pro-drug. The pro-drug would be activated when the bis-(β-chloroethyl)amine residue was separated from the phosphoryl residue as a consequence of phosphoroamidase-catalysed hydrolysis. Selectivity would be achieved because of the purported relatively greater activity of phosphoroamidase in tumour tissue.

Arnold and coworkers (Arnold and Bourseaux, 1958; Arnold *et al.*, 1961) synthesized many hundreds of phosphorus-containing compounds; one of these was cyclophosphamide (Figure 1). Actually, the concept had been formulated and pursued earlier by Seligman and coworkers (Seligman *et al.*, 1949; Rutenburg *et al.*, 1954; Friedman & Seligman, 1954); while not designing any agents that ultimately became clinically useful, these investigators did, ironically, synthesize phosphoramide mustard (Friedman and Seligman, 1954), which, as we shall see, is now recognized as the cytotoxic metabolite of cyclophosphamide.

Cyclophosphamide proved to be relatively selectively toxic to tumour cells. Moreover, as expected, it was without cytotoxic activity itself, that is, it had to be "activated" (Arnold *et al.*, 1958). However, it very quickly became apparent that activation was not by the target tumour cells as had been intended according to the rationale described, since tumours that were sensitive to the drug *in vivo* were not sensitive to it *in vitro* (Arnold *et al.*, 1958).

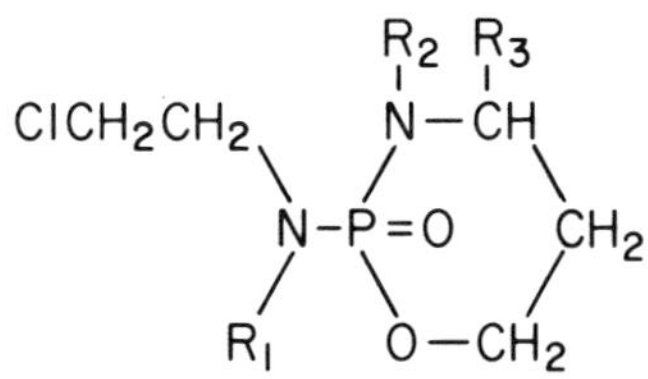

OXAZAPHOSPHORINE	R_1	R_2	R_3
CYCLOPHOSPHAMIDE			H-
4-HYDROPEROXYCYCLOPHOSPHAMIDE	$ClCH_2CH_2$-	H-	HOO-
MAFOSFAMIDE			$^{-}O_3S$-CH_2CH_2-S-
IFOSFAMIDE	H-	$ClCH_2CH_2$-	H-
4-HYDROPEROXYIFOSFAMIDE			HOO-
TROFOSFAMIDE	$ClCH_2CH_2$-	$ClCH_2CH_2$-	H-

Figure 1. Chemical structures of several oxazaphosphorines.

Hence, the metabolism of cyclophosphamide became of great research interest. Indeed, of the thousands of publications in which cyclophosphamide has been mentioned since its synthesis nearly thirty years ago, a very large fraction describe investigations directly or indirectly attempting to gain some insight as to its metabolism. This knowledge was deemed to be particularly important early on for at least four reasons: the cytotoxic action of cyclophosphamide had to be due to one or more of its metabolites, the untoward effects of cyclophosphamide were very likely produced by one or more of its metabolites, the basis for cyclophosphamide's relatively favourable therapeutic index was very likely related to its metabolism, and there was great potential for modulating, whether favourably or unfavourably, its metabolism.

Chemically, cyclophosphamide is classified by the generic term oxazaphosphorine. Other oxazaphosphorines (Figure 1) are also emerging as potentially useful therapeutic agents. Included are ifosfamide and trofosfamide which, like cyclophosphamide, are pro-drugs that require enzyme-mediated activation, and mafosfamide and 4-hydroperoxycyclophosphamide which are also pro-drugs but are quickly activated without the necessity for any enzyme involvement.

A symposium held in London, England and published in *Cancer Treatment Reports* (Cox *et al.*, 1976 a), and reviews by Hill (1975), Brock and Hohorst (1977), Friedman *et al.*, (1979), Colvin and Hilton (1981), Zon (1982) and Brock (1983) summarize much of what is known about the chemistry and pharmacology of the oxazaphosphorines.

Zon (1982) in his excellent review of cyclophosphamide analogues concludes by saying, "Friedman, Myles and Colvin (1979) have rightly emphasized the need for additional studies of (*a*) the role of the primary metabolites. . . in the transport of phosphoramide into target cells, (*b*) the role of intracellular detoxification in the control of specificity, and (*c*) the pharmacokinetics. . . of cyclophosphamide. These factors have a direct bearing on the rational design of new cyclophosphamide analogues, and until they are clarified, significant developments with analogue structures must rely upon numerous heuristic assumptions and a considerable amount of good fortune".

Many of these studies have now been conducted. The present review, in large part, summarizes the results of these investigations. Particular emphasis is placed on the metabolism of cyclophosphamide as it relates to the therapeutic efficacy of this agent.

Metabolism

Once it was recognized that cyclophosphamide itself was without alkylating or cytotoxic activity, an understanding of its metabolism was vigorously pursued. The results of these efforts have led to the abridged scheme of cyclophos-

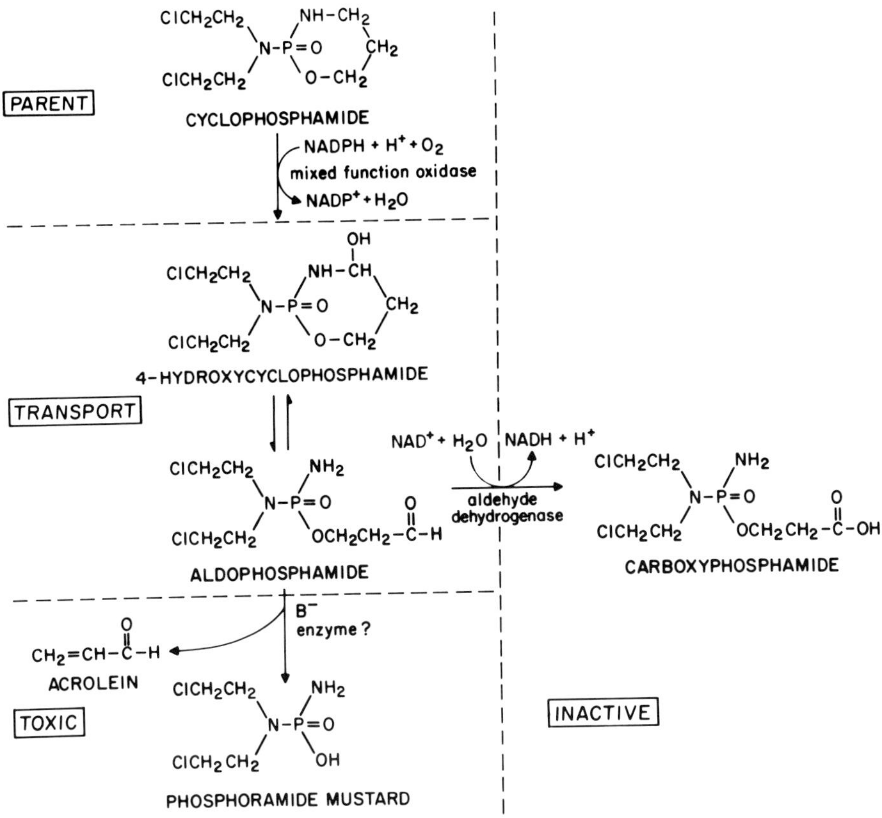

Figure 2. Metabolism of cyclophosphamide: an abridged scheme showing only the currently recognized biologically important reactions and metabolites.

phamide metabolism presented in Figure 2; only the currently recognized biologically important metabolites and reactions are presented. Thus, cyclophosphamide is first hydroxylated to yield 4-hydroxycyclophosphamide, which exists in equilibrium with its ring-opened tautomer aldophosphamide. The tautomers are themselves also without cytotoxic activity and undergo one of two fates: hydrolysis to phosphoramide mustard and acrolein, each of which is cytotoxic, or oxidation to carboxyphosphamide, a non-cytotoxic metabolite.

Hydroxylation to the 4-hydroxy intermediate is catalysed largely by the mixed-function oxidases present in the endoplasmic reticulum of liver.

Foley *et al.* (1961) were the first to demonstrate hepatic enzyme involvement in the activation of cyclophosphamide. They found cyclophosphamide to be without cytotoxic activity when added directly to cultured mammalian cells. However, incubation of cyclophosphamide with liver homogenates gave rise to a substance (or substances) that inhibited the growth of these cells.

Catalysis by microsomal mixed-function oxidases was strongly suspected when it was observed that phosphatases and phosphoroamidases were incapable of activating cyclophosphamide, that, of various hepatic subcellular fractions, microsomes were most active in activating cyclophosphamide, and that the reaction required NADPH and O_2; moreover, *in vivo*, pretreatment with SKF 525A, a known inhibitor of these enzymes, inhibited cyclophosphamide metabolism whereas pretreatment with phenobarbital, a known inducer of microsomal mixed-function oxidase activity, stimulated its metabolism (Brock & Hohorst, 1963, 1967; Brock, 1967).

Subsequently, several laboratories contributed extensively to conclusively establishing and characterizing hepatic microsomal mixed-function oxidase-catalysed oxidation of cyclophosphamide (Cohen and Jao, 1970; Connors *et al.*, 1970, 1972; Sladek, 1971, 1972 a,b; Short and Gibson, 1971; Hill *et al.*, 1972). K_m values for cyclophosphamide were between 0·5 and 1·5 mM when hepatic microsomes were obtained from rodents; the pH optimum was about 7·4 (Sladek, 1971).

The identity of the metabolite resulting from hepatic microsomal mixed-function oxidase-catalysed oxidation of cyclophosphamide was not immediately apparent. Identification of carboxyphosphamide as the most abundant cyclophosphamide metabolite in the urine of sheep (Bakke *et al.*, 1971, 1972), dogs (Struck *et al.*, 1971), and humans (Struck *et al.*, 1971), provided an important clue, as did the fact that other urinary metabolites included 4-oxocyclophosphamide and one that yielded β-hydroxypropionamide on hydrolysis. The presence of these metabolites suggested to Struck *et al.*, (1971), Hohorst *et al.* (1971) and Takamizawa *et al.* (1972) that the initial oxidative step was to 4-hydroxycyclophosphamide; that, in solution, 4-hydroxycyclophosphamide would exist in equilibrium with its acyclic tautomer now known by the trivial name aldophosphamide; and that these tautomers were intermediates in the generation of carboxyphosphamide (and 4-oxocyclophosphamide). Such a scheme had been considered earlier by Norpoth and co-workers (Norpoth, 1969; Norpoth *et al.* 1970) but, after investigating the possibility, these investigators rejected it. Ultimately, isolation and chemical and pharmacological characterization of the relevant (derivatized) metabolites, namely 4-hydroxycyclophosphamide and aldophosphamide, and the observation that, under appropriate conditions, they gave rise to carboxyphosphamide, established the correctness of the proposed route (Hill *et al.*, 1972; Sladek, 1973 a,b; Connors *et al.*, 1974; Struck, 1974, 1976; Völker *et al.*, 1974; Takamizawa *et al.*, 1975; Myles *et al.*, 1977; Fenselau *et al.*, 1977).

Hill *et al.*, (1972) were the first to demonstrate that at least two enzymes, *viz.*, purified aldehyde oxidase (EC 1.2.3.1) and a commercial preparation of NAD-linked aldehyde dehydrogenase (EC 1.2.1.3), could catalyse the oxidation of aldophosphamide to carboxyphosphamide. They and others demonstrated that hepatic cytosol could also catalyse this reaction (Hill *et al.*, 1972; Sladek, 1973 a,b; Connors *et al.*, 1974; Cox *et al.*, 1975 b, 1976 b).

Further investigation with cell-free systems revealed that the reaction could be catalysed by either cytosolic or particulate fractions of several tissues (Cox *et al.*, 1975 b, 1976 b; Domeyer and Sladek, 1980 b). Aldehyde dehydrogenase activity is known to be present in both fractions of most tissues; aldehyde oxidase activity is confined to the soluble fraction of a few tissues.

Although both may be operative, aldehyde dehydrogenase rather than aldehyde oxidase is thought to be the predominating enzyme activity *in vivo* (Domeyer and Sladek, 1980 b). Several observations are consistent with this contention. Thus, (1) experiments in which surrogate aldehydes such as acetaldehyde, butyraldehyde and benzaldehyde were used as substrates, showed that, in addition to dehydrogenase activity being virtually ubiquitous whereas oxidase activity is confined to only a few tissues, dehydrogenase activity far exceeds oxidase activity in those tissues where both activities are found, (2) as judged by K_m values, surrogate aldehydes are generally much better substrates for dehydrogenase, (3) oxidation of aldophosphamide to carboxyphosphamide by hepatic cytosol could not be demonstrated in the absence of NAD even when incubation conditions were made optimal for the expression of aldehyde oxidase activity (Domeyer and Sladek, 1980 b), (4) the phenotypic basis for the acquired resistance exhibited by mouse L1210 and P388 tumour cells to cyclophosphamide is increased aldehyde dehydrogenase activity (Hilton, 1984 a,b; Sladek and Landkamer, 1985; Manthey and Sladek, 1986), (5) the phenotypic basis for the relative insensitivity of murine pluripotent haematopoietic stem cells to cyclophosphamide is aldehyde dehydrogenase activity (Kohn and Sladek, 1985), and (6) inhibitors of aldehyde dehydrogenase activity, e.g., disulfiram or cyanamide, inhibited the conversion of aldophosphamide to carboxyphosphamide *in vivo* and potentiated the anti-tumour, leukopaenic and lethal action of cyclophosphamide, as would be expected if the dehydrogenase was operative and catalysed a detoxifying reaction (see below) (Donelli *et al.*, 1976; Cox *et al.*, 1976 b; Domeyer and Sladek, 1981; Habs *et al.*, 1981; Hacker *et al.*, 1982). The finality of this conclusion must be held in abeyance however because of reports that pyridoxal, an inhibitor of the oxidase but not of the dehydrogenase, also potentiated the cyotoxic action of cyclophosphamide (Hill *et al.*, 1972), and disulfiram and other inhibitors of aldehyde dehydrogenase did not potentiate the anti-tumour action of cyclophosphamide in some *in vivo* experiments (Montgomery and Struck, 1973; Cox *et al.*, 1976 b; Domeyer, 1977).

A number of aldehyde dehydrogenase isozymes have been identified in the mitochondria, cytosol and microsomes of normal mammalian cells (Pietruszko, 1983). The relative efficacy of these isozymes in catalysing the oxidation of aldophosphamide to carboxyphosphamide is not known. A comparison of kinetic parameters obtained when mouse hepatic soluble and particulate fractions were used to catalyse the reaction (Table 1) suggests that an isozyme located in the soluble fraction predominates in this organ and species (Manthey and Sladek, 1986).

Table 1. NAD-linked aldehyde dehydrogenase catalysis of the oxidation of aldophosphamide to carboxyphosphamide by mouse hepatic soluble and particulate fractions.†

Parameter	Particulate	Soluble
K_m (μM)	72	22
V_{max} (μmol/min/g wet tissue)	1·1	2·8
V_{max} (nmol/min/mg protein)	5	36
E_a (kcal/mol)	6·1	15·8
pH optimum	8·2	8·2

† From Manthey and Sladek (1986).

Although he did not pursue the possibility, Norpoth (1969) was the first to propose that cyclophosphamide could ultimately give rise to phosphoramide mustard. Alarcon and Meienhofer's (1971) observation that acrolein was ultimately formed when cyclophosphamide was incubated with liver microsomes, together with the knowledge that the initial metabolite was 4-hydroxycyclophosphamide in equilibrium with its acyclic tautomer aldophosphamide (see above) led Colvin *et al.* (1973) and Connors *et al.* (1974) to suggest the formation of phosphoramide mustard as a consequence of the β-elimination of acrolein from aldophosphamide. Each group isolated phosphoramide mustard after incubating cyclophosphamide with the relevant rodent hepatic subcellular fraction to buttress this notion. Conclusive to establishing its validity was the isolation of phosphoramide mustard from biological fluids of mice (Struck *et al.*, 1975) and humans (Fenselau *et al.*, 1975) given cyclophosphamide.

"Spontaneous" β-elimination of acrolein from aldophosphamide to yield phosphoramide mustard has been examined in considerable detail (Völker *et al.*, 1974; Low *et al.*, 1982, 1983; Borch *et al.*, 1984). In fact, the reaction is not spontaneous but rather is catalysed by various bases, such as hydroxyl ion, carbonate ion and dianionic phosphate. The mechanism is apparently one of general base catalysis, although specific base–general acid catalysis cannot be ruled out (Low *et al.*, 1983).

Enzymes, e.g., 3′,5′-exonucleases, may also catalyse the conversion of aldophosphamide to phosphoramide mustard and acrolein (Bielicki *et al.*, 1983, 1984; Sladek *et al.*, 1984 b). 3′,5′-Exonucleases linked to DNA polymerases may be particularly active in this regard (Bielicki *et al.*, 1983). These enzymes may be producing their effect via a general base catalytic mechanism.

Only the salient features of cyclophosphamide metabolism are presented in Figure 2. Additional, though not all, aspects are presented in Figures 3 and 4. Thus, the transport forms of cyclophosphamide are not simply 4-hydroxycyclophosphamide and aldophosphamide, but rather *cis-* and *trans-*4-hydroxycyclophosphamide, iminocyclophosphamide, aldophosphamide and aldophosphamide hydrate (Figure 4) (Borch and Getman, 1984; Borch *et al.*, 1984; Zon *et al.*, 1984). Iminocyclophosphamide is present only transiently

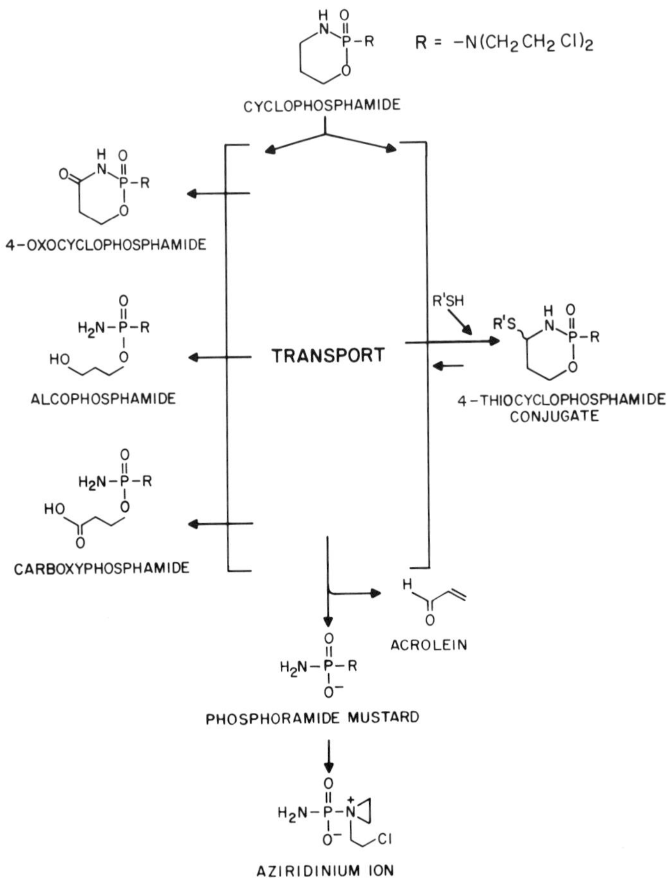

Figure 3. Metabolism of cyclophosphamide.

(Fenselau *et al.*, 1982, Borch and Getman, 1984); approximate relative amounts of the transport forms at pseudoequilibrium are given in Table 2.

The transport forms of cyclophosphamide may be converted to metabolites other than carboxyphosphamide, phosphoramide mustard and acrolein (Figure 3). Thus the transport forms may conjugate with various sulphydryls to form a 4-thiocyclophosphamide adduct (Draeger *et al.*, 1976, Hohorst *et al.*, 1976; Peter *et al.*, 1976; Peter and Hohorst, 1979; Brock, 1983; Zon *et al.*, 1984). This reaction is reversible and proceeds without benefit of enzyme involvement. Alternatively, 4-hydroxycyclophosphamide may be oxidized to 4-oxocyclophosphamide, a minor urinary metabolite of cyclophosphamide (Hohorst *et al.*, 1971; Bakke *et al.*, 1971, 1972; Struck *et al.*, 1975). This reaction is probably catalysed by aldehyde oxidase (Hohorst *et al.*, 1971). Also,

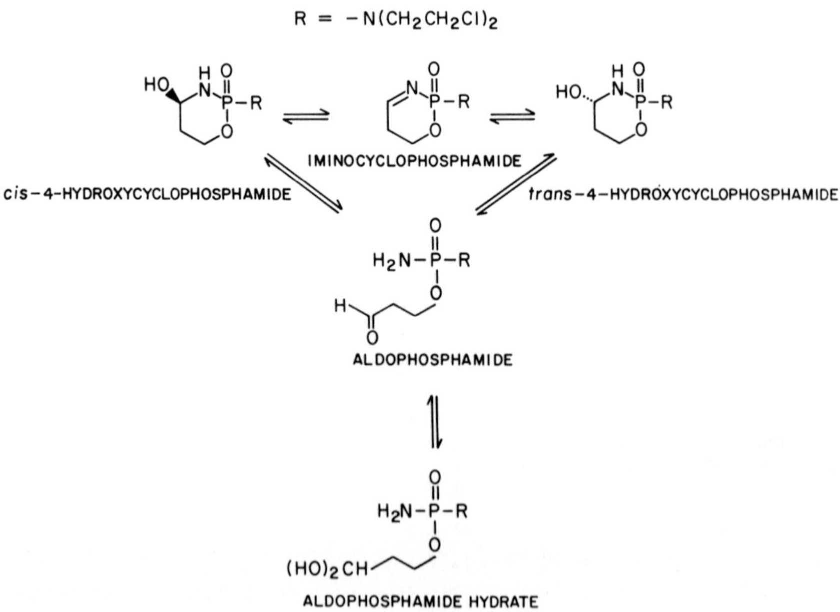

Figure 4. Transport forms of cyclophosphamide.

aldophosphamide may be reduced to alcophosphamide, yet another minor urinary metabolite (Bakke *et al.*, 1972; Connors *et al.*, 1974; Struck *et al.*, 1975; Domeyer and Sladek, 1980 b). This reaction is catalysed by alcohol dehydrogenase (Domeyer and Sladek, 1980 b).

A variety of other metabolites have also been identified (Torkelson *et al.*, 1974; Hill, 1975; Cox *et al.*, 1976 a; Friedman *et al.*, 1979; Gurtoo *et al.*, 1985). Among these is bis-(β-chloroethyl)amine (norHN2). Originally thought

Table 2. Approximate relative amounts of the transport forms of cyclophosphamide at pseudo-equilibrium in aqueous solutions.

Transport form	Borch *et al.* (1984)†	Zon *et al.* (1984) ‡
cis-4-Hydroxycyclophosphamide	13·8	14·3
trans-4-Hydroxycyclophosphamide	6·8	7·5
Iminocyclophosphamide	N.D.	N.D.
Aldophosphamide	1·0	1·0
Aldophosphamide hydrate	3·5	2·3

† Phosphate or cacodylate buffer, 0·1 M, pH 7·0; 25°C.
‡ 2,6-Dimethylpyridine buffer, 1·0 M, pH 7·4; 37°C.
N.D.: None detectable.

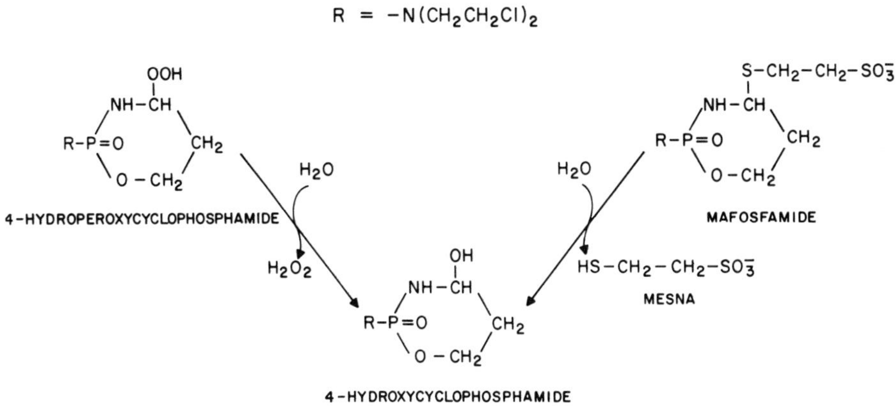

Figure 5. Mafosfamide and 4-hydroperoxycyclophosphamide: relatively stable oxazaphosphorines that, under physiological conditions, readily give rise to 4-hydroxycyclophosphamide without benefit of enzymatic involvement.

to arise principally from phosphoramide mustard (Struck, 1974; Struck *et al.*, 1975; Colvin *et al.*, 1976) and to be, perhaps, the penultimate cytotoxic metabolite (Brock & Hohorst, 1967), subsequent experimentation revealed that it is not particularly cytotoxic at physiological pH (see below) and that its apparent presence in the systemic circulation of animals and humans given cyclophosphamide may be largely artifactual since it probably is produced principally from the decomposition of carboxyphosphamide during sample collection, storage and preparation (Jardine *et al.*, 1978).

4-Hydroxycyclophosphamide can also be generated from mafosfamide and 4-hydroperoxycyclophosphamide (Figure 5). Such conversion occurs fairly rapidly under physiological conditions and without benefit of enzymatic involvement (van der Steen *et al.*, 1973; Völker *et al.*, 1974; Low *et al.*, 1982; Borch and Getman, 1984; Niemeyer *et al.*, 1984). Thus the three oxazaphosphorines are, in most respects, essentially pharmacologically equivalent (Takamizawa *et al.*, 1975; Sladek *et al.*, 1985). This equivalence and the relatively greater chemical stability of mafosfamide and 4-hydroperoxycyclophosphamide (as compared to that of 4-hydroxycyclophosphamide) make them useful in investigations and applications where it is desired to examine the effects of, or utilize, 4-hydroxycyclophosphamide, i.e., to bypass cyclophosphamide hydroxylation to 4-hydroxycyclophosphamide.

Cyclophosphamide analogues that show clinical promise include ifosfamide and trofosfamide. The metabolism of these oxazaphosphorines, particularly that of ifosfamide, has also been studied though not nearly as exhaustively (Allen and Creaven, 1972; Hill *et al.*, 1973; Cox *et al.*, 1976 a; Low *et al.*, 1983). Essentially, metabolism of these analogues is identical to that of cyclophosphamide (Figure 6).

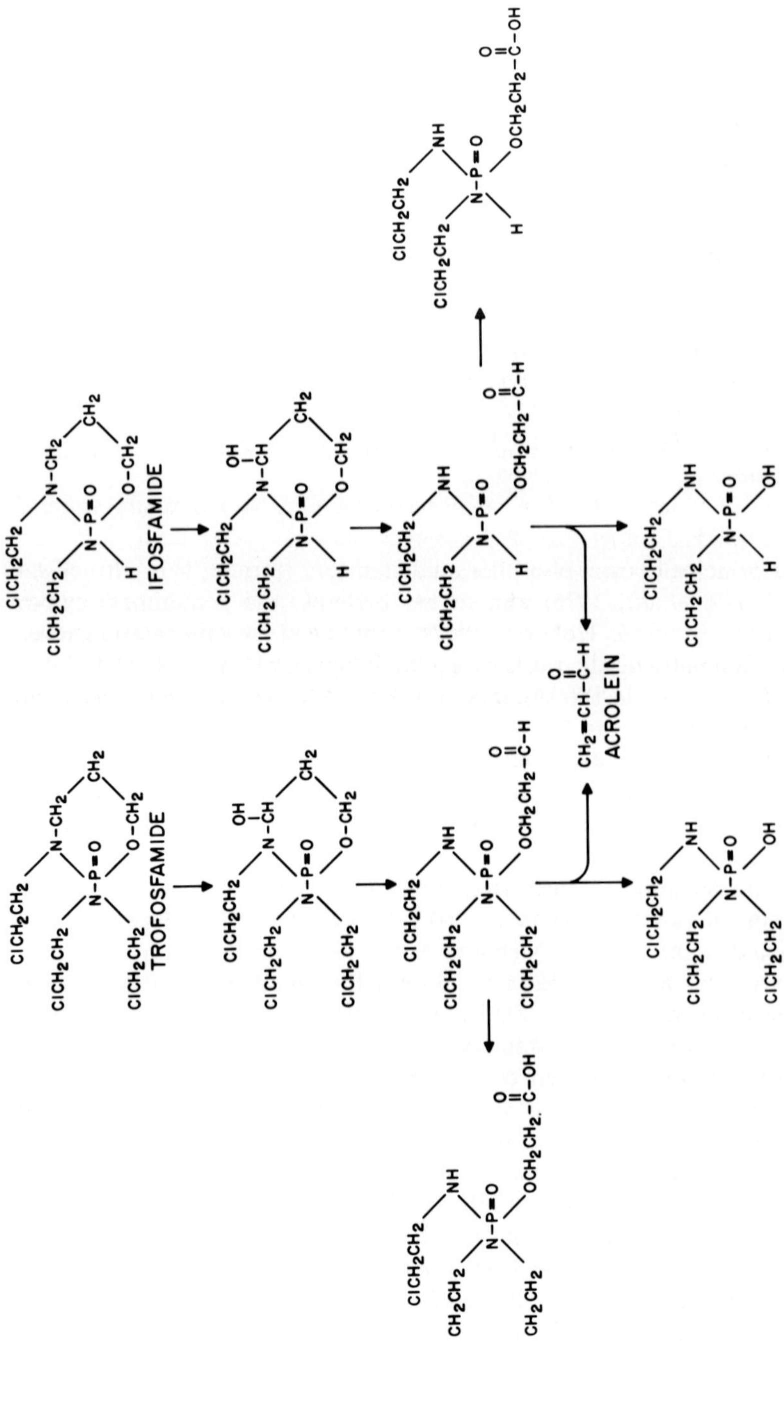

Figure 6. Metabolism of trofosfamide and ifosfamide.

Pharmacokinetics in humans

The clinical pharmacokinetics of cyclophosphamide itself have been intensely investigated. Grochow and Colvin (1980) have reviewed and summarized most of the large amount of information dealing with this subject. Much less is known about the pharmacokinetics of the clinically important circulating metabolites of cyclophosphamide, namely 4-hydroxycyclophosphamide and, to a lesser extent, phosphoramide mustard (see below).

Cyclophosphamide is given both parenterally and orally. Systemic availability after oral administration is greater than 74% and may be nearly total (D'Incalci *et al.*, 1979 a; Juma *et al.*, 1979 a; Wagner and Fenneberg, 1984). The distribution volume is approximately 0·69 l/kg (Grochow and Colvin, 1980; Juma *et al.*, 1979 a,b, 1980, 1981, 1984; Juma and Ogada, 1983; Sladek *et al.*, 1980), a value consistent with distribution of the drug in total body water.

Plasma elimination half-life values for cyclophosphamide vary considerably in adult humans (range 108–960 min); the mean value is about seven hours (Grochow and Colvin, 1980; D'Incalci *et al.*, 1979 b; Juma *et al.*, 1979 a,b, 1980, 1981; Edwards *et al.*, 1980; Ottolenghi *et al.*, 1980). Children and young adults apparently metabolize cyclophosphamide somewhat faster; the mean plasma elimination half-life in this population is about four hours (range: 145–390 min) (DeVita and Adamson, 1970; Sladek *et al.*, 1980, 1984 a; Juma *et al.*, 1984).

Total body clearance of cyclophosphamide occurs at a mean rate of about 82 ml/min (range: 35–200 ml/min) but only about 13% of total body clearance is effected by the kidney (Juma *et al.*, 1979 a, 1980, 1981; Bramwell *et al.*, 1979; Edwards *et al.*, 1980; Wagner *et al.*, 1980 a,b). Excretion in the faeces or by the lungs is insignificant (Cohen *et al.*, 1971; Bagley *et al.*, 1973) and removal of cyclophosphamide from the body is primarily by hepatic metabolism.

Cyclophosphamide metabolites are ultimately eliminated primarily by renal mechanisms. Thus, in humans given radiolabelled cyclophosphamide, 62% of the injected radioactivity was recovered in the urine within 24 to 48 hours; recovery of radiolabel from stool and expired air was less than 4%. The major urinary metabolite is carboxyphosphamide; minor urinary metabolites include 4-oxocyclophosphamide, alcophosphamide, 4-hydroxycyclophosphamide/aldophosphamide and phosphoramide mustard (see above). Less than 4% of the dose is excreted as 4-hydroxycyclophosphamide/aldophosphamide or as phosphoramide mustard (Jardine *et al.*, 1978; Wagner *et al.*, 1981; Sladek *et al.*, 1982).

The apparent plasma elimination half-life values for 4-hydroxycyclophosphamide/aldophosphamide and phosphoramide mustard in humans given cyclophosphamide have also been determined (Table 3). Elimination of the

Table 3. Apparent plasma elimination half-lives of cyclophosphamide, 4-hydroxycyclophosphamide/aldophosphamide and phosphoramide mustard after parenteral administration of cyclophosphamide to humans.

	Apparent half-life (min)						
	Cyclophosphamide		HA†		Phosphoramide mustard		
Age (yrs)	Mean	Range	Mean	Range	Mean	Range	Reference
≥19	533	382–607	—	—	521	334–756	Juma *et al.* (1980)
≥19	493	358–743	—	—	500	346–620	Juma *et al.* (1981)
≤18	88	45–150	118	70–190	182	75–320	Sladek *et al.* (1984 a)

† 4-Hydroxycyclophosphamide/aldophosphamide.

two metabolites as well as the parent compound is approximately first-order. Maximum plasma concentrations of 4-hydroxycyclophosphamide/aldophosphamide and phosphoramide mustard were about 6–16% and 9–18%, respectively, of those of cyclophosphamide (Sladek *et al.*, 1984 a). Apparent plasma elimination half-life values for 4-hydroxycyclophosphamide/aldophosphamide and phosphoramide mustard increased approximately linearly with an increase in plasma half-life values for the parent compound. These observations, and a comparison in male rats of the actual plasma half-life values for cyclophosphamide (29 min), 4-hydroxycyclophosphamide/aldophosphamide (14 min) and phosphoramide mustard (14 min) with the apparent plasma half-life values obtained for 4-hydroxycyclophosphamide/aldophosphamide (34 min) and phosphoramide mustard (55 min) following cyclophosphamide administration (Sladek *et al.*, 1984 b), strongly indicate that the major determinant with regard to the apparent plasma half-life of 4-hydroxycyclophosphamide/aldophosphamide is its rate of formation whereas in the case of phosphoramide mustard, an additional determinant, perhaps efflux from the cell, is operative.

As expected, AUC values for 4-hydroxycyclophosphamide/aldophosphamide increase approximately linearly with an increase in the amount of cyclophosphamide administered (Wagner *et al.*, 1980 b; Sladek *et al.*, 1984 b). AUC values, obtained for 4-hydroxycyclophosphamide/aldophosphamide and phosphoramide mustard following the administration of cyclophosphamide to humans, are given in Table 4.

Also as expected, at any given dose, AUC values for cyclophosphamide increase approximately linearly with an increase in its plasma half-life (Sladek *et al.*, 1984 a,b). However, AUC values for 4-hydroxycyclophosphamide/aldophosphamide and phosphoramide mustard remain essentially constant with an increase in their respective apparent plasma half-life values (Sladek *et al.*, 1984 a,b). Since the apparent plasma half-lives of the metabolites increase as the plasma half-life of cyclophosphamide increases (see above), it follows that the AUC values for 4-hydroxycyclophosphamide/aldophosphamide and

Table 4. Area under the serum concentration versus time curve (AUC, normalized for dose) for 4-hydroxycyclophosphamide/aldophosphamide and phosphoramide mustard in patients given cyclophosphamide.

Cyclophosphamide (mg/kg)	AUC/dose, mM min/(mg/kg) † HA‡	Phosphoramide mustard	Reference
6·4–12·5	—	0·38 (0·20–0·60)	Juma *et al.* (1980)
10	0·06	—	Wagner *et al.* (1980 a)
10–20	0·06 (0·02–0·09)	—	Wagner *et al.* (1980 b)
20	0·05	—	Wagner *et al.* (1981)
50–60	0·10 (0·05–0·15)	0·29 (0·24–0·36)	Sladek *et al.* (1984a)

† Figures in parentheses are ranges.
‡ 4-Hydroxycyclophosphamide/aldophosphamide

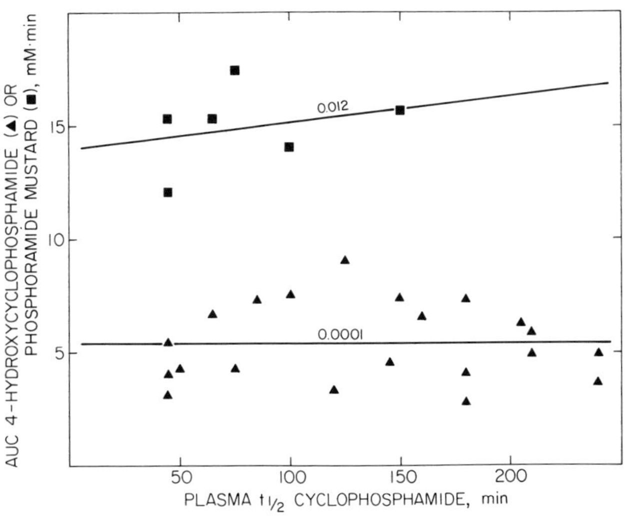

Figure 7. Plasma AUC values for 4-hydroxycyclophosphamide/aldophosphamide and phosphoramide mustard as a function of the respective plasma half-life values for cyclophosphamide. Cyclophosphamide (50–60 mg/kg) was given by i.v. infusion over a one to two hour period to children and young adults (< 19 years of age). Constructed from data published in Sladek *et al.* (1984 a). The number associated with each line is the slope of that line.

phosphoramide mustard remain essentially constant as the plasma half-life of cyclophosphamide increases (Figure 7). Others (Bagley *et al.*, 1973; Juma *et al.*, 1980; Wagner *et al.*, 1980 a,b) have also provided evidence in support of this contention and/or have reached the same conclusion.

These results are as predicted by theoretical considerations (Jao *et al.*, 1972; Bagley *et al.*, 1973; Sladek, 1972 a,b; Goldstein *et al.*, 1974) and have also been obtained in animal experiments (Sladek *et al.*, 1984 b). Thus assuming first-order kinetics, if the only change is to alter the rate at which the parent compound (e.g., cyclophosphamide) is converted to its metabolite (e.g., 4-hydroxycyclophosphamide/aldophosphamide or phosphoramide mustard), and if the parent compound is eliminated from the body primarily by

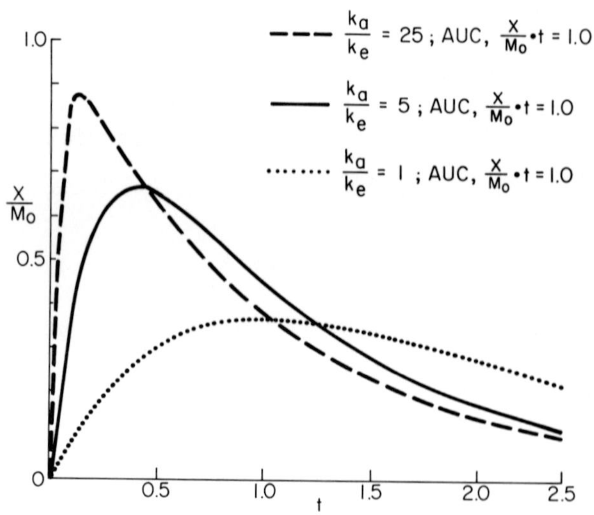

For $k_a = k_e$: $\frac{X}{M_o} = k_e t \left[e^{-k_e t}\right]$

For $k_a \neq k_e$: $\frac{X}{M_o} = \frac{k_a}{(k_e - k_a)} \left[e^{-k_a t} - e^{-k_e t}\right]$

Where:

M_o = *amount of drug introduced*
X = *amount of activated drug present at time t*
k_a = *rate constant of activation*
k_e = *rate constant of elimination*
t = *time*

Figure 8. Predicted plasma concentrations and AUC values for the active metabolite of a pro-drug, assuming that first-order kinetics describe its rate of formation (k_a) as well as its rate of removal (k_e) whether by excretion and/or further metabolism. The amount of metabolite (X) in the body is shown as a fraction of the total amount of pro-drug (M_0) placed into the body at time zero. The family of curves was generated by successively increasing k_a five-fold while keeping k_e constant. Only the first part of the relationship between X/M_0 and t is shown here; the entire relationship was taken into account when AUC values were calculated. AUC values are expressed as $(X/M_0)(t)$. Modified from Goldstein *et al.* (1974).

metabolism (i.e., only a small fraction of it is eliminated by excretion, so that regardless of the rate at which the parent compound is converted to its metabolite, ultimately almost all of it is), AUC values for the metabolite should remain constant. The point is illustrated in Figure 8. The systemic experience of cyclophosphamide (see above) is consistent with this construct.

The absorption, distribution and excretion of ifosfamide have also been intensely investigated (Allen & Creaven, 1975 a,b; McNeil & Morgan, 1981; Wagner *et al.*, 1981; Colvin, 1982). The metabolic transformations which ifosfamide undergoes are qualitatively the same as those which cyclophosphamide undergoes. However, the relative rates at which these transformations occur differ, resulting in a somewhat different overall pharmacokinetic picture. Thus, hydroxylation of ifosfamide occurs at a substantially slower rate, at least at higher doses, resulting in a longer plasma half-life. Moreover, as a consequence, another pathway, dechloroethylation, becomes quantitatively important; dechloroethylation is ordinarily insignificant in the case of cyclophosphamide. Since this pathway produces inactive metabolites, the net result is that a smaller proportion of ifosfamide, as compared to cyclophosphamide, is converted to cytotoxic metabolites.

The cytotoxic metabolite—phosphoramide mustard

Bifunctional alkylating agents of the nitrogen mustard type are all thought to effect their cytotoxic action primarily by cross-linking the two strands of DNA, although ring cleavage and depurination may also be important (Calabresi and Parks, 1985). Accordingly, the cytotoxic action of cyclophosphamide is thought to result from such actions effected by phosphoramide mustard, or more accurately, the aziridinium ion thereof. The proposed primary mechanism is schematically presented in Figure 9. Intermediates analagous to phosphoramide mustard are thought to be the therapeutically important cytotoxic metabolites of other oxazaphosphorines.

Consistent with this notion is that DNA cross-linking is observed following the administration of cyclophosphamide to rodents (Colvin and Hilton, 1981; Hilton, 1984 b). Similarly, inter-strand DNA cross-linking is observed after exposure of cultured tumour cells to 4-hydroxycyclophosphamide/aldophosphamide or surrogates thereof (Erickson *et al.*, 1980; Ramonas *et al.*, 1981; Hilton, 1984 a,b; Cairney *et al.*, 1984).

The contention that phosphoramide mustard, rather than some other metabolite or cyclophosphamide itself, is the active anti-tumour (cross-linking) agent is supported by a number of observations and considerations.

Cyclophosphamide itself is without alkylating or cytotoxic activity (see above) and thus can be ruled out.

Carboxyphosphamide, 4-oxocyclophosphamide and alcophosphamide can be ruled out because at physiological pH and temperature they are not

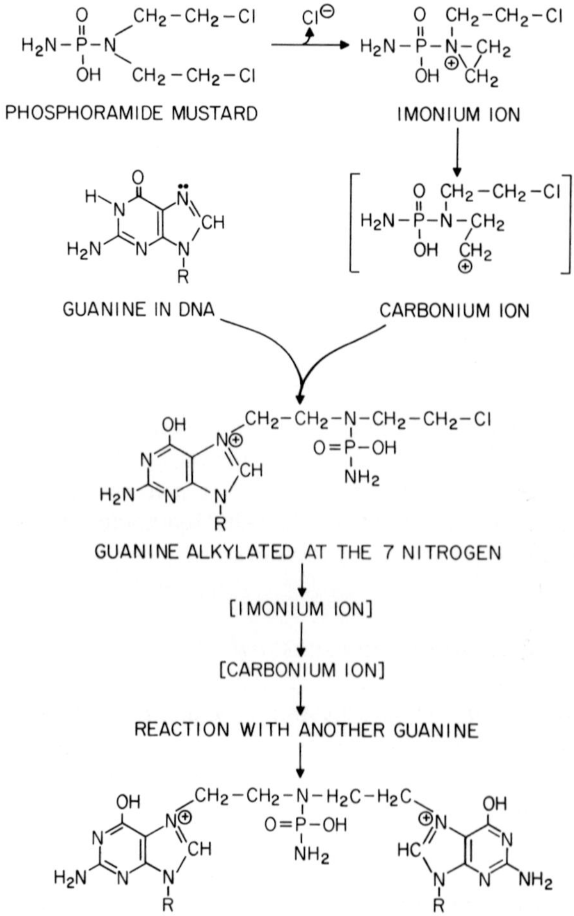

Figure 9. Primary mechanism of cyclophosphamide's cytotoxic action: cross-linking of guanine residues residing in different chains of DNA by phosphoramide mustard.

alkylating species; moreover, they do not exhibit significant cytotoxic activity *ex vivo* or *in vivo* (Norpoth *et al.*, 1970; Hohorst *et al.*, 1971; Struck *et al.*, 1971, 1975; Sladek, 1973 b; Connors *et al.*, 1974; Montgomery and Struck, 1976; Brock and Hohorst, 1977).

Acrolein, although highly cytotoxic to cultured tumour cells (Connors *et al.*, 1974; Sladek *et al.*, 1985), can be ruled out as the active cytotoxic cyclophosphamide metabolite or even as contributing to the cytotoxic action of cyclophosphamide upon its intracellular release, because it produces single-strand DNA breaks but not inter-strand DNA cross-links (Erickson *et al.*, 1980; Cairney *et al.*, 1984) and because an analogue of cyclophosphamide, dechlorocyclophosphamide, in which the bis-(β-chloroethyl)amine group has been replaced by diethylamine, readily produces acrolein on microsomal metabolism (Alarcon *et al.*, 1972) but lacks anti-tumour activity (Arnold *et al.*, 1961). Moreover, 4-hydroperoxycyclophosphamide and an analogue of it, 4-hydroperoxy-dechlorocyclophosphamide, in which the bis-(β-chloroethyl)amine group has again been replaced by diethylamine, spontaneously produce, at approximately the same rates, acrolein at physiological pH and temperature, but only the former decreased the viability of L1210 leukaemia cells (Wrabetz *et al.*, 1980). Although both compounds give rise to acrolein, only 4-hydroperoxycyclophosphamide can give rise to a bifunctional alkylating metabolite, namely phosphoramide mustard.

Bis-(β-chloroethyl)amine has been shown to arise from both carboxyphosphamide and phosphoramide mustard upon hydrolysis *in vitro* (Levins and Rogers, 1965; Jardine *et al.*, 1978). However, there is little or no evidence indicating that significant amounts of bis-(β-chloroethyl)amine are generated *in vivo* following cyclophosphamide administration. Also, at physiological pH and temperature, bis-(β-chloroethyl)amine is, relative to phosphoramide mustard, a weak alkylating agent (Struck *et al.*, 1975; Colvin *et al.*, 1976; Hohorst *et al.*, 1976; Brock and Hohorst, 1977). Moreover, bis-(β-chloroethyl)amine does not effect inter-strand DNA cross-links; rather, it effects DNA–protein cross-links (Hilton, 1984 a).

That leaves 4-hydroxycyclophosphamide/aldophosphamide and phosphoramide mustard as the remaining contenders. At physiological pH and temperature, phosphoramide mustard is an alkylating species, whereas 4-hydroxycyclophosphamide/aldophosphamide and surrogates thereof are not (Struck *et al.*, 1975; Colvin *et al.*, 1976; Hohorst *et al.*, 1976; Draeger *et al.*, 1976; Brock and Hohorst, 1977). Although usually not as potent as 4-hydroxycyclophosphamide/aldophosphamide or surrogates thereof, phosphoramide mustard is cytotoxic to tumour cells *ex vivo* and *in vivo* (Maddock *et al.*, 1966; Struck *et al.*, 1975; Hohorst *et al.*, 1976; Peter *et al.*, 1976; Friedman *et al.*, 1976; Brock and Hohorst, 1977; Sladek, 1977 a,b; Peter & Hohorst, 1979; Erickson *et al.*, 1980; Sladek *et al.*, 1985). Inter-strand DNA cross-links are found after exposure of cultured tumour cells to phosphoramide mustard (Surya *et al.*, 1978; Erickson *et al.*, 1980; Ramonas *et al.*, 1981; Hilton, 1984 a). The time course of DNA cross-link appearance in general, as well as of inter-strand DNA cross-links specifically, following exposure of cultured tumour cells to phosphoramide mustard is similar to that obtained when these cells are exposed to 4-hydroxycyclophosphamide/aldophosphamide or surrogates thereof (Erickson *et al.*, 1980; Ramonas *et al.*, 1981; Hilton, 1984 a; Cairney *et al.*, 1984). Alkylation of target molecules, such as the N-7 position of guanosine, by phosphoramide mustard proceeds directly via an aziridinium intermediate rather than after cleavage to bis-(β-chloroethyl)amine or other metabolites (Colvin *et al.*, 1976; Mehta *et al.*, 1980; Vu *et al.*, 1981; Chetsanga *et al.*, 1982; Kallama and Hemminki, 1984; Hemminki, 1985). A cross-linked dimer, *N,N*-bis-[2-(5′-phospho-7-guanosinyl)ethyl]phosphorodiamidic acid, has been isolated following the incubation of phosphoramide mustard and guanosine 5′-monophosphate (Vu *et al.*, 1981). The instability of phosphoramide mustard–guanosine adducts, potentially leading to ring cleavage and/or depurination, has been repeatedly reported (Mehta *et al.*, 1980; Vu *et al.*, 1981; Chetsanga *et al.*, 1983; Kallama and Hemminki, 1984; Hemminki, 1985).

That phosphoramide mustard, and not 4-hydroxycyclophosphamide/aldophosphamide, a 4-thiocyclophosphamide conjugate, carboxyphosphamide, 4-oxocyclophosphamide, alcophosphamide, or bis-(β-chloroethyl)amine, should be the cytotoxic species is as expected from chemical considerations (Friedman, 1967; Colvin *et al.*, 1976; Friedman *et al.*, 1979; Brock, 1983).

The significant circulating metabolite—4-hydroxycyclophosphamide/aldophosphamide

While it has been generally agreed for some time that phosphoramide mustard is the active cytotoxic species, the identity of the pharmacologically important, circulating (transport) form of cyclophosphamide and other oxazaphosphorines had been, until recently, controversial. Thus, some (Montgomery and Struck, 1973; Struck *et al.*, 1975, 1979, 1983; Friedman *et al.*, 1976; Hipkins *et al.*, 1981) favoured phosphoramide mustard, whereas others (Connors *et al.*, 1974; Brock and Hohorst, 1977; Domeyer and Sladek, 1980 a; Powers and Sladek, 1983; Sladek *et al.*, 1984 a, 1985; Hilton, 1984 b) favoured 4-hydroxycyclophosphamide/aldophosphamide. It now appears that the latter is in fact the pharmacologically important circulating form of cyclophosphamide.

The individual contribution of 4-hydroxycyclophosphamide/aldophosphamide and phosphoramide mustard to the cytotoxic effect of cyclophosphamide will depend on their relative potency and AUC values.

The sensitivities of several cultured human tumour cell lines to 4-hydroxycyclophosphamide/aldophosphamide and phosphoramide mustard are presented in Table 5. In all cases, tumour cells were much more sensitive to 4-hydroxycyclophosphamide/aldophosphamide. This is not always so. Thus, Struck *et al.* (1975) reported that cultured H. Ep.-2 tumour cells are approximately equisensitive to the two metabolites.

The sensitivities of several mouse normal and cultured tumour cells to 4-hydroxycyclophosphamide/aldophosphamide and phosphoramide mustard have been determined in a similar manner and are presented in Table 6. With the exception of pluripotent bone marrow haematopoietic cells (CFU-s), all cells were again more sensitive to 4-hydroxycyclophosphamide/aldophosphamide.

The apparent discrepancy between the belief that phosphoramide mustard is the ultimate cytotoxic species and the observations that the cytotoxic

Table 5. Sensitivity of cultured human tumour cells to 4-hydroxycyclophosphamide/aldophosphamide and phosphoramide mustard. (N. E. Sladek and G. L. Landkammer, unpublished observations).

Cell Line	Differentiation stage according to Minowada *et al.* (1981)	LC_{99} (μM)† HA‡	LC_{99} (μM)† PDA¶	PDA/HA
HPB-Null	Pre-B-blast	7·3	110	15
Molt-4	T-Blast II	16	433	27
Raji	B-Blast I	48	740	15
K-562	Pre-erythroid blast	79	620	8
U-937	Monoblast	46	700	15
KG-1	Pre-myeloid-blast	54	335	6

† Concentration required to kill 99% of the cells. LC_{99} values were determined as described by Sladek *et al.* (1985). Mafosfamide was used as a surrogate for 4-hydroxycyclophosphamide/aldophosphamide. Drug exposure was for 30 minutes.
‡ 4-Hydroxycyclophosphamide/aldophosphamide.
¶ Phosphoramide mustard.

potency of 4-hydroxycyclophosphamide/aldophosphamide is usually much greater than is that of phosphoramide mustard, can be explained by the knowledge that phosphoramide mustard, because it is largely ionized at physiological pH (Engle *et al.*, 1979, 1982), does not get into cells as readily as does 4-hydroxycyclophosphamide/aldophosphamide (Lenssen and Hohorst, 1979).

Plasma AUC values for 4-hydroxycyclophosphamide/aldophosphamide and

Table 6. Sensitivity of mouse normal and cultured tumour cells to 4-hydroxycyclophosphamide/aldophosphamide and phosphoramide mustard (from Kohn and Sladek, 1985; Smith and Sladek, 1985; Sladek *et al.*, 1985).

Cells	HA‡	PDA¶	PDA/HA
	LC_{99} (μM)†		
P388/0	6·5	107	16
L1210/0	24	178	7
	LC_{50} (μM)†		
B-Cells (LPS)	7·6	295	39
T-Cells (PHA)	16	262	16
T-Cells (ConA)	17	312	18
CFU-GM	17	73	4
CFU-s	55	60	1

† Concentration required to kill 50% or 99% of the cells. Mafosfamide was used as a surrogate for 4-hydroxycyclophosphamide/aldophosphamide. Drug exposure was for 30 minutes.
‡ 4-Hydroxycyclophosphamide/aldophosphamide.
¶ Phosphoramide mustard.

Table 7. Plasma AUC values for 4-hydroxycyclophosphamide/aldophosphamide and phosphoramide mustard in mice, rats and humans given cyclophosphamide. (From Powers and Sladek, 1983; Sladek *et al.*, 1984 a,b).

Species	Cyclophosphamide (mg/kg)	AUC (mM min) HA†	AUC (mM min) PDA ‡	PDA/HA
Mice	65	2·3	1·5	0·7
Rats	50	1·5	2·5	1·7
Humans	50–60	5·4	15·4	2·9

† 4-Hydroxycyclophosphamide/aldophosphamide.
‡ Phosphoramide mustard.

phosphoramide mustard in mice, rats and humans given cyclophosphamide are presented in Table 7. The relative amount of the two metabolites is species-dependent. In humans and rats, AUC values for phosphoramide mustard exceed those for 4-hydroxycyclophosphamide/aldophosphamide; the opposite is the case in mice. Since AUC values for 4-hydroxycyclophosphamide/aldophosphamide and phosphoramide mustard increase approximately linearly with an increase in the amount of cyclophosphamide administered (see above), it follows that the relative amount of the two metabolites would be independent of the dose of cyclophosphamide. Since AUC values for 4-hydroxycyclophosphamide/aldophosphamide and phosphoramide mustard are independent of the rate at which cyclophosphamide is converted to 4-hydroxycyclophosphamide/aldophosphamide (see above), it follows also that the relative amount of the two metabolites will be independent of this parameter.

The general relationship between AUC values and the cytotoxic potencies of any two metabolites as it pertains to determining which of the two is the most important circulating metabolite can be expressed as:

$$[\mathrm{AUC}/P]_{\mathrm{X}}/[\mathrm{AUC}/P]_{\mathrm{Y}}$$

In this relationship, AUC is the area under the plasma concentration curve for each of the two metabolites X and Y under consideration, and P is the potency of each metabolite. P is expressed as the concentration of drug required to kill a certain fraction, e.g., 50 or 99%, of the target cell population when exposure to the drug is for an exact amount of time, e.g., 30 minutes. For the relationship to have meaning, the amount of cell-kill must be determined during a time period in which cell survival decreases in an approximately log-linear manner during the period of drug exposure. When the value for the above relationship substantially exceeds 1·0, the important circulating metabolite is X. For example, when the value is greater than 4·0, more than 80% of the cell-kill can be attributed to X. Conversely, when the value is substantially less than 1·0, Y is the important circulating metabolite. For example, when the value is less than 0·25, more than 80% of the cell-kill can

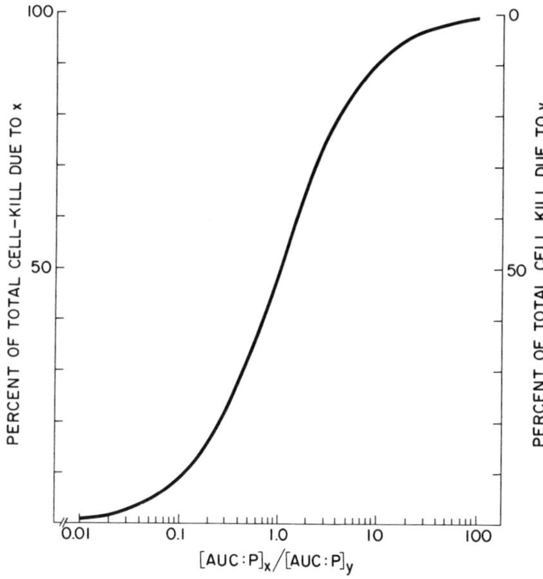

Figure 10. Predicted individual contributions of active metabolites X and Y, generated from a pro-drug, to the total cytotoxic effect of the pro-drug as a function of the relationship $[AUC/P]_X/[AUC/P]_Y$ where AUC is the area under the plasma concentration curve and P is the potency, expressed as the concentration of drug required to kill a certain fraction of the target cell population (see text), for each of the two metabolites.

be attributed to Y. Values around 1·0 indicate that both X and Y are important (Figure 10).

When the potency and AUC values presented in Tables 5, 6 and 7 are substituted into the relationship presented above, values exceeding 1·0 are always obtained and the percentage of total cell-kill hypothetically effected by circulating 4-hydroxycyclophosphamide/aldophosphamide always exceeds 66% and usually exceeds 80% (Table 8).

Thus, on the basis of the foregoing considerations, it seems clear that in the vast majority of cases, 4-hydroxycyclophosphamide/aldophosphamide will be the circulating metabolite of major importance. Occasionally, as for example when tumour cells become resistant specifically to oxazaphosphorines, phosphoramide mustard could be the circulating metabolite of major importance.

Supporting the notion that 4-hydroxycyclophosphamide/aldophosphamide is usually the circulating metabolite of importance are several additional observations. All of the cytotoxic activity (towards cultured rat W256 tumour cells) found in the plasma of cyclophosphamide-treated rats could be accounted for by the 4-hydroxycyclophosphamide/aldophosphamide found there; conversely, only a very small amount of the cytotoxic activity could be accounted for by the phosphoramide mustard present (Powers and Sladek, 1983).

Table 8. Relationship between AUC values and cytotoxic potencies of 4-hydroxycyclophosphamide/aldophosphamide and phosphoramide mustard.

Species	Type	Cells	$[AUC/LC]_{HA}/[AUC/LC]_{PDA}$†	% Cell-kill‡	
				HA	PDA
Mouse	Malignant	P388/0	25	96	4
		L1210/0	11	92	8
	Normal	B-Cells (LPS)	60	98	2
		T-Cells (PHA)	25	96	4
		T-Cells (ConA)	28	97	3
		CFU-GM	4	80	20
		CFU-s	2	67	33
Human	Malignant	HPB-Null	5	83	17
		Molt 4	9	90	10
		Raji	5	83	17
		K-562	3	75	25
		U-937	5	83	17
		KG-1	2	67	33

† Calculated from data presented in Tables 5, 6 and 7.
‡ Percentage of total cell-kill hypothetically due to circulating 4-hydroxycyclophosphamide/aldophosphamide (HA) and phosphoramide mustard (PDA). Calculated from $[AUC/LC]_{HA}/[AUC/LC]_{PDA}$ values and Figure 10.

In vivo, antibody-forming cells in mice are much more sensitive to cyclophosphamide than they are to phosphoramide mustard, indicating that a precursor, *viz.*, 4-hydroxycyclophosphamide/aldophosphamide, of the latter was the significant circulating agent (Sensenbrenner *et al.*, 1979; Colvin and Hilton, 1981). Thiosulphate, a strong nucleophile that does not readily enter cells, prevents the cytotoxic action of phosphoramide mustard against cultured tumour cells but not that of 4-hydroxycyclophosphamide/aldophosphamide (Powers and Sladek, 1978); it does not prevent the cytotoxic action of plasma taken from cyclophosphamide-treated rats against cultured tumour cells (N. E. Sladek, unpublished observations). There are examples of cyclophosphamide-resistant tumour cell lines that are fully cross-resistant to other oxazaphosphorines such as 4-hydroxycyclophosphamide/aldophosphamide, but that remain fully, or at least partially, sensitive to non-oxazaphosphorine nitrogen mustards, e.g., phosphoramide mustard (Wampler *et al.*, 1978; Gerhartz *et al.*, 1979; Schmid *et al.*, 1980; Struck *et al.*, 1983; Schabel *et al.*, 1983; Hilton, 1984 b; Sladek *et al.*, 1985). Finally, the anti-tumour potency *in vivo* and the therapeutic index of 4-hydroxycyclophosphamide/aldophosphamide approach those of cyclophosphamide; those of phosphoramide mustard do not (Brock, 1976; Brock & Hohorst, 1977).

Two observations are seemingly at odds with the conclusion that 4-hydroxycyclophosphamide/aldophosphamide is usually the circulating metabolite of major importance. Thus, *in vivo*, phosphoramide mustard is sometimes as potent as, or even more potent than, cyclophosphamide (Friedman *et al.*, 1976; Struck *et al.*, 1979, 1983), and decreasing the plasma AUC value for 4-hydroxycyclophosphamide/aldophosphamide by administering phenobarbital, an inducer of hepatic NAD-linked aldehyde dehydrogenase activity, did not alter the therapeutic response to cyclophosphamide in two strains of mice (Hipkins *et al.*, 1981).

As to the reports that phosphoramide mustard is sometimes as potent as or even more potent than, cyclophosphamide, a meaningful conclusion regarding the question at hand could have been made only if the relative AUC values for phosphoramide mustard had been determined; they were not. Relative to the investigation of Hipkins *et al.* (1981), only one dose of cyclophosphamide, 150 mg/kg, was used, and the first determination of the plasma concentration of 4-hydroxycyclophosphamide/aldophosphamide was made at 10 min after cyclophosphamide injection in one strain and at 15 min in the other. It is possible that 150 mg/kg of cyclophosphamide is much more than is needed to give the maximum therapeutic response and/or that the peak of the 4-hydroxycyclophosphamide/aldophosphamide concentration was missed in the phenobarbital-treated mice.

The bladder toxicity-inducing metabolite—acrolein

The clinical usefulness of cyclophosphamide (as well as of ifosfamide) is frequently limited by its urotoxic effects, in the form of a haemorrhagic cystitis. It was shown early on (Philips *et al.*, 1961; Bellin *et al.*, 1974) that the bladder damage was most likely effected locally by cyclophosphamide metabolites present in the urine. Phosphoramide mustard and bis-(β-chloroethyl)amine were quickly eliminated as candidate toxicants because, relative to cyclophosphamide, they were essentially without bladder toxicity when given in approximately equimolar doses to rats (Philips *et al.*, 1961; Maddock *et al.*, 1966; Cox, 1979; Brock *et al.*, 1981). Moreover, cyclophosphamide, phosphoramide mustard and bis-(β-chloroethyl)amine were relatively non-toxic to the bladder when instilled directly into it (Brock *et al.*, 1979, 1981; Sladek *et al.*, 1982). Subsequently, several observations led to the presently held view that acrolein, released in the newly-formed urine from 4-hydroxycyclophosphamide/aldophosphamide, is the primary causative urotoxic agent. Thus, direct instillation of 4-hydroxycyclophosphamide or acrolein into rat bladder induced toxicity to that organ; the urotoxic potency of acrolein was about 5–10 times that of 4-hydroxycyclophosphamide (Brock *et al.*, 1979, 1981; Sladek *et al.*, 1982). Urotoxicity was not induced by an analogue of cyclophosphamide, 5,5-dimethylcyclophosphamide, which is hydroxylated *in vivo* in position 4 of the oxazaphosphorine ring but which cannot give rise to acrolein (Brock *et al.*, 1979, 1981; Cox, 1979). Urotoxicity was induced by another analogue of cyclophosphamide, dechlorocyclophosphamide, in which the bis-(β-chloroethyl)amine group has been replaced by diethylamine (Brock *et al.*, 1979, 1981; Cox, 1979). Dechlorocyclophosphamide is not an alkylating agent nor does it give rise to one; however, it readily produces acrolein on microsomal metabolism (Alarcon *et al.*, 1972). Direct instillation of 4-hydroxy-cyclophosphamide-dechloro into rat bladder also induced toxicity in that organ (Brock *et al.*, 1981). Following i.p. administration of cyclophosphamide to rats, about 3·5% of the dose was excreted in the urine as 4-hydroxycyclophosphamide/aldophosphamide. This amount of 4-hydroxycyclophosphamide/aldophosphamide, upon conversion to acrolein, was found to be sufficient to account for the urotoxic effects of cyclophosphamide (Sladek *et al.*, 1982).

Acrolein may be generated from 4-hydroxycyclophosphamide/aldophosphamide both before and after urine formation. It is likely that only the acrolein generated in newly-formed urine contributes to the urotoxic action of cyclophosphamide. This is because acrolein is highly reactive and thus has a relatively short biological half-life, especially in an environment where there are numerous macro-, and other, molecules, e.g., proteins, with which to react. Urine is comparatively free of such molecules.

Favourable therapeutic index resides with 4-hydroxycyclophosphamaide/aldophosphamide

The underlying strategy of chemotherapy is to injure the uneconomic species without injuring the economic species. In the case of cancer chemotherapy, the goal is to selectively poison cancer cells. Relative to other nitrogen mustards, indeed, most other cancer chemotherapeutic agents, cyclophosphamide exhibits greater selectivity towards a number of animal and human tumours.

The basis for the selective cytotoxic action of cyclophosphamide cannot reside with the parent compound as was originally intended (see above) since it is itself without cytotoxic activity and is converted to 4-hydroxycyclophosphamide/aldophosphamide largely as a consequence of hepatic (non-target cell) enzyme activity (see above). It could, however, reside with either 4-hydroxycyclophosphamide/aldophosphamide, the pharmacologically important circulating (transport) form of cyclophosphamide, and/or with phosphoramide mustard, the ultimate cytotoxic species. In fact, the evidence (Brock, 1976; Brock and Hohorst, 1977) clearly points to 4-hydroxycyclophosphamide/aldophosphamide as the metabolite with which the basis for the favourable therapeutic index of cyclophosphamide resides. These investigators reported that, in rats bearing the Yoshida ascites sarcoma, the therapeutic index of 4-hydroxycyclophosphamide/aldophosphamide approached that of cyclophosphamide, whereas that of phosphoramide mustard (and acrolein, bis-(β-chloroethyl)amine, 4-oxocyclophosphamide and carboxyphosphamide) did not. Also strongly supporting the notion that the basis for the selective cytotoxic action of cyclophosphamide resides with 4-hydroxycyclophosphamide/aldophosphamide rather than with phosphoramide mustard are the experiments of Colvin and Hilton (1981). They found that when cyclophosphamide was given to L1210 tumour-bearing mice, more DNA was cross-linked in the L1210 leukaemic cells than in the bone marrow cells obtained from these animals. This was in contrast to the results obtained with phosphoramide mustard; it produced similar degrees of DNA cross-linking in the leukaemia and bone-marrow cells.

Cellular basis for favourable therapeutic index

The phenotypic basis for the relatively favourable cytotoxic selectivity exhibited by cyclophosphamide and other 2-chloroethylamido-oxazaphosphorines has, until recently, remained obscure. Obviously, those events that would influence sensitivity to all alkylating agents, e.g., DNA repair and sulphydryl content, cannot account for this selectivity. That is not to say that these determinants of cellular sensitivity to alkylating agents are not operative, only that they cannot account for the oxazaphosphorine-specific selectivity.

Given, as detailed above, that 4-hydroxycyclophosphamide/aldophosphamide is the pharmacologically important circulating metabolite; that the cytotoxic action of cyclophosphamide is effected largely by phosphoramide mustard released from 4-hydroxycyclophosphamide/aldophosphamide within cells; and that the cytotoxic selectivity of cyclophosphamide resides with 4-hydroxycyclophosphamide/aldophosphamide; oxazaphosphorine-specific selectivity must, in some way, be accounted for by the micro-pharmacokinetic behaviour of 4-hydroxycyclophosphamide/aldophosphamide, i.e., the way that this metabolite is handled by cells. Several scenarios can be envisaged: differentially greater uptake and/or trapping by the sensitive species, differentially greater activation by the sensitive species, and differentially greater inactivation by the insensitive species. While all may be operative, and operating in concert, only the latter has been clearly demonstrated to be so.

Differentially greater uptake and/or trapping by the sensitive species

Little is known about the permeation of 4-hydroxycyclophosphamide/aldophosphamide into cells. At a minimum, passive diffusion would be expected since 4-hydroxycyclophosphamide/aldophosphamide is a neutral species. Additionally, an active transport system may be operative (Redwood *et al.*, 1982). Supporting this notion, although of no apparent pharmacological significance in itself, is the observation that cyclophosphamide itself gains entry into cells, at least in part, by a carrier-mediated process (Goldenberg *et al.*, 1974).

Incubation of 4-hydroxycyclophosphamide/aldophosphamide with thiols has been shown to give rise to 4-thiocyclophosphamide conjugates (Peter *et al.*, 1976; Voelcker *et al.*, 1976; Draeger and Hohorst, 1976; Draeger *et al.*, 1976; Hohorst *et al.*, 1976; Brock and Hohorst, 1977; Peter and Hohorst, 1979; Zon *et al.*, 1984). These conjugates are themselves incapable of alkylation (or exerting a cytotoxic action) but they do retain the potential to do so since the conjugating reactions are readily and fully reversible. "Trapping" of an, effectively, latent cytotoxic agent within the cell would occur if the conjugate was ionized and/or if it was of sufficient size. Retardation of 4-hydroxycyclophosphamide/aldophosphamide efflux from cells has been reported (Draeger and Hohorst, 1976). Alternatively, differentially greater uptake by the uneconomic species of a conjugated thiol generated extracellularly could be operative.

There is, however, currently no evidence that differential uptake or efflux of 4-hydroxycyclophosphamide/aldophosphamide accounts for all or any part of the differential sensitivity that cells exhibit towards cyclophosphamide and other oxazaphosphorines.

Differentially greater activation by the sensitive species

According to this scenario, conversion of 4-hydroxycyclophosphamide/aldophosphamide to phosphoramide mustard would occur more readily in the sensitive species.

Conversion of 4-hydroxycyclophosphamide/aldophosphamide to phosphoramide mustard can be the result of "spontaneous", general base-catalysed β-elimination of acrolein from the former (see above). Candidate intracellular general base catalysts of the reaction under consideration include carbonate, and inorganic and organic phosphates (Low *et al.*, 1982, 1983). There are at present, however, no known examples of differential rates of base-catalysed activation accounting for the differential sensitivity that cells exhibit towards cyclophosphamide and other oxazaphosphorines.

Recent observations (Hohorst *et al.*, 1982; Bielicki *et al.*, 1983, 1984; Sladek *et al.*, 1984 b) indicate that conversion of 4-hydroxycyclophosphamide/aldophosphamide, and thiol conjugates thereof, to phosphoramide mustard may also be enzyme-catalysed. Catalytic activity of this type was found in serum, lymphocytes and lymphatic tissues (spleen and thymus). It was not found in liver, muscle, heart, brain or erythrocytes. The identity of the enzyme(s) catalysing this reaction was not established but 3′,5′-exonucleases were shown to do so (Hohorst *et al.*, 1982; Bielicki *et al.*, 1983, 1984).

Again, however, there is, at this time, no evidence that the differential sensitivity that cells exhibit towards cyclophosphamide and other oxazaphosphorines can be accounted for, in part or totally, by differential rates of enzyme-catalysed activation, although Hohorst *et al.* (1982) and Bielicki *et al.* (1983, 1984) have made the suggestion as part of a hypothesis that radically departs from current thinking about the mechanism of oxazaphosphorine-mediated cytotoxic action. According to these investigators, 4-hydroxycyclophosphamide/aldophosphamide is first "trapped" in cells when it conjugates with thiol groups of various molecules, one of which is a macromolecule that contains both 3′,5′-exonuclease and DNA polymerase activities. The 3′,5′-exonuclease then catalyses the release of phosphoramide mustard which alkylates, and thus inactivates, DNA polymerase, thereby preventing cell proliferation.

Differentially greater inactivation by the insensitive species

"Selective detoxification" was first offered more than ten years ago as a possible explanation for the relatively favourable therapeutic index exhibited by cyclophosphamide (Sladek, 1973 b; Domeyer and Sladek, 1974; Connors *et al.*, 1974). It has now been clearly established that, with regard to the differential sensitivity exhibited by various cell populations to cyclophosphamide, differentially greater inactivation of 4-hydroxycyclophosphamide/aldophosphamide by the relatively insensitive cells may be a major determinant, and that this inactivation is catalysed by NAD-linked aldehyde dehydrogenase(s). Several observations support this conclusion.

First, one or more of the NAD-linked aldehyde dehydrogenase isozymes is (are) capable of detoxifying 4-hydroxycyclophosphamide/aldophosphamide by catalysing its oxidation to carboxyphosphamide (see above).

Second, both indirect and direct studies have shown that most tumour cells lack the relevant aldehyde dehydrogenase activity, whereas some critical normal cells (ordinarily sensitive to alkylating agents) do not (see above).

Thus, Cox *et al.* (1975 b, 1976 b) studied the enzymatic deactivation of "activated" cyclophosphamide by the cytosol of liver, kidney, intestinal mucosa and Walker 256 tumour cells, and found greater deactivating activity in the normal tissues; deactivating activity in these tissues was proportional to aldehyde dehydrogenase activity, as determined with acetaldehyde used as the substrate. Direct assay of cellular extracts obtained from six different cultured human tumour cell lines revealed the absence of detectable aldehyde dehydrogenase-catalysed oxidation of 4-hydroxycyclophosphamide/aldophosphamide to carboxyphosphamide (C. L. Manthey and N. E. Sladek, unpublished observations). Aldehyde dehydrogenase-catalysed oxidation of 4-hydroxycyclophosphamide/aldophosphamide to carboxyphosphamide was minimal or absent in cellular extracts obtained from two primary human tumour samples (a neuroblastoma and a B-cell lymphoma) (C. L. Manthey and N. E. Sladek, unpublished observations). It was also minimal in cultured mouse oxazaphosphorine-sensitive L1210 and P388 cells; inhibitors of aldehyde dehydrogenase activity only minimally increased the sensitivity of these cell lines to 4-hydroxycyclophosphamide/aldophosphamide (Hilton, 1984 a,b; Sladek and Landkamer, 1985; C. L. Manthey and N. E. Sladek, unpublished observations). Minimal aldehyde dehydrogenase activity (test substrates were butyraldehyde and benzaldehyde) was found in cultured rat

Walker 256 carcinosarcoma cells, in cultured Novikoff rat hepatoma cells, and in mouse MC-79 and MBE sarcomas grown subcutaneously (Domeyer and Sladek, 1980 b).

In contrast, but lending additional credence to the conclusion given above, significant aldehyde dehydrogenase-catalysed oxidation of 4-hydroxycyclophosphamide/aldophosphamide to carboxyphosphamide was observed when cellular extracts obtained from two mouse tumours (L1210/0AP and P388/CLA) that exhibited an acquired resistance to the oxazaphosphorines, were examined for this activity; inhibitors of aldehyde dehydrogenase activity essentially fully restored the sensitivity of these tumour cells to the oxazaphosphorines (Hilton, 1984 a,b; Sladek *et al.*, 1985; Sladek and Landkamer, 1985; C. L. Manthey and N. E. Sladek, unpublished observations). Moreover, Hilton and Colvin (1984) reported an approximately inverse correlation between aldehyde dehydrogenase activity and the sensitivity of several rodent tumour cell lines, six human leukaemia cell lines, and leukaemic cells derived from marrow aspirates of several patients, to "activated" cyclophosphamide (4-hydroxycyclophosphamide/aldophosphamide); disulfiram, an inhibitor of aldehyde dehydrogenase activity, potentiated the cytotoxic action of "activated" cyclophosphamide against those cells with relatively high amounts of aldehyde dehydrogenase activity.

Cyclophosphamide's relatively favourable therapeutic index is the result, at least in part, of its relative haematopoietic stem cell- and platelet-sparing effects. Thus, most important to the contention presented above, aldehyde dehydrogenase-catalysed oxidation of 4-hydroxycyclophosphamide/aldophosphamide to carboxyphosphamide is observed in two cell types, namely committed megakaryocytoid progenitor cells (F. R. Kohn and N. E. Sladek, unpublished observations) and pluripotent haematopoietic cells (Kohn and Sladek, 1985), that are critical normal cells and ordinarily highly sensitive to the cytotoxic action of nitrogen mustards but which are relatively insensitive to cyclophosphamide. Inhibitors of aldehyde dehydrogenase activity increase the sensitivity of these cells to 4-hydroxycyclophosphamide/aldophosphamide (Figure 11).

Third, 4-methylcyclophosphamide exhibits a lower therapeutic index than cyclophosphamide (Cox *et al.*, 1975 a, 1976 b). 4-Methylcyclophosphamide, like cyclophosphamide, is first converted to the 4-hydroxy metabolite which then, analogously to the formation of phosphoramide mustard and acrolein from 4-hydroxycyclophosphamide/aldophosphamide, gives rise to phosphoramide mustard and methyl vinyl ketone. It cannot, however, give rise to a metabolite corresponding to carboxyphosphamide, i.e., aldehyde dehydrogenase activity cannot play a role in its metabolic fate and thus in any selective toxicity that it might exhibit. All else being the same then, cyclophosphamide and 4-methylcyclophosphamide should exhibit the same therapeutic index if aldehyde dehydrogenase activity is not an important determinant with regard to the selectivity toxicity exhibited by cyclophosphamide;

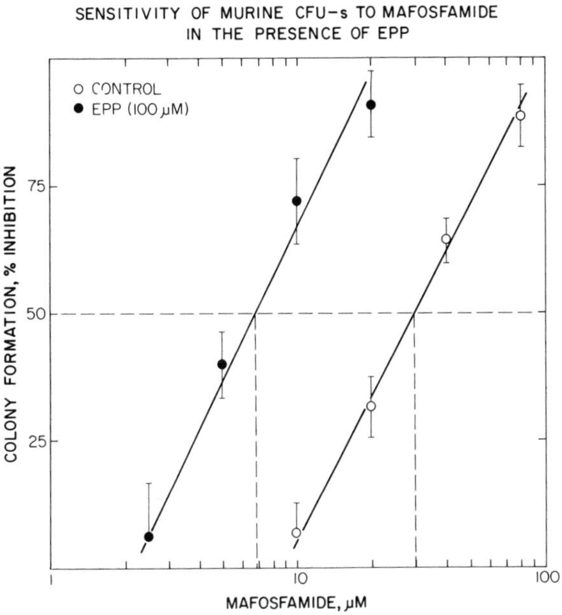

Figure 11. Sensitivity of murine pluripotent haematopoietic cells to 4-hydroxycyclophosphamide/aldophosphamide in the presence of the aldehyde dehydrogenase inhibitor ethylphenyl-(2-formylethyl)phosphinate (EPP). Mouse bone marrow cells were incubated for 60 min at 37°C in the presence (•) and absence (○) of 100 μM EPP. Vehicle or mafosfamide was then added and incubation was continued at 37°C for an additional 30 min. Following incubation, the cells were harvested, resuspended in drug-free medium, and assayed for viable pluripotent haematopoietic stem cells (CFU-s assay). Points are means ± S. D. of observations made in 4–5 mice. Modified from Kohn and Sladek (1985).

if this enzyme activity is an important determinant, the therapeutic index exhibited by cyclophosphamide should exceed, as was the case, that of 4-methylcyclophosphamide.

Fourth, the therapeutic index of cyclophosphamide is lowered when an inhibitor of aldehyde dehydrogenase activity is also given (Cox *et al.*, 1976 b). This would be as expected if differentially greater inactivation by aldehyde dehydrogenase activity in the economic species accounted for a part of the favourable therapeutic index.

Clearly, then, consideration of the foregoing observations leads inexorably to the conclusion that the relatively favourable margin of safety exhibited by cyclophosphamide and other oxazaphosphorines is largely due to differential aldehyde dehydrogenase activity which favourably affects differences in the balance between the formation of cytotoxic metabolites and the conversion to inactive metabolites in neoplastic and critical normal cells such as haematopoietic stem cells.

Future directions

Despite the wealth of knowledge already accumulated with regard to the metabolism of the oxazaphosphorines and the important role that biotransformation plays in the therapeutic efficacies of these agents, several important questions have yet to be satisfactorily answered.

Many of these revolve around aldehyde dehydrogenase-catalysed oxidation of 4-hydroxycyclophosphamide/aldophosphamide to carboxyphosphamide. Thus, next to nothing is currently known about which of the several isozymes that are found in mammalian cells catalyse this reaction, or about the tissue distribution, substrate specificity, sensitivity to various inhibitors, and inducibility, of these isozymes.

Yet to be determined also is whether conversion of 4-hydroxycyclophosphamide/aldophosphamide to phosphoramide mustard is enzymatically mediated *in vivo*, as has been suggested by at least two laboratories (Bielicki *et al.*, 1983; Sladek *et al.*, 1984 b). Should enzymatic involvement be established, a whole new set of questions concerning the potential modulation of such catalysis would have to be addressed as well.

Rodent tumour cell populations that exhibit an acquired resistance to the oxazaphosphorines are often not cross-resistant to other cross-linking agents (Wampler *et al.*, 1978; Gerhartz *et al.*, 1979; Schmid *et al.*, 1980; Schabel *et al.*, 1983; Sladek *et al.*, 1985). In at least two such instances, the phenotypic basis for the acquired resistance was increased detoxification due to increased aldehyde dehydrogenase activity (Sladek *et al.*, 1985). Not known is the genotypic basis for the increased enzyme activity.

Unfortunately, acquired resistance to the oxazaphosphorines also often occurs in humans. Whether it is occasionally or inevitably due to increased aldehyde dehydrogenase activity remains to be determined.

The *ex vivo* use of the oxazaphosphorines for the purpose of purging bone marrow of neoplastic cells in autologous bone marrow transplantation procedures has yet to be optimized, and the *ex vivo* use of these agents for the purpose of purging bone marrow of the cells that give rise to graft-versus-host disease in allogenic transplantation has yet to be fully explored. Modulation of the relevant non-enzymatic and enzymatic reactions could be useful in either case.

Cyclophosphamide is therapeutically efficacious not only in the treatment of certain malignancies but also when used for immunosuppressive purposes in bone marrow transplantation protocols and in the treatment of various autoimmune disorders (see above). Relative to other cross-linking agents, cyclophosphamide seems to be more useful in that regard. Why is not known. The fact that cellular elements of the humoral and cell-mediated immune systems are differentially sensitive to the cytotoxic action of the oxazaphosphorines may be important (Hilgard *et al.*, 1985; Smith and Sladek, 1985). So could the fact that differentiated blood cells seem to be more sensitive to the cytotoxic action of the oxazaphosphorines than are pluripotent or committed progenitor haematopoietic cells (N. E. Sladek, unpublished observations). Differential sensitivity could be the resullt of differential rates of biotransformation. Seemingly paradoxical is the fact that low doses of the oxazaphosphorines may effect an augmentation of the cell-mediated immune response; this may be because T-suppressor cells are apparently more sensitive to these agents than are other T-cell subsets (Hilgard *et al.*, 1985). More information is needed.

Cancer prevention is still a goal that is far from being realized. Organ and tissue transplantation is likely to become even more common in future years. Increasingly, newly emerging evidence suggests that the aetiology of many of the so-called chronic disorders, e.g., rheumatoid arthritis, insulin-dependent diabetes, multiple sclerosis, myasthenia gravis, systemic lupus erythaematosus, alopecia areata, etc., includes an autoimmune component. Cyclophosphamide is of demonstrated, but limited, value in the treatment of certain neoplasms and chronic disorders, and in transplant protocols. Its biggest drawback is that it is carcinogenic. All DNA–DNA cross-linking agents probably are. Thus, pursuit of an "improved cyclophosphamide" would not seem wise. However, advantage could be taken of the fact that some critical normal cell populations, e.g., pluripotent haematopoietic cells, contain aldehyde dehydrogenase activity, whereas some undesired cell populations, malignant or normal depending on the therapeutic goal, may not. Aldehydes or non-cytotoxic precursors thereof should be sought which, (1) as aldehydes

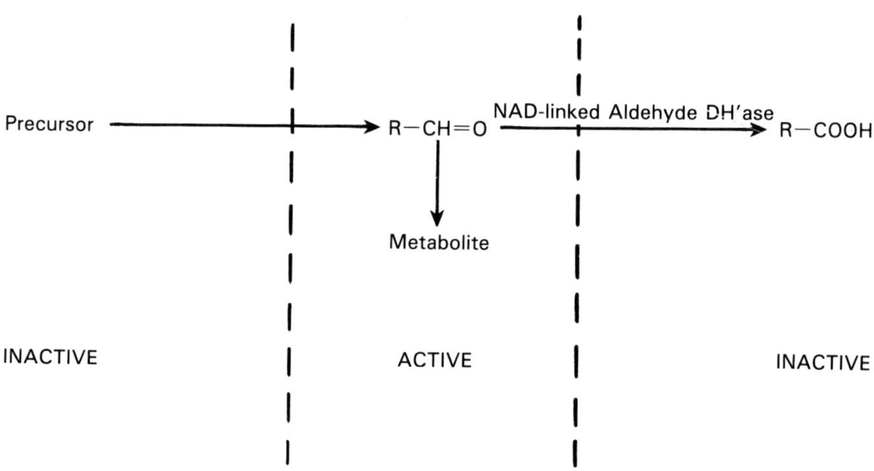

Figure 12. The design of cytotoxic agents that are selectively toxic to the uneconomic species because of a differentially greater aldehyde dehydrogenase activity in the economic species: general considerations.

or metabolites (other than the corresponding acids) thereof, are cytotoxic, and (2) as aldehydes, are substrates for the relevant aldehyde dehydrogenase isozyme(s) (Figure 12). In this scenario, the oxidized products of aldehyde dehydrogenase catalysis, i.e., the corresponding acids, would be without cytotoxic activity. Cytotoxicity could be by any mechanism that does not lead to malignancy. Cytotoxic aldehydes are not unheard of (Schauenstein and Esterbauer, 1979; Hauptlorenz *et al.*, 1985).

Fruitful also may be the design of agents that selectively (1) induce the activity of the relevant aldehyde dehydrogenase isozymes in the economic species or (2) inhibit/depress the activity of the relevant isozyme in the uneconomic species when it is present in this species.

References

Alarcon, R. A. and Meienhofer, J., 1971, Formation of the cytotoxic aldehyde acrolein during *in vitro* degradation of cyclophosphamide. *Nature, New Biology*, **233**, 250–252.

Alarcon, R. A., Meienhofer, J. and Atherton, E., 1972, Isophosphamide as a new acrolein-producing antineoplastic isomer of cyclophosphamide. *Cancer Research*, **32**, 2519–2523.

Allen, L. M. and Creaven, P. J., 1972, In vitro activation of isophosphamide (NSC-109724), a new oxazaphosphorine, by rat liver microsomes. *Cancer Treatment Reports*, **56**, 603–610.

Allen, L. M. and Creaven, P. J., 1975 a, Pharmacokinetics of ifosfamide. *Clinical Pharmacology and Therapeutics*, **17**, 492–498.

Allen, L. M. and Creaven, P. J., 1975 b, Human pharmacokinetic model for isophosphamide (NSC-109724). *Cancer Chemotherapy Reports*, **59**, 877–882.

American Medical Association, 1983, Antineoplastic agents. In *AMA Drug Evaluations*, 5th edition, edited by D. R. Bennett (Chicago: American Medical Association), pp. 1481–1513.

Arnold, H. and Bourseaux, F., 1958, Synthese und Abbau cytostatisch wirksamer cyclischer N-Phosphamidester des Bis-(β-chloräthyl)-amins. *Angewandte Chemie*, **70**, 539–544.

Arnold, H., Bourseaux, F. and Brock, N., 1958, Chemotherapeutic action of a cyclic nitrogen mustard phosphamide ester (B 518-ASTA) in experimental tumours of the rat. *Nature*, **181**, 931.

Arnold, H., Bourseaux, F. and Brock, N., 1961, Über Beziehungen zwischen chemischer Konstitution and cancertoxischer Wirkung in der Reihe der Phosphamidester des Bis-(β-choräthyl)-amins. *Arzneimittel-Forschung, Drug Research*, **11**, 143–158.

Bagley, C. M., Jr., Bostick, F. W. and DeVita, V. T., Jr., 1973, Clinical pharmacology of cyclophosphamide. *Cancer Research*, **33**, 226–233.

Bakke, J. E., Feil, V. J. and Zaylskie, R. G., 1971, Characterization of the major sheep urinary metabolites of cyclophosphamide, a defleecing chemical. *Journal of Agricultural and Food Chemistry*, **19**, 788–790.

Bakke, J. E., Feil, V. J., Fjelstul, C. E. and Thacker, E. J., 1972, Metabolism of cyclophosphamide by sheep. *Journal of Agricultural and Food Chemistry*, **20**, 384–388.

Bellin, H. J., Cherry, J. M. and Koss, L. G., 1974, Effects of a single dose of cyclophosphamide. V. Protective effect of diversion of the urinary stream on dog bladder. *Laboratory Investigation*, **30**, 43–47.

Bielicki, L., Voelcker, G. and Hohorst, H. J., 1983, Enzymatic toxicogenation of "activated" cyclophosphamide by 3′-5′ exonucleases. *Journal of Cancer Research and Clinical Oncology*, **105**, 27–29.

Bielicki, L., Voelcker, G. and Hohorst, H. J., 1984, Activated cyclophosphamide: an enzyme-mechanism-based suicide inactivator of DNA polymerase/3′-5′ exonuclease. *Journal of Cancer Research and Clinical Oncology*, **107**, 195–198.

Borch, R. F. and Getman, K. M., 1984, Base-catalyzed hydrolysis of 4-hydroperoxycyclophosphamide: evidence for iminocyclophosphamide as an intermediate. *Journal of Medicinal Chemistry*, **27**, 485–490.

Borch, R. F., Hoye, T. R. and Swanson, T. A., 1984, *In situ* preparation and fate of *cis*-4-hydroxycyclophosphamide and aldophosphamide: ^{1}H and ^{31}P NMR evidence for equilibration of *cis*- and *trans*-4-hydroxycyclophosphamide with aldophosphamide and its hydrate in aqueous solution. *Journal of Medicinal Chemistry*, **27**, 490–494.

Bramwell, V., Calvert, R. T., Edwards, G., Scarffe, H. and Crowther, D., 1979, The disposition of cyclophosphamide in a group of myeloma patients. *Cancer Chemotherapy and Pharmacology*, **3**, 253–259.

Brock, N., 1967, Pharmacologic characterization of cyclophosphamide (NSC-26271), and cyclophosphamide metabolites. *Cancer Chemotherapy Reports*, **51**, 315–325.

Brock, N., 1976, Comparative pharmacologic study in vitro and in vivo with cyclophosphamide (NSC-26271), cyclophosphamide metabolites, and plain nitrogen mustard compounds. *Cancer Treatment Reports*, **60**, 301–307.

Brock, N., 1983, Oxazaphosphorine cytostatics: structure–activity relationships, selectivity and metabolism, regional detoxification. In *Structure–activity Relationships of Anti-tumor Agents*, edited by D. N. Reinhoudt, T. A. Connors, H. M. Pinedo and K. W. van de Poll (Boston: Martinus Nijhoff Publishers), pp 239–267.

Brock, N. and Hohorst, H. J., 1963, Über die Aktivierung von Cyclophosphamid in vivo und in vitro. *Arzneimittel-Forschung, Drug Research*, **13**, 1021–1031.

Brock, N. and Hohorst, H. J., 1967, Metabolism of cyclophosphamide. *Cancer*, **20**, 900–904.

Brock, N. and Hohorst, H. J., 1977, The problem of specificity and selectivity of alkylating cytostatics: studies on N-2-chloroethylamido-oxazaphosphorines. *Zeitschrift für Krebsforschung und Klinische Onkologie*, **88**, 185–215.

Brock, N., Stekar, J., Pohl, J., Niemeyer, U. and Scheffler, G., 1979, Acrolein, the causative factor of urotoxic side-effects of cyclophosphamide, ifosfamide, trofosfamide and sufosfamide. *Arzneimittel-Forschung, Drug Research*, **29**, 659–661.

Brock, N., Pohl, J. and Stekar, J., 1981, Studies on the urotoxicity of oxazaphosphorine cytostatics and its prevention. I. Experimental studies on the urotoxicity of alkylating compounds. *European Journal of Cancer*, **17**, 595–607.

Cairney, A. E., Sladek, N. E. and Woods, W. G., 1984, DNA crosslinking by 4-hydroperoxycyclophosphamide in sensitive and resistant mouse leukemia cells. *Proceedings of the American Association for Cancer Research*, **25**, 339.

Calabresi, P. and Parks, R. E., Jr., 1985, Chemotherapy of neoplastic diseases. In *The Pharmacological Basis of Therapeutics*, 7th edition, edited by A. G. Gilman, L. S. Goodman, T. W. Rall and F. Murad (New York: Macmillan Publishing Co.), pp. 1240–1258.

Chetsanga, C. J., Polidori G. and Mainwaring, M., 1982, Analysis and excision of ring-opened phosphoramide mustard-deoxyguanine adducts in DNA. *Cancer Research*, **42**, 2616–2621.

Cohen, J. L. and Jao, J. Y., 1970, Enzymatic basis of cyclophosphamide activation by hepatic microsomes of the rat. *Journal of Pharmacology and Experimental Therapeutics*, **174**, 206–210.

Cohen, J. L., Jao, J. Y. and Jusko, W. J., 1971, Pharmacokinetics of cyclophosphamide in man. *British Journal of Pharmacology*, **43**, 677–680.

Colvin, M., 1982, The comparative pharmacology of cyclophosphamide and ifosfamide. *Seminars in Oncology*, **9** (Suppl. 1), 2–7.

Colvin, M., Padgett, C. A. and Fenselau, C., 1973, A biologically active metabolite of cyclophosphamide. *Cancer Research*, **33**, 915–918.

Colvin, M., Brundrett, R. B., Kan M. N. N., Jardine, I. and Fenselau, C., 1976, Alkylating properties of phosphoramide mustard. *Cancer Research*, **36**, 1121–1126.

Colvin, M. and Hilton, J., 1981, Pharmacology of cyclophosphamide and metabolites. *Cancer Treatment Reports*, **65**, 89–95.

Connors, T. A., Grover, P. L. and McLoughlin, A. M., 1970, Microsomal activation of cyclophosphamide in vivo. *Biochemical Pharmacology*, **19**, 1533–1535.

Connors, T. A., Foster, A. B., Gilsenan, A. M., Jarman, M. and Tisdale, M. J., 1972, Observations on the metabolism of cyclophosphamide. *Biochemical Pharmacology*, **21**, 1373–1376.

Connors, T. A., Cox, P. J., Farmer, P. B., Foster, A. B. and Jarman, M., 1974, Some studies of the active intermediates formed in the microsomal metabolism of cyclophosphamide and isophosphamide. *Biochemical Pharmacology*, **23**, 115–129.

Cox, P. J., 1979, Cyclophosphamide cystitis—identification of acrolein as the causative agent. *Biochemical Pharmacology*, **28**, 2045–2049.

Cox, P. J., Farmer, P. B. and Jarman, M., 1975 a, The microsomal metabolism of some analogues of cyclophosphamide: 4-methylcyclophosphamide and 6-methylcyclophosphamide. *Biochemical Pharmacology*, **24**, 599–606.

Cox, P. J., Phillips, B. J. and Thomas, P., 1975 b, The enzymatic basis of the selective action of cyclophosphamide. *Cancer Research*, **35**, 3755–3761.

Cox, P. J., Farmer, P. B. and Jarman, M. (editors), 1976 a, Proceedings of the Symposium on the Metabolism and Mechanism of Action of Cyclophosphamide. *Cancer Treatment Reports*, **60**, 299–525.

Cox, P. J., Phillips, B. J. and Thomas, P., 1976 b, Studies on the selective action of cyclophosphamide (NSC-26271): inactivation of the hydroxylated metabolite by tissue-soluble enzymes. *Cancer Treatment Reports*, **60**, 321–326.

DeVita, V. T. and Adamson, R. H., 1970, The metabolism of ^{14}C-cyclophosphamide: comparative drug metabolism studies on African and American patients with lymphosarcoma and Burkitt's tumor. *Progress in Antimicrobial and Anticancer Chemotherapy*, **2**, 218–225.

D'Incalci, M., Bolis, G., Facchinetti, T., Mangioni, C., Morasca, L., Morazzoni, P. and Salmona, M., 1979 a, Decreased half life of cyclophosphamide in patients under continual treatment. *European Journal of Cancer*, **15**, 7–10.

D'Incalci, M., Facchinetti, T., Bolis, G., Mangioni, C. and Morasca, L., 1979 b, Pharmacokinetics of cyclophosphamide after prolonged low dose treatment in ovarian cancer patients. *European Journal of Drug Metabolism and Pharmacokinetics*, **4**, 83–85.

Domeyer, B. E., 1977, Biotransformation of "activated" cyclophosphamide. Minneapolis, Ph.D. Thesis, University of Minnesota.

Domeyer, B. E. and Sladek, N. E., 1974, Potential for *in vivo* inactivation of a cyclophosphamide metabolite (aldophosphamide) by tumor enzymes. *Federation Proceedings*, **33**, 581.

Domeyer, B. E. and Sladek, N. E., 1980 a, Kinetics of cyclophosphamide biotransformation *in vivo*. *Cancer Research*, **40**, 174–180.

Domeyer, B. E. and Sladek, N. E., 1980 b, Metabolism of 4-hydroxycyclophosphamide/aldophosphamide *in vitro*. *Biochemical Pharmacology*, **29**, 2903–2912.

Domeyer, B. E. and Sladek, N. E., 1981, Inhibition by cyanamide of 4-hydroxycyclophosphamide/aldophosphamide oxidation to carboxyphosphamide. *Biochemical Pharmacology*, **30**, 2065–2973.

Donelli, M. G., Bartośek, I., Guaitani, A., Martin, A., Colombo, T., Pacciarini, M. A. and Modica, R., 1976, Importance of pharmacokinetic studies on cyclophosphamide (NSC-26271) in understanding its cytotoxic effect. *Cancer Treatment Reports*, **60**, 395–401.

Draeger, U. and Hohorst, H. J., 1976, Permeation of cyclophosphamide (NSC-26271) metabolites into tumor cells. *Cancer Treatment Reports*, **60**, 423–427.

Draeger, U., Peter, G. and Hohorst, H. J., 1976, Deactivation of cyclophosphamide (NSC-26271) metabolites by sulfhydryl compounds. *Cancer Treatment Repots*, **60**, 355–359.

Edwards, G., Calvert, R. T., Crowther, D., Bramwell, V. and Scarffe, H., 1980, Repeated investigations of cyclophosphamide disposition in myeloma patients receiving intermittent chemotherapy. *British Journal of Clinical Pharmacology*, **10**, 281–285.

Engle, T. W., Zon, G. and Egan, W., 1982, ^{31}P NMR kinetic studies of the intra- and intermolecular alkylation chemistry of phosphoramide mustard and cognate N-phosphorylated derivatives of N,N-bis(2-chloroethyl)amine. *Journal of Medicinal Chemistry*, **25**, 1347–1357.

Engle, T. W., Zon, G. and Egan, W., 1982, ^{31}P NMR kinetic studies of the intra- and inermolecular alkylation chemistry of phosphoramide mustard and cognate N-phosphorylated derivatives of N,N-bis(2-chloroethyl)amine. *Journal of Medicinal Chemistry*, **25**, 1347–1357.

Erickson, L. C., Ramonas, L. M., Zaharko, D. S. and Kohn, K. W., 1980, Cytotoxicity and DNA cross-linking activity of 4-sulfidocyclophosphamides in mouse leukemia cells in vitro. *Cancer Research*, **40**, 4216–4220.

Fenselau, C., Kan, M. N. N., Billets, S. and Colvin, M., 1975, Identification of phosphorodiamidic acid mustard as a human metabolite of cyclophosphamide. *Cancer Research*, **35**, 1453–1457.

Fenselau, C., Kan, M.-N. N., Rao, S. S., Myles, A., Friedman, O. M. and Colvin, M., 1977, Identification of aldophosphamide as a metabolite of cyclophosphamide in vitro and in vivo in humans. *Cancer Research*, **37**, 2538–2543.

Fenselau, C., Lehman, J. P., Myles, A., Brandt, J., Yost, G. S., Friedman, O. M. and Colvin, O. M., 1982, Iminocyclophosphamide as a chemically reactive metabolite of cyclophosphamide. *Drug Metabolism and Disposition*, **10**, 636–640.

Foley, G. E., Friedman, O. M. and Drolet, B. P., 1961, Studies on the mechanism of action of cytoxan—evidence of activation *in vivo* and *in vitro*. *Cancer Research*, **21**, 57–63.

Friedman, O. M., 1967, Studies of some newer phosphoramide mustards. *Cancer Chemotherapy Reports*, **51**, 1967.

Friedman, O. M. and Seligman, A. M., 1954, Preparation of N-phosphorylated derivatives of bis-β-chloroethylamine. *Journal of American Chemical Society*, **76**, 655–658.

Friedman, O. M., Wodinsky, I. and Myles, A., 1976, Cyclophosphamide (NSC-26271)-related phosphoramide mustards—recent advances and historical perspective. *Cancer Treatment Reports*, **60**, 337–346.

Friedman, O. M., Myles, A. and Colvin, M., 1979, Cyclophosphamide and related phosphoramide mustards. Current status and future prospects. *Advances in Cancer Chemotherapy*, **1**, 143–204.

Gerhartz, H. H., Liss, E. and Schmidt, H., 1979, Cyclophosphamide-resistant Yoshida ascites tumor cells and their cross resistance to some alkylating agents. *Journal of Cancer Research and Clinical Oncology*, **94**, 257–263.

Goldenberg, G. J., Land, H. B. and Cormack, D. V., 1974, Mechanism of cyclophosphamide transport by L5178Y lymphoblasts in vitro. *Cancer Research*, **34**, 3274–3282.

Goldstein, A., Aronow, L. and Kalman, S. M., 1974, *Principles of Drug Action: The Basis of Pharmacology*, 2nd edition, (New York: John Wiley), pp. 333–338.

Gomori, G., 1948, Histochemical demonstration of sites of phosphamidase activity. *Proceedings of the Society for Experimental Biology and Medicine*, **69**, 407–409.

Grochow, L. B. and Colvin, M., 1980, Clinical pharmacokinetics of cyclophosphamide. *Clinical Pharmacokinetics*, **4**, 380–394.

Gurtoo, H. L., Bansal, S. K., Pavelic, Z. and Struck, R. F., 1985, Effects of the induction of hepatic microsomal metabolism on the toxicity of cyclophosphamide. *British Journal of Cancer*, **51**, 67–75.

Habs, H., Habs, M. and Schmähl, D., 1981, Influence of pretreatment with disulfiram on the acute toxicity of cyclophosphamide in male Sprague–Dawley rats. *Arzneimittel-Forschung, Drug Research*, **31**, 530–531.

Hacker, M. P., Ershler, W. B., Newman, R. A. and Gamelli, R. L., 1982, Effect of disulfiram (tetraethylthiuram disulfide) and diethyldithiocarbamate on the bladder toxicity and antitumor activity of cyclophosphamide in mice. *Cancer Research*, **42**, 4490–4494.

Hauptlorenz, S., Esterbauer, H., Moll, W., Pumpel, R., Schauenstein, E. and Puschendorf, B., 1985, Effects of the lipid peroxidation product 4-hydroxynonenal and related aldehydes on proliferation and viability of cultured Ehrlich ascites tumor cells. *Biochemical Pharmacology*, **34**, 3803–3809.

Hemminki, K., 1985, Binding of metabolites of cyclophosphamide to DNA in a rat liver microsomal system and in vitro in mice. *Cancer Research*, **45**, 4237–4243.

Hilgard, P., Pohl, J., Stekar, J, and Voegeli, R., 1985, Oxazaphosphorines as biological response modifiers—experimental and clinical perspectives. *Cancer Treatment Reviews*, **12**, 155–162.

Hill, D. L., 1975, *A Review of Cyclophosphamide* (Springfield, IL: Charles C. Thomas).

Hill, D. L., Laster, W. R., Jr., Kirk, M. C., El Dareer, S. and Struck, R. F., 1973, Metabolism of iphosphamide [2-(2-chloroethylamino)-3-(2-chloroethyl)tetrahydro-2H-1,3,2-oxazaphosphorine 2-oxide] and production of a toxic iphosphamide metabolite. *Cancer Research*, **33**, 1016–1022.

Hill, D. L., Laster, W. R., Jr., Struck, R. F., 1972, Enzymatic metabolism of cyclophosphamide and nicotine and production of a toxic cyclophosphamide metabolite. *Cancer Research*, **32**, 658–665.

Hilton, J., 1984 a, Deoxyribonucleic acid crosslinking by 4-hydroperoxycyclophosphamide in cyclophosphamide-sensitive and -resistant L1210 cells. *Biochemical Pharmacology*, **33**, 1867–1872.

Hilton, J., 1984 b, Role of aldehyde dehydrogenase in cyclophosphamide-resistant L1210 leukemia. *Cancer Research*, **44**, 5156–5160.

Hilton, J. and Colvin, M., 1984, The role of aldehyde dehydrogenase activity in cyclophosphamide sensitivity of hematopoetic and leukemic cell populations. *Proceedings of the American Association of Cancer Research*, **25**, 339.

Hipkens, J. H., Struck, R. F. and Gurtoo, H. L., 1981, Role of aldehyde dehydrogenase in the metabolism-dependent biological activity of cyclophosphamide. *Cancer Research*, **41**, 3571–3583.

Hohorst, H. J., Ziemann, A. and Brock, N., 1971, 4-Ketocyclophosphamide, a metabolite of cyclophosphamide. Formation, chemical and biological properties. *Arzneimittel-Forschung, Drug Research*, **21**, 1254–1257.

Hohorst, H. J., Draeger, U., Peter, G. and Voelcker, G., 1976, The problem of oncostatic specificity of cyclophosphamide (NSC-26271): Studies on reactions that control the alkylating and cytoxic activity. *Cancer Treatment Reports*, **60**, 309–315.

Hohorst, H. J., Bielicki, L. and Voelcker, G., 1982, Release of phosphoramide mustard from activated cyclophosphamide by DNA-polymerase linked 3′5′ exonuclease as basis for cytotoxic specificity. *Proceedings of Thirteenth International Cancer Congress*, p. 384.

Jao, J. Y., Jusko, W. J. and Cohen, J. L., 1972, Phenobarbital effects on cyclophosphamide pharmacokinetics in man. *Cancer Research*, **32**, 2761–2764.

Jardine, I., Fenselau, C., Appler, M., Kan, M. N., Brundrett, R. B., and Colvin, M., 1978, Quantitation by gas chromatography–chemical ionization mass spectrometry of cyclophosphamide, phosphoramide mustard, and nornitrogen mustard in the plasma and urine of patients receiving cyclophosphamide therapy. *Cancer Research*, **38**, 408–415.

Juma, F. and Ogada, T., 1983, Pharmacokinetics of cyclophosphamide in Kenyan Africans. *British Journal of Clinical Pharmacology*, **16**, 61–63.

Juma, F. D., Rogers, H. J. and Trounce, J. R., 1979 a, Pharmacokinetics of cyclophosphamide and alkylating activity in man after intravenous and oral administration. *British Journal of Clinical Pharmacology*, **8**, 209–217.

Juma, F. D., Rogers, H. J. and Trounce, J. R., 1979 b, The kinetics of salivary elimination of cyclophosphamide in man. *British Journal of Clinical Pharmacology*, **8**, 455–458.

Juma, F. D., Rogers, H. J. and Trounce, J. R., 1980, The pharmacokinetics of cyclophosphamide, phosphoramide mustard and nor-nitrogen mustard studied by gas chromatography in patients receiving cyclophosphamide theraphy. *British Journal of Clinical Pharmacology*, **10**, 327–335.

Juma, F. D., Rogers, H. J. and Trounce, J. R., 1981, Effect of renal insufficiency on the pharmacokinetics of cyclophosphamide and some of its metabolites. *European Journal of Clinical Pharmacology*, **19**, 443–451.

Juma, F. D., Koech, D. K., Kasili, E. G. and Ogada, T., 1984, Pharmacokinetics of cyclophosphamide in Kenyan African children with lymphoma. *British Journal of Clinical Pharmacology*, **18**, 106–107.

Kallama, S. and Hemminki, K., 1984, Alkylation of guanosine by phosphoramide mustard, chloromethine hydrochloride and chlorambucil. *Acta Pharmacologica et Toxicologica*, **54**, 214–220.

Kluin-Nelemans, H. C., Löwenberg, B., Martens, A. C. M. and Hagenbeek, A., 1984, In vitro chemotherapy with ASTA-Z-7557: Studies in rat and human acute lyeloid leukemia. In *Autologous Bone Marrow Transplantation and Solid Tumours*, edited by J. G. McVie, O. Dalesio and I. E. Smith (New York: Raven Press), pp. 33–39.

Kohn, F. R. and Sladek, N. E., 1985, Aldehyde dehydrogenase activity as the basis for the relative insensitivity of murine pluripotent hematopoietic stem cells to oxazaphosphorines. *Biochemical Pharmacology*, **34**, 3465–3471.

Lenssen, U. and Hohorst, H. J., 1979, Zur Frage der Permeabilität von N,N-Bis(2-chloräthyl)-phosphorsäurediamid in Tumorzellen. *Journal of Cancer Research and Clinical Oncology*, **93**, 161–164.

Levins, P. L. and Rogers, W. I., 1965, Nuclear magnetic resonance study of stability of a salt of N,N-bis(2-chloroethyl)phosphorodiamidic acid (NSC-69945) in aqueous solution. *Cancer Chemotherapy Reports*, **44**, 15–17.

Low, J. E., Borch, R. F. and Sladek, N. E., 1982, Conversion of 4-hydroperoxycyclophosphamide and 4-hydroxycyclophosphamide to phosphoramide mustard and acrolein mediated by bifunctional catalysts. *Cancer Research*, **42**, 830–837.

Low, J. E., Borch, R. F. and Sladek, N. E., 1983, Further studies on the conversion of 4-hydroxyoxazaphosphorines to reactive mustards and acrolein in inorganic buffers. *Cancer Research*, **43**, 5815–5820.

Lu, C., Braine, H. G., Kaizer, H., Saral, R., Tutschka, P. J. and Santos, G. W., 1984, Preliminary results of high-dose busulfan and cyclophosphamide with syngeneic or autologus bone marrow rescue. *Cancer Treatment Research*, **68**, 711–717.

Maddock, C. L., Handler, A. H., Friedman, O. M., Foley, G. E. and Farber, S., 1966, Primary evaluation of alkylating agent cyclohexylamine salt of N,N-bis(2-chloroethyl)phosphorodiamidic acid (NSC 69945; OMF-59) in experimental antitumor assay systems. *Cancer Chemotherapy Reports*, **50**, 629–638.

Manthey, C. L. and Sladek, N. E., 1986, Characterization of NAD-linked aldehyde dehydrogenase catalysis of the oxidation of aldophosphamide by mouse liver fractions. *Proceedings of the American Association for Cancer Research*, **27**, 421.

McNeil, N. O. and Morgan, L. R., Jr., 1981, The bioavailability of oral and intravenous ifosfamide in the treatment of bronchogenic carcinoma. *International Journal of Clinical Pharmacology, Therapy and Toxicology*, **19**, 490–493.

Mehta, J. R., Przbylski, M. and Ludlum, D. B., 1980, Alkylation of guanosine and deoxyguanosine by phosphoramide mustard. *Cancer Research*, **40**, 4183–4186.

Minowada, J., Koshiba, H., Sagawa, K., Kubonishi, I., Lok, M. S., Taksumi, E., Han, T., Srivastava, B. I. S., Ohnuma, T., 1981, Marker profiles of human leukemia and lymphoma cell lines. *Journal of Cancer Research and Clinical Oncology*, **101**, 91–100.

Montgomery, J. A. and Struck, R. F., 1973, The relationship of the metabolism of anticancer agents to their activity. *Progress in Drug Research*, **17**, 320–409.

Montgomery, J. A. and Struck, R. F., 1976, Synthesis and structure–activity relationships of pre-activated analogs of cyclophosphamide (NSC-26271). *Cancer Treatment Reports*, **60**, 381–393.

Myles, A., Fenselau, C. and Friedman, O. M., 1977, Synthesis of aldophosphamide, a key cyclophosphamide metabolite. *Tetrahedron Letters*, No. 29, 2475–2478.

Niemeyer, U., Engel, J., Scheffler, G., Molge, K., Sauerbier, D., Weigert, W., 1984, Chemical characterization of ASTA Z 7557 (INN mafosfamide, *cis*-4-sulfoethylthiocyclophosphamide), a stable derivative of 4-hydroxycyclophosphamide. *Investigational New Drugs*, **2**, 133–139.

Norpoth, K., 1969, Untersuchungen zur oxydativen Umsetzung von Endoxan in vivo und in vitro. Münster, Habilitationsschrift, Fach Physiologische Chemi, Westfälischen Wilhelms-Universität.

Norpoth, K., Golovinsky, E. and Rauen, H. M., 1970, Untersuchungen an hypothetischen Metaboliten des 2-[Bis(2-chloräthyl)amino]tetrahydro-2*H*-1,3,2-oxazaphosphorin-2-oxids (Cyclophosphamide). *Hoppe-Seyler's Zeitschrift für Physiologische Chemie*, **351**, 377–383.

Ottolenghi, L., Morasca, L., Marsoni, S., Piazza, E., Soresi, E., Libretti, A. and Garattini, S., 1980, Plasma levels of cyclophosphamide in patients under polychemotherapeutic regimens. *Biomedicine*, **32**, 123–127.

Peter, G. and Hohorst, H. J., 1979, Synthesis and preliminary antitumor evaluation of 4-(SR)-sulfido-cyclophosphamides. *Cancer Chemotherapy and Pharmacology*, **3**, 181–188.

Peter, G., Wagner, T. and Hohorst, H. J., 1976, Studies on 4-hydroperoxycyclophosphamide (NSC-181815): a simple preparation method and its application for the synthesis of a new class of "activated" sulfur-containing cyclophosphamide (NSC-26271) derivatives. *Cancer Treatment Reports*, **60**, 429–435.

Philips, F. S., Sternberg, S. S., Cronin, A. P. and Vidal, P. M., 1961, Cyclophosphamide and urinary bladder toxicity. *Cancer Research*, **21**, 1577–1589.

Pietruszko, R., 1983, Aldehyde dehydrogenase isozymes. In *Isozymes: Current Topics in Biological and Medical Research. Cellular Localization, Metabolism, and Physiology*, edited by M. C. Rattazzi, J. G. Scandalios and G. S. Whitt (New York: Alan R. Liss), Vol. 8, pp. 195–217.

Powers, J. F. and Sladek, N. E., 1978, Influence of thiosulfate on the cytotoxic action of cyclophosphamide metabolites. *The Pharmacologist*, **20**, 250.

Powers, J. F. and Sladek, N. E., 1983, Cytotoxic activity relative to 4-hydroxycyclophosphamide and phosphoramide mustard concentrations in the plasma of cyclophosphamide-treated rats. *Cancer Research*, **43**, 1101–1106.

Ramonas, L. M., Erickson, L. C., Klesse, W., Kohn, K. W. and Zaharko, D. S., 1981, Differential cytotoxicity and DNA cross-linking produced by polymeric and monomeric activated analogues of cyclophosphamide in mouse L1210 leukemia cells. *Molecular Pharmacology*, **19**, 331–336.

Redwood, W. R., Hilton, J., Colvin, M. and Owens, A. H., Jr., 1982, The cellular uptake of 4-hydroperoxycyclophosphamide. *Proceedings of the American Association for Cancer Research*, **23**, 169.

Rutenburg, A. M., Persky, L., Friedman, O. M. and Seligman, A. M., 1954, Toxicity in mice of new secondary nitrogen mustards. *Journal of Pharmacology and Experimental Therapeutics*, **111**, 483–488.

Schabel, F. M., Jr., Skipper, H. E., Trader, M. W., Laster, W. R., Jr., Griswold, D. P., Jr. and Corbett, T. H., 1983, Establishment of cross-resistance profiles for new agents. *Cancer Treatment Reports*, **67**, 905–922.

Schauenstein, E. and Esterbauer, H., 1979, Formation and properties of reactive aldehydes. In *Submolecular Biology in Cancer*. Ciba Foundation Symposium (Amsterdam: Excerpta Medica), Vol. 67, pp. 225–244.

Schmid, F. A., Otter, G. M. and Stock, C. C., 1980, Resistance patterns of Walker carcinosarcoma 256 and other rodent tumors to cyclophosphamide and 1-phenylalanine mustard. *Cancer Research*, **40**, 830–833.

Seligman, A. M., Nachlas, M. M., Manheimer, L. H., Friedman, O. M. and Wolf, G., 1949, Development of new methods for the histochemical demonstration of hydrolytic intracellular enzymes in a program of cancer research. *Annals of Surgery*, **130**, 333–341.

Sensenbrenner, L. L., Marini, J. J. and Colvin, M., 1979, Comparative effects of cyclophosphamide, isophosphamide, 4-methylcyclophosphamide, and phosphoramide mustard on murine hematopoietic and immunocompetent cells. *Journal of the National Cancer Institute*, **62**, 975–981.

Sharkis, S. J., Santos, G. W. and Colvin, M., 1980, Elimination of acute myelogenous leukemic cells from marrow and tumor suspensions in the rat with 4-hydroperoxycyclophosphamide. *Blood*, **55**, 521–523.

Short, R. D. and Gibson, J. E., 1971, Development of cyclophosphamide activation and its implications in perinatal toxicity to mice. *Toxicology and Applied Pharmacology*, **19**, 103–110.

Sladek, N. E., 1971, Metabolism of cyclophosphamide by rat hepatic microsomes. *Cancer Research*, **31**, 901–908.

Sladek, N. E., 1972 a, Therapeutic efficacy of cyclophosphamide as a function of its metabolism. *Cancer Research*, **32**, 535–542.

Sladek, N. E., 1972 b, Therapeutic efficacy of cyclophosphamide as a function of inhibition of its metabolism. *Cancer Research*, **32**, 1848–1854.

Sladek, N. E., 1973 a, Evidence for an aldehyde possessing alkylating activity as the primary metabolite of cyclophosphamide. *Cancer Research*, **33**, 651–658.

Sladek, N. E., 1973 b, Bioassay and relative cytotoxic potency of cyclophosphamide metabolites generated *in vitro* and *in vivo*. *Cancer Research*, **33**, 1150–1159.

Sladek, N. E., 1977 a, Potentiation of antitumor drug action by centrophenoxine: specificity. *Journal of Pharmacology and Experimental Therapeutics*, **201**, 518–526.

Sladek, N. E., 1977 b, Cytotoxic activity of alkylating agents in the presence of centrophenoxine and its hydrolysis products. *Journal of Pharmacology and Experimental therapeutics*, **203**, 630–639.

Sladek, N. E. and Landkamer, G. L., 1985, Restoration of sensitivity to oxazaphosphorines by inhibitors of aldehyde dehydrogenase activity in cultured oxazaphosphorine-resistant L1210 and cross-linking agent-resistant P388 cell lines. *Cancer Research*, **45**, 1549–1555.

Sladek, N. E., Priest, J., Doeden, D., Mirocha, C. J., Pathre, S. and Krivit, W., 1980, Plasma half-life and urinary excretion of cyclophosphamide in pediatric patients. *Cancer Treatment Reports*, **64**, 1061–1066.

Sladek, N. E., Smith, P. C., Bratt, P. M., Low, J. E., Powers, J. F., Borch, R. F. and Coveney, J. R., 1982, Influence of diuretics on urinary general base catalytic activity and cyclophosphamide-induced bladder toxicity. *Cancer Treatment Reports*, **66**, 1889–1900.

Sladek, N. E., Doeden, D., Powers, J. F. and Krivit, W., 1984 a, Plasma concentrations of 4-hydroxycyclophosphamide and phosphoramide mustard in patients repeatedly given high doses of cyclophosphamide in preparation for bone marrow transplantation. *Cancer Treatment Reports*, **68**, 1247–1254.

Sladek, N. E., Powers, J. F. and Grage, G., 1984 b, Half-life of oxazaphosphorines in biological fluids. *Drug Metabolism and Disposition*, **12**, 553–559.

Sladek, N. E., Low, J. E. and Landkamer, G. J., 1985, Collateral sensitivity to cross-linking agents exhibited by cultured L1210 cells resistant to oxazaphosphorines. *Cancer Research*, **45**, 625–629.

Smith, P. C. and Sladek, N. E., 1985, Sensitivity of murine B- and T-lymphocytes to oxazaphosphorine and non-oxazaphosphorine nitrogen mustards. *Biochemical Pharmacology*, **34**, 3459–3463.

Struck, R. F., 1974, Isolation and identification of a stabilized derivative of aldophosphamide, a major metabolite of cyclophosphamide. *Cancer Research*, **34**, 2933–2935.

Struck, R. F., 1976, Aldophosphamide; synthesis, characterization, and comparison with "Hohorst's aldophosphamide". *Cancer Treatment Reports*, **60**, 317–319.

Struck, R. F., Kirk, M. C., Mellett, L. B., El Dareer, S. and Hill, D. L., 1971, Urinary metabolites of the antitumour agent cyclophosphamide. *Molecular Pharmacology*, **7**, 519–529.

Struck, R. F., Kirk, M. C., Witt, M. H. and Laster, W. R. Jr., 1975, Isolation and mass spectral identification of blood metabolites of cyclophosphamide: evidence for phosphoramide mustard as the biologically active metabolite. *Biomedical Mass Spectrometry*, **2**, 46–52.

Struck, R. F., Trader, M. W., Dykes, D. J., Corbett, T. H. and Laster, W. R., Jr., 1979, Synthesis and antitumor evaluation of isophosphoramide mustard, the active metabolite of the clinical antitumor agent ifosfamide. In *Current Chemotherapy and Infectious Disease. Proceedings of the Eleventh Congress of Chemotherapy*, edited by J. D. Nelson and C. Grassi (Boston: American Society for Microbiology, pp. 1520–1522.

Struck, R. F., Dykes, D. J., Corbett, T. H., Suling, W. J. and Trader, M. W., 1983, Isophosphoramide mustard, a metabolite of ifosfamide with activity against murine tumours comparable to cyclophosphamide. *British Journal of Cancer*, **47**, 15–26.

Surya, Y. A., Rosenfeld, J. M. and Hillcoat, B. L., 1978, Cross-linking of DNA in L1210 cells and nuclei treated with cyclophosphamide and phosphoramide mustard. *Cancer Treatment Reports*, **62**, 23–29.

Takamizawa, A., Tochino, Y., Hamashima, Y. and Iwata, T., 1972, Studies on cyclophosphamide metabolites and their related compounds. *Chemical and Pharmaceutical Bulletin*, **20**, 1612–1616.

Takamizawa, A., Matsumoto, S., Iwata, T., Tochino, Y., Katagiri, K., Yamaguchi, K. and Shiratori, O., 1975, Studies on cyclophosphamide metabolites and their related compounds. Preparation of an active species of cyclophosphamide and related compounds. *Journal of Medicinal Chemistry*, **18**, 376–383.

Thomas, E. D., Storb, R., Clift, R. A., Fefer, A., Johnson, F. L., Neiman, P. E., Lerner, K. G., Glucksberg, H. and Buckner, C. D., 1975, Bone-marrow transplantation. *New England Journal of Medicine*, **292**, 832–843 and 895–902.

Torkelson, A. R., LaBudde, J. A. and Weikel, J. H., Jr., 1974, The metabolic fate of cyclophosphamide. *Drug Metabolism Reviews*, **3**, 131–165.

van der Steen, J., Timmer, E. C., Westra, J. G. and Benckhuysen, C., 1973, 4-Hydroperoxidation in the Fenton oxidation of the antitumor agent cyclophosphamide. *Journal of the American Chemical Society*, **95**, 7535–7536.

Voelcker, G., Wagner, T. and Hohorst, H. J., 1976, Identification and pharmacokinetics of cyclophosphamide (NSC 26271) metabolites in vivo. *Cancer Treatment Reports*, **60**, 415–422.

Völker, G., Dräger, U., Peter, G. and Hohorst, H. J., 1974, Studien zum Spontanzerfall von 4-Hydroxycyclophosphamid und 4-Hydroperoxycyclophosphamid mit Hilfe der Dünnschichtchromatographie, *Arzneimittel-Forschung, Drug Research*, **24**, 1172–1176.

Vu, V. T., Fenselau, C. C. and Colvin, O. M., 1981, Identification of three alkylated nucleotide adducts from the reaction of guanosine 5′-monophosphate with phosphoramide mustard. *Journal of the American Chemical Society*, **103**, 7362–7364.

Wagner, T. and Fenneberg, K., 1984, Bioavailability of cyclophosphamide from oral formulations. *European Journal of Clinical Pharmacology*, **26**, 269–270.

Wagner, T., Heydrich, D., Bartels, H. and Hohorst, H. J., 1980 a, Einfluß von Leberparenchymschäden, Niereninsuffizienz und Hämodialyse auf die Pharmakokinetik von Cyclophosphamid und seinen aktiviertem Metaboliten. *Arzneimittel-Forschung, Drug Research*, **30**, 1588–1592.

Wagner, T., Heydrich, D., Voelcker, G. and Hohorst, H. J., 1980 b, Über Blutspiegel und Urin-ausscheidung von aktiviertem Cyclophosphamid und seinen Deaktivierungsprodukten beim Menschen. *Journal of Cancer Research and Clinical Oncology*, **96**, 79–92.

Wagner, T., Heydrich, D., Jork, T., Voelcker, G. and Hohorst, H. J., 1981, Comparative study on human pharmacokinetics of activated ifosfamide and cyclophosphamide by a modified fluorometric test. *Journal of Cancer Research and Clinical Oncology*, **100**, 95–104.

Wampler, G. L., Regelson, W. and Bardos, T. J., 1978. Absence of cross-resistance to alkylating agents in cyclophosphamide-resistant L1210 leukemia. *European Journal of Cancer*, **14**, 977–982.

Wrabetz, E., Peter, G. and Hohorst, J. J., 1980, Does acrolein contribute to the cytotoxicity of cyclophosphamide? *Journal of Cancer Research and Clinical Oncology*, **98**, 119–126.

Zon, G., 1982, Cyclophosphamide analogues. *Progress in Medicinal Chemistry*, **19**, 205–246.

Zon, G., Ludeman, S. M., Brandt, J. A., Boyd, V. L., Ozkan, G., Egan, W. and Shao K-l., 1984, NMR spectroscopic studies of intermediary metabolites of cyclophosphamide. A comprehensive kinetic analysis of the interconversion of *cis*- and *trans*-4-hydroxycyclophosphamide with aldophosphamide and the concomitant partitioning of aldophosphamide between irreversible fragmentation and reversible conjugation pathways, *Journal of Medicinal Chemistry*, **27**, 466–485.

4. Purine and pyrimidine biochemistry, and some relevant clinical and preclinical cancer chemotherapy research

Daniel S. Martin

Introduction

Antimetabolites are compounds that interfere in either the biosynthesis, utilization or metabolic function of normal cellular metabolites. Often they are closely related in structure to the antagonized metabolites (Figure 1). To be successfully selective in the chemotherapy of tumours, an antimetabolite should adversely affect one or more vital metabolic reactions in the tumour without seriously endangering normal tissues. Unfortunately, there are quantitative, rather than qualitative, biochemical differences between normal and neoplastic tissues. Nevertheless, these quantitative differences can be utilized as a basis for chemotherapy, and antimetabolites that interfere with purine or pyrimidine metabolism can be important components in the combination (multi-drug) chemotherapy of cancer.

Effective therapy for cancer requires the administration of multiple drugs in combination to overcome the chemotherapeutic heterogeneity that is caused by the variable tumour cell biochemistry present within the neoplastic cell population of individual tumours (Baylin, 1982; Goldie, 1983; Heppner, 1984; Martin, 1958; Martin and Gelhorn, 1951). Chemotherapeutic heterogeneity was recognized 35 years ago as mandating the need for the combination chemotherapy of cancer over single-agent treatment (Martin, 1958; Martin and Gelhorn, 1951). Heterogeneity is the basic feature of cancer because genetic instability is inherent in malignant cells (Nowell, 1976; Schnipper, 1986). It is this genetic instability of cancer cells that leads to spontaneous mutations in clonogenic cells that results in the expression of biochemical heterogeneity. Since heterogeneity (which by definition cannot be exactly reproduced) must vary, there is a variable biochemical overlap between individual tumours, as well as among all types of mammalian neoplasms (Baylin, 1982); this, in turn, results in a variable chemotherapeutic correlation between types of cancer. Because of this chemotherapeutic heterogeneity, and the fact that a single active anti-cancer agent acts primarily against only its own drug-sensitive

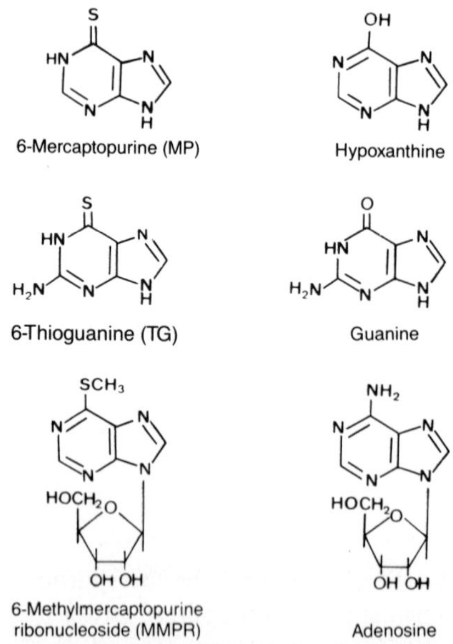

Figure 1. Structural differences between common purine antimetabolites and the related metabolite.

subset of the total neoplastic cell population of an individual tumour, multiple drugs are required for more effective therapy of the tumour's entire cell population.

Chemotherapeutic heterogeneity makes the therapeutic problem difficult, but cure of some types of cancer nevertheless can be attained by combination chemotherapy (Chabner *et al.*, 1984). Significant cure rates are now achievable in tumours of haematological and embryological origin (e.g., acute lymphocytic leukaemia, Hodgkin's disease, testicular cancer, choriocarcinoma), but cure of the more common advanced epithelial cancers (e.g., lung, breast, colon) has not been accomplished.

Selectivity is, of course, the key to all chemotherapy (Elion, 1985). However, selectivity is very difficult to achieve against cancer cells *in vivo* because the biochemical differences between cancer and normal cells are quantitative rather than qualitative. Consequently, anti-cancer agents have a narrow therapeutic index, and therefore combination chemotherapy is frequently toxic to the patient as well as to the tumour. In addition to this obstacle, and in addition to the large therapeutic problem(s) brought about by the different quantitative biochemical patterns present between the subsets of cancer cells within an individual tumour, there is the further difficulty that biochemical heterogeneity usually extends "quantitatively" *within* each subset of malignant cells. The latter condition means that a subset of cancer cells that is sensitive to a single anti-cancer agent possesses a gradient of responsiveness to that agent. Due to this gradient of sensitivity, and the *low* chemotherapeutic indices of anti-cancer agents, eradication of even slightly resistant cells of the drug-sensitive subset is impossible at the agent's *low in vivo-tolerated* dose. When this occurs, this component of the malignant population is untreated and can then grow to dominance as an apparently drug-resistant tumour. These cells are actually only pseudo-resistant, but under the described chemotherapeutic treatment conditions will appear unresponsive to chemotherapy and grow into a large tumour recurrence. This recurrence may then mutate into a new truly drug-resistant malignant cell population. To avoid this lethal eventuality, the use of new treatment strategies (e.g., biochemical modulation, as will be discussed in later sections) can be employed to create new intracellular biochemical conditions in the quasi-drug-resistant (but actually drug-sensitive) cells that then will permit their destruction by *in vivo* tolerated doses of the effector agent.

Drug resistance to antineoplastic agents is an important clinical problem. In classical "empirical" combination chemotherapy, simply adding more agents, each with single agent clinical activity directed at chemotherapeutically different subsets of cancer cells, will worsen "quantitative" drug resistance, since adding additional agents usually causes unacceptable toxicity that necessitates reducing the dose of the drugs in the combination. Quantitative biochemical differences in cells whose drug sensitivity is similar suggest that one approach to improving the selectivity of anti-cancer agents (as well as to circumvent the development of drug resistance) is to utilize selective biochemical modulation to increase the therapeutic activity of individual effector agents in a drug combination.

Improving a drug's selectivity through biochemical modulation requires an understanding of the drug's probable mechanism of action. A clinically useful anti-cancer drug that is a known antimetabolite provides the advantage that the drug has already proven itself at the clinical level, and that its competing metabolite's biochemical pathways are often understood, and therefore specific biochemical loci of potential action by the antimetabolite may be examined in experimental tumour models. The identification of specific critical loci may then provide the opportunity for improved selectivity through appropriate biochemical modulation. However, despite biochemical investigation and clinical use for almost 35 years of the purine antagonists 6-mercaptopurine (6-MP), 6-thioguanine (6-TG) and 6-methylmercaptopurine riboside (MMPR) (Burchenal *et al.*, 1953; Elion *et al.*, 1952), the *primary* biochemical determinant(s) of their activity are not agreed upon. The same may be said for the clinically utilized pyrimidine antagonists 5-fluorouracil (FUra) and cytosine arabinoside (Ara-C).

All of these antimetabolites are "pro-drugs" that become active only after conversion to the nucleotide level. The mode of action of these antimetabolites may be highly complex. In the case of the above thiopurines, they are anabolized to a multitude of inhibitors affecting all the principal branches of purine metabolism; indeed, at least 30 enzymes may be inhibited (Hitchings and Elion, 1972; Montgomery, 1970). This makes it difficult to establish the inhibitions that are most important for the anti-tumour effect. However, regardless of the specific critical loci of drug action, the anti-cancer effect depends ultimately on the amount and retention of the cytotoxic nucleotides in the target cancer cells. Thus preclinical studies have demonstrated that it is possible to increase the amount of a substrate (e.g., phosphoribosylpyrophosphate, or PRPP) that is obligatory for the optimal functioning of a pertinent anabolic enzyme (e.g., orotate phosphoribosyltransferase) in pyrimidine metabolism, and thereby to cause increased FUra activation (Martin *et al.*, 1983 b), and also that it is possible to utilize the "rescue principle" to shield normal cells at specific loci—e.g., uridine to differentially rescue (FUra)RNA in normal tissues (Klubes and Cerna, 1983; Klubes, *et al.*, 1982; Martin *et al.*, 1982; Sawyer *et al.*, 1984 b)—and thereby to improve selectivity and the therapeutic index. In clinical studies, the use of a metabolite, leucovorin, as a "rescue" agent following methotrexate treatment has led to the safe use of this antimetabolite in high doses and an improved therapeutic index for the use of this drug in some human cancers (Bertino, 1979).

It is the purpose of this chapter to present the biochemistry of certain purine and pyrimidine antimetabolites commonly used in the therapy of certain clinical cancers, along with some recent preclinical findings in experimental tumour models demonstrating the ability of biochemical modulation to improve the selectivity of these antimetabolites as anti-cancer agents.

Normal purine biosynthesis and salvage pathways

Figure 2 presents the *de novo* biosynthesis and salvage pathways of purine nucleotides in schematic outline. The pathway for *de novo* purine biosynthesis initially requires 5-phosphoribosylpyrophosphate (PRPP), and then goes through ten anabolic steps to form the parent purine compound, inosine 5′-monophosphate or inosinic acid (IMP). Synthesis of IMP requires the energy of four adenosine triphosphate (ATP) molecules and one PRPP molecule, as well as active folic acid methyl carriers, and the amino acids glutamine, glycine and aspartate. The purine nucleotide IMP then undergoes metabolic conversion to adenine and guanine nucleotides (AMP and GMP) which, after conversion to ribo- and deoxyribotriphosphates, are incorporated into nucleic acids.

In addition to the *de novo* pathway outlined for purines, Figure 2 also notes salvage pathways, or pathways that utilize intact purine bases which arise from cleavage of pre-existing nucleotides. There are two purine salvage phosphoribosyltransferase (PRTase) enzymes; one for adenine (APRTase), and another for hypoxanthine and guanine (HGPRTase), that convert purine bases to the corresponding ribonucleotide by reacting them with PRPP (e.g., the hypoxanthine to IMP salvage pathway, Figure 2).

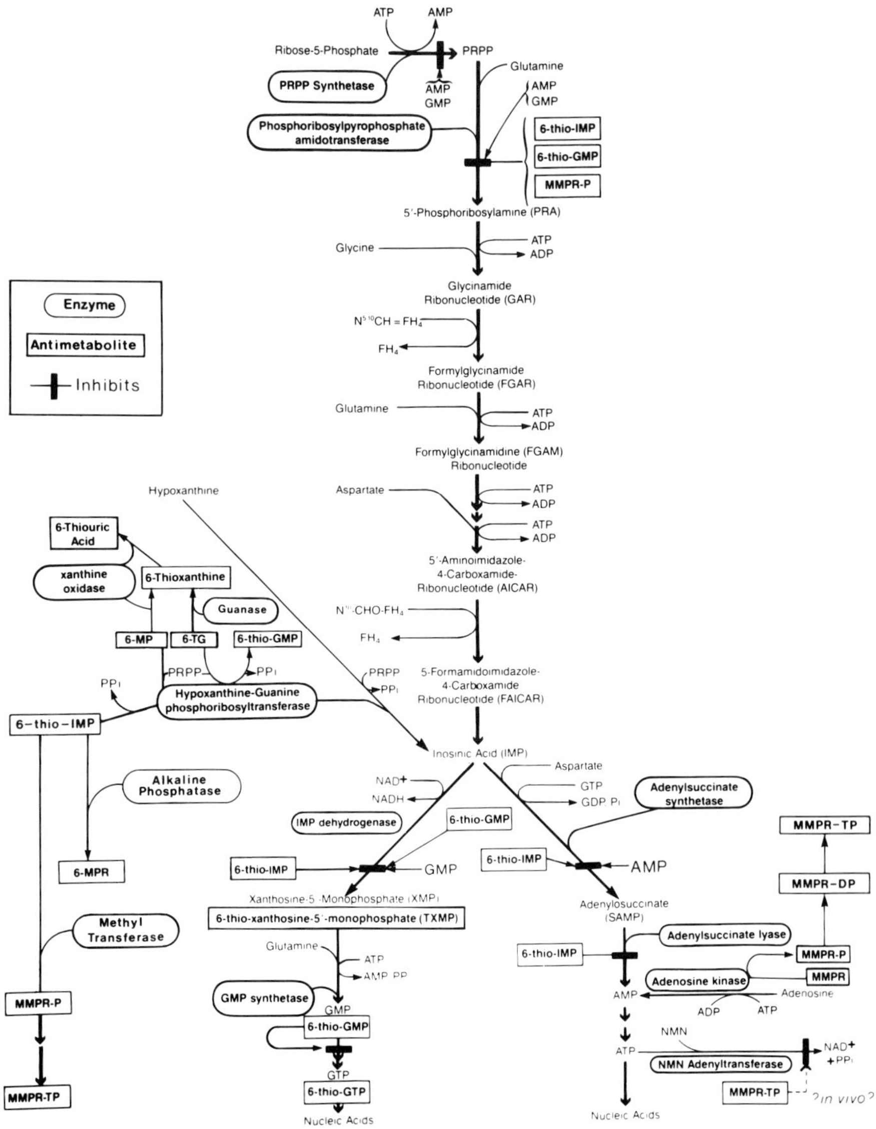

Figure 2. Purine *de novo* biosynthetic and salvage pathways. Inhibitory effects of some thiopurine antimetabolites.

Salvage formation of purine nucleotides may also occur by conversion of free bases to ribonucleosides (or deoxyribonucleosides) and subsequent phosphorylation to ribonucleotides (or deoxyribonucleotides). The first step is catalysed by nucleoside phosphorylase with base and ribose-(or desoxyribose)-1-phosphate as substrates. The second step is catalysed by a nucleoside kinase utilizing a ribonucleoside or deoxyribonucleoside triphosphate as a phosphate donor. Figure 2 outlines the enzymatic reaction of the adenine nucleoside, adenosine, with adenosine triphosphate (ATP) by adenosine kinase to yield adenylic acid, AMP, which undergoes subsequent phosphorylation to ATP and is then incorporated into nucleic acid.

PRPP is a critical substrate not only for purine biosynthesis, but also for pyrimidine and nicotinamide nucleotides (Fox and Kelly, 1971). Its synthesis is regulated in a complex manner by inorganic phosphate, ATP, magnesium, ribose-5-phosphate and end-product nucleotides (Crabtree and Henderson, 1971; Fox and Kelly, 1971; Henderson *et al.*, 1975; Hershko *et al.*, 1969; Planet and Fox, 1976). For example, PRPP synthetase is under "feedback" control by adenosine triphosphates (Atkinson and Fall, 1967; Fox and Kelly, 1971; Henderson *et al.*, 1975; Planet and Fox, 1976). In "copycat" fashion, the thiopurine nucleotide antimetabolite 6-(methylmercapto)purine ribonucleoside 5′-phosphate (MMPR-P) can inhibit PRPP synthetase when in high concentration (Planet and Fox, 1976; Yen and Becker, 1980), although not in all cell types (Henderson and Khoo, 1965; Paterson and Wang, 1970). If the inhibitor is a normally occurring purine nucleotide (e.g., AMP) it is said to act as a "feedback" inhibitor; if an analogue (e.g., MMPR-P), then a "pseudofeedback" inhibitor (McCollister *et al.*, 1964). Thus, the synthesis of purine nucleotides may be controlled by feedback and/or pseudofeedback inhibition at several sites: PRPP synthetase, PRPP amidotransferase, and at the distal branch points where IMP is converted to adenine and guanine nucleotides. AMP may inhibit the conversion of IMP into adenylosuccinate, and GMP the conversion of IMP into xanthosine-5′-monophosphate (Hershfield and Seegmiller, 1977).

The problem of understanding the biological activity of a purine antimetabolite is complicated by regulation of purine biosynthesis by feedback control of purine end products. These controls result from inhibition or activation of certain enzymes by specific purine nucleotides which modify the catalytic activity of the enzymes by combining with them at sites other than the catalytic sites. Figure 2 indicates the various sites of feedback inhibition; e.g., the earliest enzymatic step in the *de novo* pathway, phosphoribosylpyrophophate amido-transferase, by the purine nucleotide end products, AMP and GMP. Similarly, the thiopurine nucleotide anti-cancer agents 6-mercaptopurine, 6-thioguanine and MMPR can exert pseudofeedback inhibitory effects on this same enzyme, thus mimicking the effects of natural purine nucleotide modulators of purine biosynthesis.

Interaction of purine nucleotides with biosynthesis of pyrimidines

High intracellular concentrations of purine ribonucleotides can exert toxicity by inducing a depletion of pyrimidines, and the ensuing toxicity can be reversed by exogenous uridine (Bloch, 1974; Green and Chan, 1973; Ishii and

Green, 1973). These effects were attributed to interference by the purine nucleotide with the *de novo* biosynthesis of uridylate at the stage of phosphorylation of orotate (Ishii and Green, 1973). These *in vitro* studies utilized adenosine (but whether the findings were due to the inhibitory effect of an adenosine nucleotide on the activity of the PRPP-dependent enzyme OMP phosphoribosyltransferase, or to decreased availability of PRPP due to decreased synthesis of PRPP due to high levels of ATP, was not determined) (Green and Chan, 1973; Ishii and Green, 1973). Similar results were found with guanosine (Bloch, 1974) and presumably occurred because guanosine (presumably converted to its nucleotide) had been reported (Bresnick, 1962; Bresnick and Blatchford, 1964) to be a feedback inhibitor of aspartate transcarbamylase and dihydroorotase, enzymes involved in *de novo* pyrimidine synthesis. However, PRPP is necessary for pyrimidine biosynthesis, and purine nucleotides are known to be feedback inhibitors of PRPP synthetase (Fox and Kelly, 1971; Jackson *et al.*, 1980); also, an alternative or complementary explanation might be that the conversion of the purine nucleosides to nucleotides may deplete the cellular pool of inorganic phosphate which is an obligatory activator of PRPP synthetase (Crabtree and Henderson, 1971; Henderson *et al.*,1975; Hershko *et al.*, 1969; Planet and Fox, 1976).

Metabolic activation of the major purine anti-cancer agents is a requirement for their cytotoxic effects

The major purine anti-cancer drugs are thiopurines: 6-mercaptopurine (6-MP, an analogue of hypoxanthine), 6-thioguanine (6-TG, an analogue of guanine), and 6-methylmercaptopurine ribonucleoside (MMPR, an analogue of adenosine) (Figure 1). All three thiopurines are "pro-drugs" that become active only after intracellular conversion to the nucleotide level. Since these drugs have to be converted by intracellular metabolism to an active form, it cannot be assumed that the concentration of drug in the blood is the same as the concentration of drug at the subcellular target site (Powis, 1985). Thus their intracellular biochemical pharmacology is more important than their plasma pharmacokinetic data, for their anti-cancer effect depends ultimately on the amount and persistence of thiopurine nucleotides in the target cancer cells.

Both 6-MP and 6-TG are metabolically activated in drug-sensitive cells to a nucleotide via the PRPP-requiring enzyme, hypoxanthine-guanine phosphoribosyltransferase (HGPRTase). 6-MP, as an analogue of hypoxanthine, is anabolized to 6-thioinosinate (6-thio-IMP, or MPRP), and 6-TG, as a derivative of guanine, to 6-thioguanylate (6-thio-GMP). 6-Methylmercaptopurine riboside (MMPR), as an analogue of adenosine, is activated by adenosine kinase (utilizing ATP as the phosphate donor) to 6-methylthio-IMP (MMPR-P) (Figure 2).

Once the fraudulent purine nucleotides are formed, there are three general mechanisms by which they may cause cytotoxicity:

1. Appreciable concentrations of purine nucleotide analogues may act as pseudofeedback inhibitors, or allosteric inhibitors of metabolic processes in the biosynthesis of purines, their nucleotides, and their incorporation into nucleic acids.
2. As fraudulent purine nucleotides, they may successfully compete with normal purine nucleotides for enzymes that catalyse the normal anabolic steps or interconversions of normal purine nucleotides and form an inhibitory analogue–enzyme complex that prevents the synthesis of an essential intermediate.
3. They may be converted to nucleoside triphosphates and then be incorporated into the nucleic acids where they may cause damage as fraudulent nucleic acids.

Anabolism and multiple biochemical loci of action of 6-MP

The PRPP-dependent HGPRTase-derived 6-MP ribonucleotide, 6-thio-IMP or MPRP, is a pseudofeedback inhibitor of phosphoribosylpyrophosphate amidotransferase, the enzyme controlling the first reaction step unique to the *de novo* purine nucleotide pathway (Figure 2). This locus of inhibition may be primarily responsible for the cytotoxic activity *in vivo* of all three thiopurines (Bennett *et al.*, 1963; McCollister *et al.*, 1964). However, the importance of this pseudofeedback inhibition has been questioned by the observation of these effects in preclinical studies in *both* purinethiol-susceptible and -resistant tumours (Hitchings and Elion, 1972; LePage and Jones, 1961 a). Although 6-thio-ITP has been identified *in vitro* (Kawahata *et al.*, 1983) the formation of 6-thio-ITP *in vivo* has never been demonstrated (G.B. Elion, personal communication; Paterson and Tidd, 1975).

6-Thio-IMP inhibits, in addition to phosphoribosylpyrophosphate amidotransferase, a number of other enzymes. For example, the purine nucleotide interconversions (Figure 2): IMP dehydrogenase, the conversion of inosinic acid (IMP) to xanthosine 5′-monophosphate (XMP), a necessary step in the formation of guanosine-5′-monophosphate (GMP) (Atkinson *et al.*, 1963; Elion, 1975; Salser *et al.*, 1960); also, adenylsuccinate synthetase, the conversion of IMP to adenylosuccinate (SAMP) (Atkinson *et al.*, 1964; Salser *et al.*, 1960); and adenylosuccinate lyase, the conversion of adenylosuccinate to adenylic acid (AMP) (Atkinson *et al.*, 1964). However, inhibition of these interconversion steps of the purine ribonucleotides was either weak or absent in some 6-MP-sensitive murine tumours (Bennett *et al.*, 1963); these steps were therefore were not considered a primary site of 6-MP action.

Other enzymes inhibited by 6-thio-IMP include xanthine oxidase (Silberman and Wyngaarden, 1961), hypoxanthine–guanine phosphoribosyltransferase

(Atkinson and Murray, 1965), nicotinamide mononucleotide adenyltransferase (Atkinson *et al.*, 1961) and the exonuclease repair activity of DNA polymerase (Lee *et al.*, 1980). In addition, a possibly fraudulent NAD analogue of 6-MP, nicotinamide 6-mercaptopurine dinucleotide, has been reported (Atkinson *et al.*, 1962).

As indicated in Figure 2, in addition to being a competitive inhibitor of IMP dehydrogenase, 6-thio-IMP may also be its substrate and be oxidized to 6-thioxanthylate (TXMP) (Atkinson *et al.*, 1965), subsequently be metabolized by guanylate synthetase to 6-thioguanylate, 6-thio-GMP (Tidd and Paterson, 1974 a) and then be incorporated into DNA and RNA as the deoxy- or ribonucleotide derivative of 6-TG (Breter and Zahn, 1979; Elion, 1975; LePage and Jones, 1961 b; Nelson *et al.*, 1975; Tidd and Paterson, 1974 a, b; Zimm *et al.*, 1985). The metabolism of 6-MP to 6-TG deoxynucleotide and the subsequent incorporation into DNA, rather than the incorporation into RNA, is believed by some investigators (Nelson *et al.*, 1975; Tidd and Paterson, 1974 a,b) to be primarily responsible for the anti-cancer activity of 6-MP. Others (Elion, 1975) have been reluctant to accept this explanation because of the finding that a *greater* incorporation of 6-MP into DNA in the form of 6-TG nucleotide occurs in a 6-MP-resistant murine tumour than in a sensitive line (Bieber *et al.*, 1961; Scannel and Hitchings, 1966). However, incorporation into nucleic acids is not the final step in the action of 6-MP or 6-TG, and it has been suggested that this MP-resistant tumour may be a mutant in which the toxic effects of the DNA-incorporated analogue were suppressed in some manner (Tidd and Paterson, 1974 a). Although there is evidence that the incorporation of 6-TG nucleotides into DNA induces DNA strand breaks (Christie *et al.*, 1984), little is known about the functional properties of DNA-containing 6-TG analogues. The cytotoxic effect of 6-TG is delayed, and associated with a block in cell cycle progression in the G2 phase, which may be due to inhibition of RNA transcription or the production of defective RNAs (Wotring and Roti, 1980). The incorporation of 6-TG into all major species of RNA (Kwan *et al.*, 1973), inhibition of the maturation of rRNA in Novikoff hepatoma cells by 6-thioguanosine (Weiss and Pitot, 1974) and a (6-TG)RNA-induced decrease in enzyme activities of regenerating rat liver (Carrico and Sartorelli, 1977) have been reported. Thus, the incorporation of 6-MP into RNA in the form of 6-TG nucleotides may also contribute to 6-MP cytotoxicity. The formation of 6-thio-ITP *in vitro*, and inhibition of RNA transcription by 6-thio-ITP, has been reported as one of the mechanisms of the cytotoxic action of 6-MP in cultured human tumour cells (Kawahata *et al.*, 1983).

Studies on the primary mechanism of action of 6-MP are further complicated by the fact that its anabolic product, 6-thio-IMP, is metabolized by methylation to 6-methylmercaptopurine ribonucleotide (MMPR-P) (Remy, 1963) and subsequently to the MMPR triphosphate (Elion, 1975). MMPR-P, and its higher nucleotides, are formed slowly intracellularly, over 20 hours (Breter and Zahn, 1979; Elion, 1975; Zimmerman *et al.*, 1974). It is possible that MMPR-P may be the most important metabolic product of 6-MP because it is the most potent inhibitor of phosphoribosylpyrophosphate amidotransferase (Hill and Bennett, 1969) and therefore a powerful inhibitor of purine biosynthesis *de novo*.

Thus, the important ribonucleotides of 6-MP formed intracellularly include 6-thio-IMP, 6-thio-GMP and MMPR-P. Differences in the effects of 6-MP in various experimental systems may reflect differences in the proportion of 6-MP metabolites, as well as differences in the intrinsic sensitivities of their sites of action (Paterson and Tidd, 1975).

Anabolism and multiple biochemical loci of action of 6-TG

6-TG, like 6-MP, requires activation to the nucleotide level to exert cytotoxicity (Brockman, 1963). Also, like 6-MP and the natural purine bases hypoxanthine and guanine, 6-TG may be converted to its nucleotide, 6-thioguanylate (6-thio-GMP), by the PRPP-dependent enzyme, hypoxanthine-guanine phosphoribosyltransferase (Sartorelli *et al.*, 1958). Although 6-TG may be converted by a purine nucleoside phosphorylase to 6-thioguanosine, the kinase activity of a kinase which would convert the 6-thioguanosine to 6-thio-GMP appears to be, at best, minimal (Lee and Sartorelli, 1981). And, as indicated in Figure 2, 6-thio-GMP, like 6-thio-IMP, is a pseudofeedback inhibitor of phosphoribosylpyrophosphate amidotransferase, the first enzyme in the *de novo* purine biosynthetic pathway (Brockman, 1964; Hill and Bennett, 1969; LePage and Jones, 1961; McCollister *et al.*, 1964). As in the case of 6-thio-IMP, the importance of this inhibition of *de novo* purine synthesis in the inhibition of tumour growth is open to question, since these feedback effects were observed in both 6-TG-susceptible and -resistant tumours (LePage and Jones, 1961 a). A methylated metabolite of 6-TG, 6-methylthioguanylic acid, can inhibit phosphoribosylpyrophosphate amidotransferase, but it is not considered to contribute to the inhibition by TG of *de novo* purine biosynthesis (Allan and Bennett, 1971; Paterson and Tidd, 1975).

6-TG also can inhibit purine ribonucleotide interconversions. Like 6-thio-IMP, 6-thio-GMP can inhibit IMP dehydrogenase (Paterson and Tidd, 1975; Miech *et al.*, 1967). However, 6-thio-GMP also inhibits guanylate kinase (Miech *et al.*, 1969). Thus 6-TG can have a greater effect on GTP formation than ATP formation by lowering the formation of all purine nucleotides through its allosteric pseudofeedback effect on phosphoribosylpyrophosphate amidotransferase, along with inhibition of IMP dehydrogenase and guanylate kinase (Nelson and Parks, 1972). (The opposite—a greater effect on ATP formation than on GTP—may be found with 6-MP; Nelson and Parks, 1972; Scholar *et al.*, 1972). While 6-thio-GMP is a relatively poor substrate for guanylate kinase, it is phosphorylated by this enzyme to the di- and triphosphates (6-thio-GTP) and incorporated into both DNA and RNA (Carrico and

Sartorelli, 1977; Kwan *et al.*, 1973; LePage, 1960; LePage and Jones, 1961 b; Nelson *et al.*, 1975; Sartorelli *et al.*, 1958) (Figure 2). 6-TG has also had inhibitory effects on glycoprotein synthesis (Lazo *et al.*, 1977, 1979).

It was initially hypothesized that the incorporation of 6-TG into the nucleic acids, particularly DNA, is essential for its tumour inhibition (LePage, 1960). Although some early findings were not consistent with this hypothesis (Bieber *et al.*, 1961; Scannel and Hitchings, 1966), the more recent findings that DNA synthesis inhibitors may protect from the cytoxicity of 6-TG (Lee and Sartorelli, 1981; Nelson *et al.*, 1975), that inhibition of RNA synthesis did not protect from 6-TG toxicity (Nelson *et al.*, 1975), and that TG-induced specific chromosome deformation (Maybaum and Mandel, 1983 b) and DNA strand breaks (Christie *et al.*, 1984) correlate with 6-TG incorporation into DNA and cytotoxicity, offer support for the suggestion that incorporation of TG into DNA is the critical event. On the other hand, in a different cell line, incorporation of 6-TG into RNA may contribute to 6-TG toxicity, since methotrexate pretreatment of cells before 6-TG administration resulted in the suppression of 6-TG incorporation into DNA, with a large increase in both the rate of incorporation into RNA and cytotoxicity (Armstrong *et al.*, 1982). As noted earlier, there are a number of other reports indicating that the presence of 6-TG in RNA may contribute to toxicity (Carrico and Sartorelli, 1977; Kwan *et al.*, 1973; Weiss and Pitot, 1974; Wotring and Roti, 1980).

In general, 6-MP and 6-TG behave similarly in producing similar biochemical lesions, although there may be some quantitative differences from one cell line to another, and sometimes there may be clear differences in the apparent mechanisms of cytotoxicity in a single cell line (Maybaum *et al.*, 1985). Since the thiopurines produce multiple biochemical lesions which are interactive, it has been difficult to assign a primary mechanism of toxicity (e.g., inhibition of *de novo* purine biosynthesis, inhibition of purine nucleotide interconversion, and/or incorporation of TG into nucleic acids, or a reinforcing combination of all three of these mechanisms. Very recently, an additional anti-cancer mechanism—the induction of differentiation in cancer cells—has been suggested (Maybaum *et al.*, 1985).

A variety of compounds (hormones, vitamins, tumour promoters, anti-cancer agents, cryoprotective agents) promote the differentiation of various cell types in culture; indeed, the chemical structures and biological activities are so diverse that no unifiable concept on the underlying mechanisms of induction has been reached (Sartorelli, 1985). It is conceivable that some of the antineoplastic agents may exert their therapeutic effects through a mixture of cytodestructive and differentiation-inducing actions (Sartorelli, 1985). Among the chemotherapeutic agents, 6-TG has been shown to be a potent inducer of differentiation of both the Friend murine erythroleukaemia (Gusella and Housman, 1976) and HL-60 human acute promyelocytic leukaemia (Gallagher *et al.*, 1984; Ishiguro *et al.*, 1984) cell lines in culture which lack HGPRTase activity. Studies (Ishiguro *et al.*, 1984; Ishiguro and Sartorelli, 1985) have provided evidence that the free base 6-TG is the form of this drug that induces differentiation while the formation of 6-TG nucleotides leads to cytotoxicity and inhibits differentiation. The simultaneous administration of hypoxanthine prevents the cytoxicity and allows expression of the differentiation-inducing properties of HL-60 cells treated with 6-TG. Sartorelli (1985) has noted that, since it is probable that all cells in a malignant cell population will not have the capacity to respond to inducers of maturation to generate end-stage cells with no proliferative capacity, mixtures of agents appear necessary that would function through both differentiation and cytotoxic actions without mutual antagonism.

Anabolism and biochemical loci of action of MMPR

MMPR (6-methylmercaptopurine ribonucleoside) is considered an analogue of adenosine (Figure 1). Like 6-MP and 6-TG, MMPR requires activation to the nucleotide level to exert cytotoxicity, but unlike 6-MP and 6-TG, which are activated by the PRPP-dependent enzyme HGPRTase, MMPR is converted to its active nucleotide inhibitor, MMPR-P (the 5′-phosphate of 6-methylmercaptopurine ribonucleoside, or 6-methyl-thio-IMP), by the ATP-dependent enzyme adenosine kinase (Bennett *et al.*, 1965; Caldwell *et al.*, 1966; Shantz *et al.*,1973). MMPR-P may then be converted to the di- and triphosphates (Elion, 1975; Paterson and Tidd, 1975) (Figure 2), though these forms are generally present only in small amounts relative to the monophosphate.

MMPR-P is a strong inhibitor of the *de novo* pathway of purine synthesis (Henderson and Khoo, 1965) and is the most potent inhibitor of phosphoribosylpyrophosphate amidotransferase (Hill and Bennett, 1969; Tay *et al.*, 1969). The latter inhibition is believed to be its primary mechanism of action (Bennet *et al.*, 1965; Bennett and Adamson, 1970). However, all facets of the metabolism and inhibitory actions of MMPR may not be known. There is evidence that certain additional effects (e.g., inhibition of pyrimidine synthesis (Woods *et al.*, 1978); inhibition of PRPP synthetase (Planet and Fox, 1976; Yen and Becker, 1980); inhibition of IMP dehydrogenase (Shantz, *et al.*, 1972); inhibition of adenylosuccinate synthetase (Hershfield and Seegmiller, 1977) may be seen if high concentrations of the drug are employed. Perhaps the observed effects of the agent depend not only on the particular concentrations, but on the biological system used. For example, the mechanism for toxicity due to the related compound 6-MP may vary depending on the cell type studied, because the levels of incorporation of thioguanylate into the DNA varies markedly in different cell lines (Drake *et al.*, 1982; Maybaum *et al.*, 1985; Maybaum and Mandel, 1983). Thus, the differences in the effects of MMPR in various experimental systems may reflect differences in the amounts of anabolites (MMPR-P, di- and triphosphates) produced in the particular cell line, as well as differences in the intrinsic sensitivities of the enzymatic site(s) of action. The abovementioned additional potential inhibitory sites of MMPR activity may depend on the importance of the particular enzymic inhibition to the individual target cells, the concentration of the enzyme in the cells, the relative pool sizes of enzyme and metabolite and inhibitor, and on the binding affinities of the metabolite and inhibitor for the enzyme (Elion, 1967; Roy-Burman, 1970). Also, enzymes that may be affected *in vitro* by a very high concentration of MMPR may not be *in vivo* if the required high level of MMPR is not employed, or cannot be either achieved or tolerated *in vivo*. Since there is general agreement that the primary mechanism of action of MMPR is inhibition of phosphoribosylpyrophosphate amidotransferase, only this site of inhibition by MMPR is indicated in Figure 2.

It is of interest that methylation of the sulphur of 6-MP-ribonucleoside (MPR) to MMPR completely changes its substrate specificity for some of the enzymes of purine metabolism. Thus, unlike MPR, MMPR is not a substrate for nucleoside purine phosphorylase, and is a substrate for a nucleoside kinase (adenosine kinase) that does not act on MPR (Bennett *et al.*, 1965; Lee and Sartorelli, 1981 b). Further, although both compounds are potent pseudofeedback inhibitors of purine biosynthesis, the 6-methylthio-IMP of MMPR is a much more potent inhibitor of the PRPP-amidotransferase enzyme than the 6-thio-IMP of 6-MP (Hill and Bennett, 1969; Tay *et al.*, 1969), and can have inhibitory activity against both 6-MP-sensitive and 6-MP-resistant experimental tumours (Bennett *et al.*, 1965).

Biochemical modulation of purine metabolism by administration of MMPR before either 6-MP or 6-TG can augment their cytoxic activity (Scholar *et al.*, 1972). MMPR-P, by its inhibition of the purine *de novo* pathway, spares the utilization of PRPP required for the *de novo* synthesis of purine nucleotides. Increased PRPP supplies are then available for increased anabolism of the thiopurines, 6-MP and 6-TG, to their cytoxic nucleotides, 6-thio-IMP and 6-thio-GMP. In addition, the nucleotide of MMPR may protect 6-thiopurine nucleotides from catabolic dephosphorylation by alkaline phosphatase (Nelson and Parks, 1972), serving as an alternate substrate for this catabolic enzyme. And, although purine nucleoside phosphorylase (PNPase) can convert 6-TG to 6-thioguanosine (6-TGuo), 6-TGuo cannot proceed to 6-thio-GMP as the activity of 6-TGuo kinase is at best minimal (Lee and Sartorelli, 1981 b). Under these circumstances, this conversion of 6-TG to 6-TGuo could serve as a trap to limit the availability of 6-TG for conversion to 6-thio-GMP by HPRTase. However, *pre*incubation with MMPR blocks the efflux of this 6-TGuo and thereby affects the equilibrium of the PNPase reaction and reduces the intracellular accumulation of 6-TG as 6-TGuo because the rate of nucleoside formation is considerably reduced due to inhibition of the constant removal (efflux) of the nucleoside from the cell. Thus, MMPR enhances the formation of 6-thio-GMP, not only by increasing levels of PRPP and preventing its dephosphorylation, but also by making more 6-TG available for HPRTase conversion to 6-thio-GMP by preventing the trapping of 6-TG as

6-TGuo, which is otherwise destined to be largely lost from the cell (Lee and Sartorelli, 1981 b). It is of interest that the administration of MMPR before 6-TG conferred sensitivity to a tumour normally resistant to 6-TG (Nelson and Parks, 1972). Therapeutic synergism has been observed in various experimental tumour systems for combinations of MMPR before 6-TG, or before 6-MP (Nelson and Parks, 1972; Paterson and Morivaki, 1969; Paterson and Tidd, 1975; Paterson and Wang, 1970; Scholar *et al.*, 1972). At the clinical level, however, MMPR did not improve the 6-MP response rate in acute myelogenous leukaemia (Hewlett, 1979).

The toxicity of MMPR is associated with the general depletion of purine nucleotides resulting in growth inhibition and the inhibition of RNA and DNA synthesis (Bennett *et al.*, 1965; Warnick and Paterson, 1973; Woods *et al.*, 1978). However, resumption of DNA synthesis was found to be dependent on the return to normal of guanine nucleotide levels, but not of adenine nucleotide levels (Cohen and Sadie, 1983; Nguyen *et al.*, 1984). In these studies, the biological consequences of purine starvation appeared primarily mediated by the *depletion* of guanine nucleotides rather than that of either deoxyguanine triphosphates (dGTP) or adenine nucleotides; however, adenine starvation measurably contributed (i.e., was synergistic) to the overall toxicity of MMPR (Nguyen *et al.*, 1984). It was suggested that DNA synthesis inhibition appeared to result from the interruption of a process essential for DNA synthesis which uses either GTP or some nucleotide or cofactor, other than dGTP, which is derived from guanine ribonucleotides (Cohen and Sadie, 1983). In contrast, however, in other studies (Sidi *et al.*, 1985; Sidi and Mitchell, 1984), guanine ribonucleotide *accumulation* was found to be associated with inhibition of *de novo* purine biosynthesis, a moderate decline in adenine nucleotide pools, and inhibition of cellular proliferation. It should be noted that there is increasing evidence that guanine ribonucleotides may be important regulators of cell growth (Gilman, 1984; Hugles, 1984). It is also of interest that UTP pools were depressed in the face of GTP elevation (Sidi *et al.*, 1985), suggesting an additional inhibitory effect of GTP elevation on pyrimidine biosynthesis; however, the addition of uridine did not prevent growth inhibition, making it unlikely that pyrimidine starvation played a role in inhibiting cell growth (Sidi *et al.*, 1985).

Interaction of MMPR with pyrimidine biosynthesis

When guanosine nucleosides were shown to dramatically potentiate the *in vitro* anti-tumour effects of the adenosine analogue MMPR, a metabolic study indicated that the locus of action was an early step in purine biosynthesis, and therefore probably due to synergistic feedback inhibitory effects by the simultaneous binding of the phosphorylated guanosine, GMP, and MMPR-P to phosphoribosylpyrophosphate amidotransferase (Grindey *et al.*, 1976). (It had been shown previously that the enzyme has separate binding sites for purine ribonucleotides and that different types may act simultaneously upon the enzyme molecule (Caskey *et al.*, 1964).) Since hypoxanthine had previously been reported (Bennett and Adamson, 1970; Hershfield and Seegmiller, 1977; Shantz *et al.*, 1972) to reverse the cytotoxicity of MMPR, although not at very high concentrations of MMPR, hypoxanthine (in place of GR) was found to partially reverse the anti-tumour effects of MMPR (indicating that the site of synergistic interaction involved *de novo* purine biosynthesis); moreover, the further addition of uridine to hypoxanthine provided still higher protection, indicating that MMPR must also have an additional site(s) of action concerned with pyrimidine metabolism (Grindey *et al.*, 1976). Other studies (Woods *et al.*, 1978) also have demonstrated that high concentrations of MMPR as a single agent can reduce pyrimidine concentrations (in addition, of course, to lowering the level of purine nucleotides).

In studies *in vitro* (Thomas *et al.*, 1981) with a high concentration of the purine precursor aminoimidazole carboxamide ribonucleoside (AICAR; see Figure 2), growth inhibition was produced as a consequence of inhibition of the pyrimidine biosynthesis enzymes, orotate phosphoribosyltransferase-orotidylylic decarboxylase (OPRT-ODC), as evidenced by a depletion of UTP and CTP, accumulation of orotate, and reversal by uridine. The findings of concomitant reduction of intracellular PRPP and a large increase in the concentration of purine nucleotides were believed responsible (as a combination) for this inhibition of the OPRT-ODC (Thomas *et al.*, 1981). It is known that the activity of the OPRT-ODC complex can be inhibited by purine nucleotides (Traut and Jones, 1977). Also, PRPP is an obligatory substrate in *de novo* pyrimidine synthesis, and as noted in several reports (Planet and Fox 1976; Yen and Becker, 1980), MMPR-P can inhibit PRPP synthetase when in high concentration, although not in all cell types (Henderson and Khoo, 1965; Paterson and Wang, 1970). The potency of a feedback effector and the relative intensity of the inhibition seem to depend on the tissue of origin of the enzyme (Grindey *et al.*, 1976).

Resistance to the major thiopurines

Resistance to 6-MP and 6-TG in cultured murine tumour cells has been associated with markedly decreased levels of HGPRTase (Brockman, 1963), the enzyme which activates them to their cytotoxic nucleotides. A deficiency of adenosine kinase, which activates MMPR, has also been found in some MMPR-resistant cell lines (Bennett *et al.*, 1966).

However, *in vitro* mechanisms of resistance do not necessarily parallel *in vivo* findings. Study of HPRTase activity in 6-MP-sensitive and -resistant human leukaemias showed that decreased enzyme activity occurred only in one of fifteen resistant leukaemias (Davidson and Winter, 1964). Therefore, the lack of HPRTase as a basis for resistance in human leukaemic cells *in vivo* appears to be rare (Rosman and Williams, 1973).

Resistance to 6-thiopurines in preclinical studies also has been associated with an elevation in the activity of a membrane-bound alkaline phosphatase that involves an increased rate of degradation of the active mononucleotides to inactive 6-thioinosine and inorganic phosphate (Lee *et al.*, 1978, 1980; Wolpert *et al.*, 1971). In leukaemia patients, a similar correlation between increases in alkaline phosphatase activity and 6-thiopurine resistance has been reported (Rosman *et al.*, 1974; Scholar and Calabresi, 1979).

Resistance to 6-TG also may be contributed to by higher intracellular purine nucleoside phosphorylase activity, which can convert a portion of the 6-TG to 6-thioguanosine that is destined to be largely lost from the cell. 6-TG levels are thereby diminished and unavailable for conversion by HPRTase to the cytotoxic nucleotide of 6-TG (Lee and Sartorelli, 1981).

A decrease in the intracellular levels of PRPP, and an alteration in the properties of PRPP amidotransferase which included significant loss of sensitivity to feedback inhibition by 6-thio-GMP, also has been reported as a mechanism for 6-TG resistance (Ishiguro and Sartorelli, 1984). Decreased feedback inhibition of an altered PRPP amidotransferase by MMPR nucleotide also has been reported for a MMPR-resistant cell line (Henderson *et al.*, 1967).

Catabolism of thiopurines

6-MP is oxidized to 6-thioxanthine and then to 6-thiouric acid by xanthine oxidase, and eliminated in the urine (Figure 2); sulphate is also a primary excretion product (Montgomery, 1970). The concurrent administration of 6-MP and allopurinol, a potent inhibitor of xanthine oxidase, diminishes 6-MP's catabolism and potentiates its toxicity (Elion *et al.*, 1963). Allopurinol does not alter the therapeutic index of 6-MP, but a substantial dose reduction (75%) is recommended for patients receiving both 6-MP and allopurinol (Calabresi and Parks, 1985).

6-TG is deaminated by the enzyme guanase to 6-thioxanthine, and then oxidized by xanthine oxidase to 6-thiouric acid (Figure 2). After methylation of the sulphur substituent, there is oxidation with elimination of the sulphate (Roy-Burman, 1970). Although 6-TG is catabolized by xanthine oxidase, dosage reductions are not necessary if allopurinol is given concomitantly. The reason is that, in order for 6-TG to be a substrate for xanthine oxidase, it must first be converted to 6-thioxanthine, which is an inactive compound and therefore does not contribute to 6-TG toxicity.

MMPR, in man, is quickly taken up by blood cells, particularly erythrocytes, and completely transformed to the nucleotide which persists intracellularly for a long time; accordingly, its urinary excretion is slow and sustained (Loo *et al.*, 1969).

Clinical use of thiopurines

The principal clinical role for 6-MP is in maintenance therapy in acute lymphoblastic leukaemia. The major role for 6-TG is in combination chemotherapy regimens for the induction and maintenance of remission in acute non-lymphocytic leukaemias. Both drugs are usually administered p.o. in tablet form, and an i.v. preparation of 6-TG is available. Details of the clinical use of these two thiopurines may be obtained in any of the current textbooks of oncology. In leukaemias, these two thiopurines are useful agents. Their major toxicity is myelosuppression, although there is also gastrointestinal toxicity, liver dysfunction and occasional hepatic necrosis.

MMPR has not exhibited any appreciable activity against acute myelocytic leukaemia. Its clinical toxicities are primarily mucositis with occasional myelosuppression and gastrointestinal toxicity (Freireich *et al.*, 1967; Luce *et al.*, 1967).

These three thiopurines have received limited clinical trials as single agents against solid tumours because very little therapeutic activity has been discerned, and there is some toxicity (Britell *et al.*, 1981; Esterhay *et al.*, 1978; Konits *et al.*, 1982; Pandya *et al.*, 1980; Presant *et al.*, 1980; Regelson *et al.*, 1967).

The indication for biochemical modulation of thiopurines

Although the thiopurines are considered effective anti-cancer agents in human leukaemias, the therapeutic results leave much room for improvement. In acute myeloid leukaemia, the predominant type of leukaemia in adults, complete remission is achieved in only two thirds of cases, and combination chemotherapy (including a thiopurine) cures only 15–20% (Freireich, 1986).

In contrast, in human solid tumours, the apparent failure of thiopurines to effect a discernible response may be more apparent than real. In the laboratory, the thiopurines are active against advanced solid tumours because the criteria of response include inhibition of tumour growth, a criterion not employed clinically; in the clinic, even complete cessation of growth (i.e., "stable disease") is not considered indicative of drug activity. In the laboratory, combination chemotherapy with a thiopurine can effect solid tumour regression. However, in solid tumours in patients, the thiopurines were evaluated only as single agents, and largely in patients who had been heavily pretreated with combination chemotherapy (Britell *et al.*, 1981; Esterhay *et al.*, 1978; Konits *et al.*, 1982; Pandya *et al.*, 1980; Presant *et al.*, 1980; Regelson *et al.*, 1967).

It seems clear that in the human leukaemias it is necessary to extend the therapeutic efficacy of present chemotherapy (Freireich, 1986). In human solid tumours such as colon carcinoma, there is the possibility that thiopurines have a degree of anti-cancer activity—e.g., 33%, 40% and 55% "stable disease" (Britell *et al.*, 1981; Konits *et al.*, 1982; Presant *et al.*, 1980), respectively, along with a 24% partial response rate (Presant *et al.*, 1980)—that might be expanded to a discernible tumour regression rate by the appropriate application of biochemical modulation. This approach is feasible because so much is known about the biochemical loci of action of the thiopurines.

Although there are some differences between the three major thiopurines, in general they have overlapping mechanisms of action and similar therapeutic effects (Maybaum, *et al.*, 1985; Maybaum and Mandel, 1983). And since our research group had previous positive experience with MMPR (Martin *et al.*, 1980, 1981) on a difficult-to-treat murine spontaneous mammary carcinoma (Martin *et al.*, 1975; Stolfi *et al.*, 1971), we selected MMPR as the thiopurine to manipulate with biochemical modulation.

The rationale for biochemical modulation of MMPR

The anti-tumour toxicity of MMPR is known to be associated with the general depletion of purine nucleotides resulting in the inhibition of macromolecular synthesis and tumour growth (Bennett *et al.*, 1965; Nelson and Parks, 1972; Scholar *et al.*, 1972; Warnick and Paterson, 1973; Woods *et al.*, 1978). The thiopurine-induced decrease in ATP levels, along with the overall decrease in the total adenine nucleotides of the cell, has previously been considered as a mechanism having an adverse effect on cellular energy metabolism due to a decrease in the adenylate energy charge of the tumour cell (Atkinson, 1969; Scholar *et al.*, 1972). It was noted that the metabolic consequences of decreases in the concentrations of adenine nucleotides might be reflected in decreases in a number of key enzymic reactions for which these nucleotides serve as substrates, and particularly since a number of important enzymes in energy metabolism appear to be regulated by the adenylate charge of the cell (Atkinson, 1969). If so, a possible way to biochemically modulate the MMPR-induced lowering of the adenylate energy charge of the tumour cell would be to interfere with high-energy phosphate generation, and thereby further decrease the rate of synthesis of high-energy phosphate bonds relative to their consumption.

Oxidative phosphorylation, the major source of ATP in mammals, is the process in which ATP is formed as electrons are transferred from NADH (or $FADH_2$) to O_2 by a series of electron carriers. Oxidation and phosphorylation are coupled processes. Fraudulent NAD-dependent dehydrogenases are incapable of undergoing normal oxidation reactions (Dietrich, 1975; Dietrich *et al.*, 1958 a,b); if oxidative phosphorylation does not occur, the result is impaired ATP synthesis, and ATP is then consumed faster than it is regenerated. Since the concentration of NAD-dependent enzymes in neoplastic tissue is lower than in normal tissues (Glock and McLean, 1957; Jediken and Weinhouse, 1955; Martin *et al.*,1957; Morton, 1958), it should be possible to inhibit more selectively these enzymes present in cancer tissue in small amounts, while producing much less inactivation of the same enzymes in normal tissues containing larger amounts (Ackerman and Potter, 1949). Moreover, metabolic antagonists do not antagonize all systems dependent on the metabolite to the same degree, and a particular antagonist could be more selective in inhibiting the same enzyme in the tumour tissue than in normal tissue (Dietrich *et al.*, 1958 b; Martin *et al.*, 1957). Thus, in *in vivo* studies with a solid experimental tumour (Dietrich *et al.*, 1958; Martin *et al.*, 1957), we previously demonstrated that a potent nicotinamide antagonist, 6-aminonicotinamide (6-AN) (Johnson and McColl, 1955), preferentially inhibited in tumour tissue certain NAD-dependent enzymes (α-ketoglutarate dehydrogenase, 3-phosphoglyceraldehyde dehydrogenase and β-hydroxybutyrate dehydrogenase) which function in the citric acid cycle, glycolytic and fatty acid metabolic pathways to generate ATP by oxidative phosphorylation. We also found that this *in vivo* 6-AN treatment resulted in markedly lower ATP and ADP levels with a large increase in the concentration of AMP, and effective anti-tumour activity (Dietrich *et al.*, 1958 b; Martin *et al.*, 1957). More recently (Hunting *et al.*, 1985), 6-AN was reported to be a potent inhibitor of tumour growth *in vitro*, accompanied by a depletion of purine and pyrimidine nucleotides and NAD, as well as a reduction in the ATP to ADP ratio that suggested energy deprivation in the treated tumour cells. The depleted ATP levels might slow down the formation of pyrimidine di- and triphosphates at the kinase step, but still another inhibition of *de novo* pyrimidine biosynthesis might occur at the dihydroorotate to orotate conversion, an NAD-requiring dehydrogenase step (Figure 3). Further, 6-AN may interfere with *de novo* purine synthesis by inhibiting IMP dehydrogenase, another NAD-dependent enzyme (Figure 2).

Since MMPR, as a single agent in high dosage, can decrease pyrimidine ribonucleotide concentrations (Grindey *et al.*, 1976; Woods *et al.*, 1978) and since a pyrimidine antagonist, PALA, as a single agent in low dosage, can selectively lower pyrimidine levels in certain tumours (Martin *et al.*, 1983 a), it seems reasonable that low-dose PALA added to MMPR therapy could reinforce MMPR's inhibition of pyrimidine synthesis.

Thus, the three drugs—PALA + MMPR + 6AN—might be expected to produce synergistic inhibition of *de novo* nucleic acid precursor synthesis not possible with any pair of them.

Results of preclinical studies with PALA + MMPR + 6-AN

On the basis of the rationale outlined above, the triple combination of PALA + MMPR + 6-AN was evaluated in mice bearing advanced solid tumours, and striking tumour regression rates were demonstrated against large, well-established murine mammary carcinomas.

Table 1. Combination therapy with *N*-(phosphonacetyl)-L-aspartate (PALA) + 6-aminonicotinamide (6-AN) + 6-methyl mercaptopurine riboside (MMPR)

Treatment†		% of PR‡	Percent body weight change	Dead/ total
1.	Saline	0/29	+17	4/29
2.	$MMPR_{175}$	0/30	−3	0/30
3.	$6\text{-}AN_{25}$	0/30	−25	5/30
4. $PALA_{100}$ $\xrightarrow{18\ h}$	$6\text{-}AN_{10}$	0/30	−3	10/30
5. $PALA_{100}$ $\xrightarrow{18\ h}$	$MMPR_{150}$	2/28(7)%	−14	2/28
6.	$6\text{-}AN_{10}$ + $MMPR_{150}$	5/29(17%)	−11	0/29
7. $PALA_{100}$ $\xrightarrow{18\ h}$	$6\text{-}AN_{10}$ + $MMPR_{150}$	17/28(61%)	−22	0/28

Pooled data from three experiments in first-generation CD8F1 advanced breast tumours (Experiments 1164, 1170, 1171) averaging 150 mg when therapy was initiated.
† Three courses of the indicated treatment were administered with a one-week interval between courses. Subscripts are doses in mg/kg. Observations five days after third course of treatment.
‡ PR = partial tumour regression (≥50% of initial tumour size).

Table 1 records pooled data from three experiments with CD8F1 mice bearing CD8F1 mammary tumour first generation transplants. The tumours were advanced, averaging 150 mg when treatment was initiated. The important therapeutic endpoint is in the percent partial regressions (PR) of the treated tumours. Neither the maximum tolerated dose (MTD) of MMPR alone (group 2), nor 6-AN alone (group 3) nor the double combination of PALA and 6-AN (group 4), produced any partial regressions (although tumour growth was inhibited in each group compared to the saline-treated controls, group 1). The double combination of PALA and MMPR (group 5), and that of 6-AN and MMPR (group 6), produced relatively minor objective response rates, 7% and 17% PR rates, respectively. In marked contrast the triple combination of PALA + 6-AN + MMPR effected an impressive 61% PR rate, without mortality and with only moderate body weight loss.

It is of interest that none of the single agents and none of the double combinations evidence a tumour regression rate that would be considered "active" in the clinic. By clinical criteria of activity (i.e., the need to demonstrate at least 20% PR rate to be considered an "active" agent), these single agents would be dropped (tumour growth inhibition, even if complete, is not a clinical criterion of activity), and would not be put into combination chemotherapy trial. And in the unlikely event that pairs of the apparently "clinically negative" compounds were evaluated as a double combination, a minor objective response rate (e.g., 7% and 17% as in these experiments) would probably preclude clinical trial of the triple combination, which produced in the experimental findings the dramatic 61% PR rate. The experimental data suggest that a combination of agents with apparent "modulatory" interrelationships, and with preclinical evidence of the capability to induce tumour regressions *in vivo*, should receive clinical evaluation in the full combination that induced the tumour regressions.

Preliminary biochemical studies with PALA + MMPR + 6-AN

Table 2 records *preliminary* data on the effect of this highly active triple combination of nucleotide pools in advanced CD8F1 breast tumours. Note that the ribonucleoside triphosphates of purines and pyrimidines are substantially depressed. In particular, the lowering of ATP, when viewed as the ratio of ATP/ADP (57% of control) suggests energy deprivation in the treated tumour cells. An ATP/ADP ratio of less than 75% of control is considered indicative of impaired energy metabolism (Hunting *et al.*, 1985). Similar results were found with very high doses *in vitro* of 6-AN alone in L1210 leukaemia cells (Hunting *et al.*, 1985).

It should be noted that the biochemical rationale(s) for combining PALA plus MMPR and MMPR plus 6-AN are still only hypotheses. To summarize the biochemical rationale, MMPR is administered in high dosage to decrease both purine and pyrimidine *de novo* synthesis. PALA reinforces the block on *de novo* pyrimidine synthesis, and 6-AN may contribute the depletion of ATP (by preventing the generation of ATP via glycolytic and citric acid cycle pathways). This literature-derived hypothesis as explanation for presumed biochemical modulation of cellular energy requires further evaluation *in vivo* in the tumour–host system. The *in vivo* effect of 6-AN, MMPR and PALA, alone and in double and triple combination, at various time points on the reductions of the ATP level and the interactions with purine and pyrimidine synthesis, as well as the nucleotide levels of the tumour and various host normal tissues (e.g., brain, bone marrow, liver and intestine) need to be

Table 2 Effect of PALA + MMPR + 6-AN on CD8F1 tumour nucleotide pools.

	μg Nucleotide per mg tumour protein					
	NAD	ATP	UTP	CTP	GTP	ATP/ADP†
Saline	2·41 ± 0·15	7·10 ± 0·32	2·24 ± 0·13	0·68 ± 0·05	2·73 ± 0·24	2·1
PALA + MMPR + 6-AN						
24 h‡	2·60 ± 0·25	4·16 ± 0·31	1·27 ± 0·06	0·42 ± 0·02	1·61 ± 0·03	1·3
48 h	1·42 ± 0·35	0·89 ± 0·14	0·32 ± 0·10	0·09 ± 0·02	0·36 ± 0·13	1·2

† The ratio of ATP to ADP, a measure of energy charge in the cell.

‡ Tumour-bearing CD8F1 mice received either saline or PALA (100 mg/kg) followed 18 h later by MMPR (150 mg/kg) and 6-AN (10 mg/kg). Animals were sacrificed either 24 h or 48 h after the MMPR plus 6-AN injections. Perchloric acid extracts were prepared from tumours and the nucleotides were quantitated by HPLC.

documented. However, at the time of writing, the therapeutic results—striking regression rates of advanced, large murine solid carcinomas (Table 1)—are impressive anti-tumour effects upon which to build further. For example, the addition of FUra to this combination may provide additional therapeutic gain since both PALA and MMPR have been shown to be useful modulators of FUra (Martin *et al.*, 1980, 1981, 1983 a). And the addition of an alkylating agent may be potentiated by 6-AN due to the latter agent's inhibition of DNA repair (Berger *et al.*, 1982; Hunting *et al.*, 1985).

"Rescue" to facilitate more effective combination chemotherapy

To add additional agents to this combination, it will be desirable (and, probably, necessary) to control or ameliorate host toxicity while retaining the selectivity of anti-tumour action. The tool of "delayed rescue" to differentially rescue the host by the sequential administration of metabolites following antimetabolite therapy has been used successfully for high-dose FUra (i.e., uridine; Martin *et al.*, 1983 b), and for high dose MTX (i.e., leucovorin; (Bertino, 1981; Martin *et al.*, 1983 b). Clinically, one benefit of high-dose MTX, and perhaps the most important advantage of using LV rescue, is the relative lack of toxicity of MTX (Bertino, 1981). It is possible under the protection of appropriate rescue to give much higher doses of the anti-tumour agent with resultant greater therapeutic activity (Martin *et al.*, 1982, 1983 b). The importance of drug dose and intensity in determining tumour response to chemotherapy has been well stressed (Frei and Cannelos, 1980; Hryniuk, 1986; Hryniuk and Bush, 1984). Thus, "delayed rescue" of host toxicity with nicotinamide (for 6-AN), purine nucleosides or bases (for MMPR), and uridine (for PALA), might provide further improvement of the therapeutic index of this triple combination, as well as an opportunity for the safe addition of other anti-cancer drugs. Accordingly, we have begun such delayed rescue trials of the PALA + MMPR + 6-AN combination at the preclinical level.

Nicotinamide antagonists as anti-cancer agents

Another nicotinamide antagonist, 2-ethylamino-1,3,4-thiadiazole (A-TDA), also with recognized preclinical anti-tumour properties for some 30 years and with toxicity that is also controllable by nicotinamide, has just received a clinical phase I–II evaluation that is reported as promising (Stewart *et al.*, 1986). Moreover, these investigators have stated, "It may be anticipated that other compounds with the same mechanism of action may prove to have useful activity in patients with cancer". 6-AN certainly fits into this category. It is clear that there are qualitative differences between the action of these nicotinamide antagonists. For example, even at toxic doses, 6-AN (unlike

A-TDA) has no uricogenic properties in man, and 6-AN surprisingly can reverse the preclinical tumour-inhibitory effect of A-TDA (Krakoff and Balis, 1959; Oettgen *et al.*, 1960). And, very recently, new analogues of nicotinamide with interesting anti-tumour effects have been reported (Grassetti, 1986). Nicotinamide antagonists merit attention as anti-cancer agents with clinical potential.

Normal pyrimidine biosynthesis and salvage pathways

The pyrimidine deoxyribonucleoside triphosphates (dCTP, dTTP) and ribonucleoside triphosphates (UTP, CTP) are utilized for DNA and RNA synthesis, respectively. Thus, the four major pyrimidine nucleotides share equally with the four major purine nucleotides (as DNA and RNA) in the expression of genetic information. Figure 3 presents some pyrimidine molecular structures. The pyrimidine nucleotides, although quantitatively less important than the purine nucleoside triphosphates, also participate in the transfer of energy, as well as in the biosynthesis of a number of important biological compounds (e.g., UDP-glucose, UDP-galactose, UDP-glucuronate, UDP-xylose, UDP-*N*-acetylmuramyl-pentapeptide, CDP-choline, TDP-rhamnose, polyglycan, glycoproteins and phospholipids).

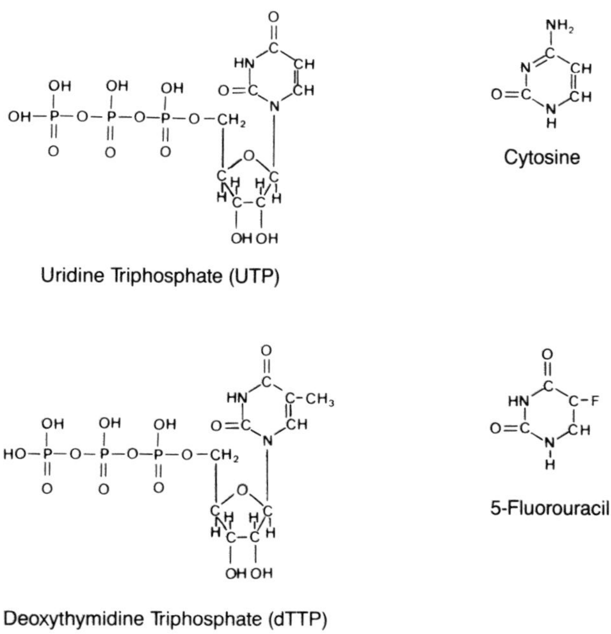

Figure 3. Major pyrimidines and 5-fluorouracil.

De novo synthesis of pyrimidines proceeds from simple compounds (HCO_3^-, glutamine and ATP) through six enzymatic steps to uridine monophosphate, or UMP (Figure 4; lower left half). UMP is the common product of both the *de novo* pathway of pyrimidine biosynthesis and of the reutilization of preformed uridine or uracil on the salvage pathways (Figure 4).

The first three enzymes in *de novo* pyrimidine biosynthesis are linked in a trifunctional complex, which contains glutamine-dependent carbamoyl-phosphate synthetase (CPS II), aspartate transcarbamylase (ATCase), and dihydro-orotase (Mally *et al.*, 1980). ATCase incorporates aspartic acid (ASP) into the pyrimidine ring as its amino acid backbone (in contrast to the glycine nucleus of the purine ring; Figure 2). The fourth enzyme, dihydroorotate (DHO) oxidase or dehydrogenase, requires the cofactor, NAD^+. A protein controlling synthesis of UMP from orotate is composed of the 5th and 6th enzymes, orotate phosphoribosyltransferase (OPRTase) and orotidine-5′-phosphate decarboxylase (OMP decarboxylase). OPRTase requires phosphoribosylpyrophosphate (PRPP) to convert orotate to OMP. The initial enzyme of the *de novo* pathway, CPS II is activated by PRPP, and is under allosteric negative feedback control by the endproduct of the pathway, UTP (Keppler *et al.*, 1970; Mally *et al.*, 1980; Roy-Burman, 1970).

The level of activity of OPRTase is dependent on the availability of PRPP in the regulation of *de novo* pyrimidine biosynthesis. For example, orotate accumulates in cultures of mammalian cells to which small amounts of adenine have been added, and the toxic effects of adenine may be removed by supplementation of cells with uridine, showing that the toxicity is caused by pyrimidine starvation (Ishii and Green, 1973).

In addition to the *de novo* pathways, "salvage" or "reutilization" pathways exist which utilize nucleosides and free bases arising from prior cleavage of nucleotides or exogenously supplied pyrimidines (Figure 4). Uracil may be converted directly to UMP by the enzyme uracil phosphoribosyltransferase and PRPP. Cytosine and thymidine are not anabolized by similar reactions. However, all four pyrimidine bases may be converted to their nucleotides by first being converted to nucleosides. This first step is catalysed by nucleoside phosphorylase (which under appropriate conditions can also cleave the nucleoside back to the pyrimidine base and deoxy-(dR-1-P) or ribose-(R-1-P) sugar), and the second step (to the nucleotide) by a kinase. Thus uridine phosphorylase catalyses reversibly the reaction between uracil and ribose-1-phosphate to form uridine (UR) and inorganic phosphates, followed by uridine kinase catalysing the conversion of uridine to uridine-5′-monophosphate (UMP).

The conversion of uridine to UMP is rate-limiting, and sensitive to feedback inhibition by uridine triphosphates (UTP) and cytidine triphosphates (CTP). The phosphorylation of cytidine by kinase is also feedback-inhibited by UTP and CTP, and that of thymidine by deoxythymidine triphosphate (dTTP) and deoxycytidine triphosphate (dCTP) (Anderson and Brockman, 1964; Bresnick

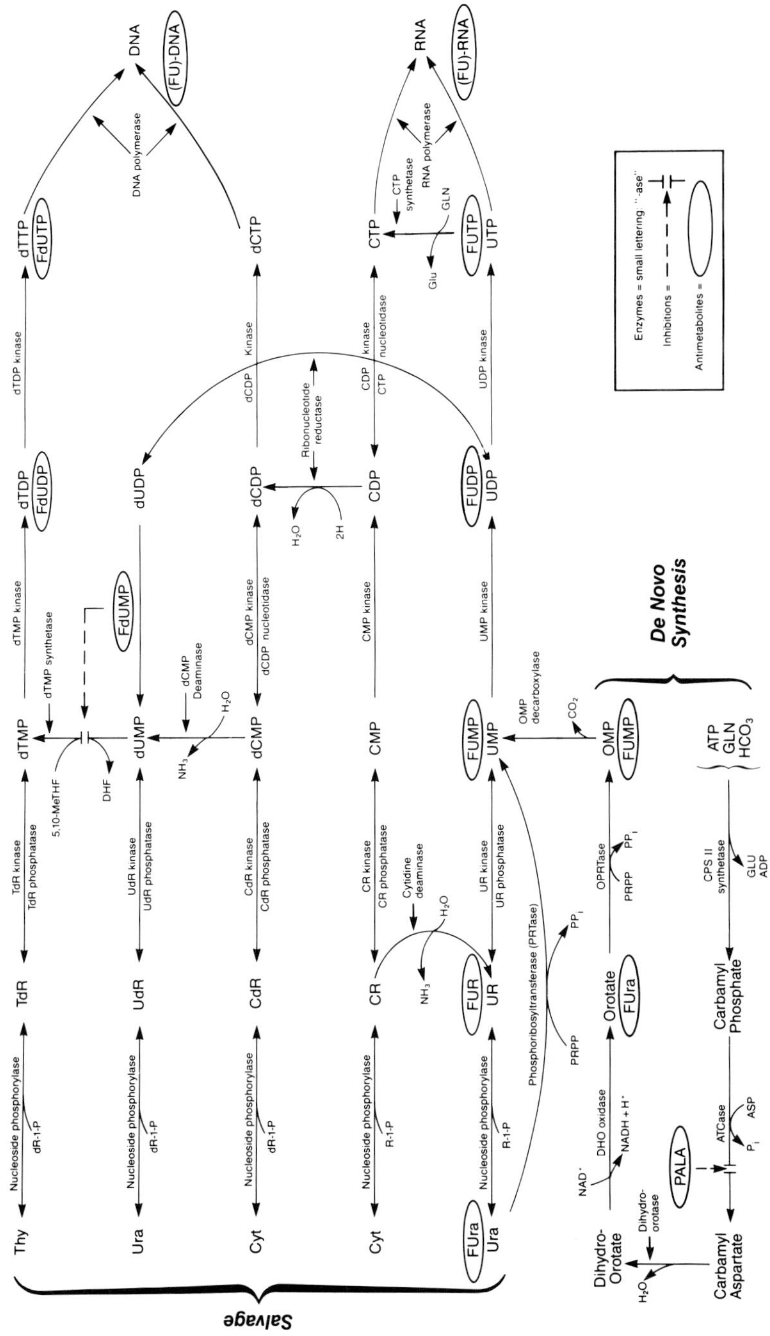

Figure 4. Pyrimidine pathways.

et al., 1964). The 5′-monophosphate nucleosides are converted to diphosphates and triphosphates by kinases which require ATP as the phosphate donor.

In the *de novo* synthesis of pyrimidines, cytidine triphosphates (CTP) are formed from UTP by the enzyme, CTP synthetase, in a reaction requiring glutamine as an amine source.

The deoxyribonucleoside triphosphates originate from the reduction of the ribonucleotide diphosphates by the enzyme, ribonucleotide reductase (R.R.), and, with the exception of dTTP, a single additional kinase step is required to provide the deoxynucleoside triphosphate. Deoxythymidine monophosphate (dTMP) arises from R.R. reduction of either UDP or CDP to dUDP. dUDP is converted to dUMP (deoxyuridine 5′-phosphate), with the subsequent introduction of the methyl group to form dTMP by the enzyme thymidylate (dTMP) synthetase. Thymidine nucleotides replace uridine in DNA synthesis. Formate serves as a source of the methyl group donated by N_5N_{10}-methylenetetrahydrofolic acid (5,10-MeTHF). dUMP is methylated in the 5-position, catalysed by combining with thymidylate synthetase and 5,10-MeTHF to form a ternary complex, followed by the oxidation of the tetrahydrofolate to dihydrofolate (DHF) and the release of dTMP (Cory and Chiba, 1985; Reichard, 1978; Santi *et al.*, 1974). (Figure 4).

In general, uridine is incorporated only into RNA and thymidine only into DNA, although there are exceptions to this rule. dUTP can be utilized by DNA polymerase and incorporated into DNA, but most cells have efficient mechanisms to remove or repair dUMP residues in DNA.

Catabolism of normal pyrimidines

Figure 4 does not indicate the degradative pathways. DNA and RNA are degraded by ribonucleases and deoxyribonucleases to nucleoside monophosphates, which are dephosphorylated to nucleosides by various specific and non-specific phosphatases. The nucleosides are then split to free bases by nucleoside phosphorylases. The catabolism is carried out exclusively through uracil and thymine. Cytosine derivatives are degraded via uracil derivatives by enzymatic deamination of dCMP to dUMP, deoxycytidine to deoxyuridine, or cytidine to uridine. Uracil and thymine both undergo a reduction step (NADPH to $NADP^+$) via the enzyme dihydrouracil dehydrogenase, with the formation of 5,6-dihydro derivatives. This is followed by ring opening to ureido derivatives, which are then cleaved to β-amino acids which may enter the citric acid cycle. Dihydrouracil dehydrogenase (also responsible for the breakdown of 5-fluorouracil) is largely located in the liver and is the rate-limiting enzyme. Although murine tumours lack the enzyme, it is present in human tumours (Naguib *et al.*, 1985; Roy-Burman, 1970).

5-Fluorouracil and its conversion to nucleotides

An analogue of uracil, 5-fluorouracil (FUra) has a fluorine atom at the 5-position in place of hydrogen (Figure 3), and is a potent pyrimidine antimetabolite. FUra is a "pro-drug" in that its cytotoxicity is dependent upon anabolism to a nucleotide. This may occur via two pathways (Figure 4). In the first, FUra may be converted to a ribonucleotide, 5-fluorouridine monophosphate (FUMP), in a two step reaction. Initially, to 5-fluorouridine (FUR) by reaction with ribose-1-phosphate (R-1-P); this enzymatic reaction is catalysed by nucleoside phosphorylase and is reversible. FUR is then phosphorylated by uridine (UR) kinase to FUMP, and subsequently phosphorylated further by kinases to the di- (FUDP) and triphosphates (FUTP), followed by incorporation of FUTP into RNA, the result being a fraudulent RNA, (FU)RNA.

In the second pathway, FUra may be directly anabolized to its ribonucleotide, FUMP, by a one-step conversion through PRPP-dependent orotate phosphoribosyltransferase (Reyes, 1969; Reyes and Guganig, 1975; Reyes and Hall, 1969). As mentioned, FUMP subsequently is converted by kinases to FUTP, and FUTP is incorporated into RNA in place of UTP to form (FU)RNA.

When FUMP is phosphorylated to FUDP, ribonucleoside reductase may convert this diphosphate ribonucleotide derivative of FUra to 5-fluoro-2′-deoxyuridine-5′-monophosphate (FdUMP) (Figure 4). FUra also may be converted directly to a deoxyribonucleotide in a two-step reaction by reacting with deoxyribose-1-phosphate (dR-1-P) via a nucleoside phosphorylase to give 5-fluoro-2′-deoxyuridine (FUdR), which is then phosphorylated by deoxyuridine (UdR) kinase to FdUMP. Thus, FUra may undergo anabolic conversion to FdUMP along either the ribonucleotide or deoxyribonucleotide pathway. FUdR may be cleaved back to FUra by both thymidine and deoxyuridine phosphorylases. FdUMP also may be phosphorylated further to 5-fluoro-2′-deoxyuridine-5′-triphosphate (FdUTP). FdUTP can serve as a substrate for DNA polymerase and be incorporated into DNA. The enzymes dUTPase and uracil DNA glycosylase, which function to prevent the incorporation of uracil into DNA by hydrolysing dUTP to dUMP and by removing dUMP residues from DNA, are thought to be similarly responsible for limiting the incorporation of FdUMP into DNA.

FdUMP also is a powerful inhibitor of the enzyme thymidylate synthetase (TS), which methylates dUMP to thymidylate (dTMP), and the resulting depletion of dTMP may limit DNA synthesis (Cory and Chiba, 1985; Heidelberger, 1975; Reichard, 1978; Santi *et al.*, 1974) (Figure 4). The rate at which FdUMP inactivates TS is dependent on the accumulated dUMP concentrations. The binding of FdUMP to TS is reversible; hence, high dUMP levels are able to lower the rate of TS inactivation, presumably via active site occupancy (Myers, 1981).

Summary of mechanism(s) of cytotoxicity of FUra.

Following activation to the nucleotide form, the cytotoxic effects of the fraudulent pyrimidine, FUra, may result from interference with the synthesis and function of either RNA or DNA. FUTP can be incorporated into cellular RNA and affect RNA maturation and processing adversely (Dolnick and Pink, 1985; Glazer and Lloyd, 1982; Heidelberger *et al.*, 1983; Mandel *et al.*, 1978; Martin *et al.*, 1978 b; Myers, 1981; Sawyer *et al.*, 1981; Spiegelman *et al.*, 1980; Washtien, 1984; Wilkinson and Pitot, 1973). FdUMP can inhibit dTMP synthetase, the result being depletion of dTTP pools and subsequent inhibition of DNA synthesis (Cory and Chiba, 1985; Heidelberger, 1975; Heidelberger *et al.*, 1983; Reichard, 1978; Santi *et al.*, 1974). Still another possible cytotoxic mechanism for FUra is the incorporation of FdUTP into cellular DNA (Cheng and Nakayama, 1983; Danenberg *et al.*, 1981; Kufe *et al.*, 1981; Lonn and Lonn, 1984; Major *et al.*, 1982; Sawyer *et al.*, 1984 a). Different degrees of sensitivity to FUra among various cell lines and experimental tumours are apparently due to cell line differences in FUra metabolism, whereby either an RNA-directed or DNA-directed action ensues (Ardalan *et al.*, 1980; Evans *et al.*, 1980; Laskin *et al.*, 1979; Lonn and Lonn, 1984; Maybaum *et al.*, 1980; Washtien, 1984).

Biochemical modulation of FUra with PALA

Regardless of whether FUra acts through a DNA or RNA mechanism, FUra must compete with uridine nucleotides at every metabolic step of its way toward its DNA- and/or RNA-target site(s). Therefore, an agent that lowers uracil nucleotide (UTP) pools (and which particularly does so in tumour tissue) will favour greater metabolic targeting of FUra-containing nucleotides and thereby enhance FUra's anti-tumour efficacy. PALA, *N*-(phosphonacetyl)-L-aspartate, an inhibitor of *de novo* pyrimidine synthesis (Figure 4), is such an agent.

PALA irreversibly inhibits aspartate transcarbamylase, the second enzyme in the *de novo* pathway for the biosynthesis of pyrimidine, by competing with its natural substrate, carbamyl phosphate (Collins and Stark, 1971; Swyrd *et al.*, 1974). Inhibition of *de novo* synthesis results in a lowering of UTP pools. When PALA is administered before FUra, the resulting decrease in pyrimidine pools favours greater utilization of FUra at its metabolic targets, resulting, for example, in increased incorporation of FUra into tumour RNA and enhanced anti-tumour activity in a number of animal tumour models (Ardalan *et al.*, 1980; Johnson *et al.*, 1980; Kufe and Egan, 1981; Kufe and Major, 1981; Martin *et al.*, 1978 a, 1980, 1981; Spiegelman *et al.*, 1980; Sawyer *et al.*, 1981).

Disappointingly, though, the results of clinical trials against advanced cancer with the PALA-before-FUra sequence were reported to be no better than the results seen in historical clinical controls receiving the maximum tolerated dose (MTD) of FUra alone (Bedikian *et al.*, 1981; Erlichman *et al.*, 1982; Meshad *et al.*, 1981; O'Connell *et al.*, 1982). However, a critique of all accumulated data, both preclinical and clinical, reveals that the probable cause for the disappointing clinical results with the PALA + FUra regimen lies in errors in the design of these clinical protocols (Martin *et al.*, 1983 a, 1985).

PALA and FUra have overlapping toxic side-effects. Combination chemotherapy with such agents with the administration of one agent in high dosage requires the dose of the other agent to be much lower than its maximum tolerated dose (MTD) as a single agent. The dose of PALA used in the initial clinical studies was *high* (1–2 g/m^2), which permitted only small doses of FUra to be given. Recent biochemical clinical research has shown that excellent inhibition of pyrimidine synthesis can be achieved in patients with only 250 mg/m^2 of PALA. A recently completed Phase I trial using this *low* dose of PALA in weekly combination with FUra, permitted employing the weekly MTD (600 mg/m^2) of FUra with only mild to moderate toxicity (Casper *et al.*, 1983).

Since a *high* dose of PALA mandates a *low* dose of FUra in combination, the resulting anti-cancer effect of such a combination cannot necessarily be expected to yield better anti-cancer results than are obtainable with the MTD of FUra alone. The reason is that, since PALA is clinically inactive as an anticancer agent (Carroll *et al.*, 1980; Rubin *et al.*, 1981; Van Echo *et al.*, 1980) whereas FUra is considered to have therapeutic activity, the anti-cancer effect of the PALA/FUra combination depends largely on the magnitude of the FUra dose. In the treatment of cancer patients, PALA is a "modulatory" agent only, whereas FUra is an "effector" anti-cancer agent. Hence, a low but biochemically active dose of PALA, followed by FUra at its MTD, as in the above low PALA–high (MTD) FUra phase I study (Casper *et al.*, 1983), might be expected to yield better therapeutic results than FUra alone at its MTD due to the pyrimidine-depleting biochemical effects of PALA. Since PALA's target enzyme, aspartate transcarbamylase, is apparently in lower concentration in tumour tissue than in normal tissues (Moore *et al.*, 1982), a low biochemically active dose of PALA may selectively and safely modulate the anti-cancer activity of a high dose of FUra in cancer patients, as it does in tumour-bearing animals (Martin *et al.*, 1983a). It is possible to inhibit more selectively an enzyme present in cancer tissue in small amounts, while producing much less inactivation of the same enzyme in normal tissues containing larger amounts (Ackerman and Potter, 1949).

Improvement in the therapeutic index of FUra by PALA would only occur if the metabolism of FUra were enhanced to a greater extent in malignant cells relative to host target tissues. The relatively high dose of PALA that has been employed in previous trials might result in equivalent intracellular biochemical perturbations in both tumour and host tissues. In contrast, a low PALA dose may be capable of selectively potentiating the effect of FUra in human tumour cells with relative sparing of host normal tissues, and thereby improve the therapeutic index. In humans, a low dose of PALA (250 mg/m^2) has been associated with prolonged (one week) inhibition of aspartate transcarbamylase (Casper *et al.*, 1983). Thus, the effects of a single dose of PALA can last long enough to result in optimal depletion of pyrimidine pools hours later. In mice, a low non-therapeutic dose of PALA (100 mg/kg), which can lower UTP pools at 24 hours in a murine breast tumour, can be administered safely 24 hours prior to the MTD of FUra alone (100 mg/kg), and the consequent low PALA/high FUra combination can produce synergistic anti-cancer activity (Martin *et al.*, 1983 a). A Phase II clinical study of the therapeutic effect of low-dose PALA followed by high-dose (MTD) FUra on human tumours has not yet been reported.

In patients with very advanced (Stage IV) breast cancer, and despite the heavily pretreated state of these patients, a relatively low (400 mg/m^2) dose of PAL plus FUra at less than its MTD produced a 28% response rate, against 14% for 5-FU alone (Mann *et al.*, 1985). These are encouraging results. The documented Phase I clinical study (Casper *et al.*, 1983), and the rationale for an appropriate ratio of the PALA–FUra combination in patients, calls for a still lower dose PALA (250 mg/m^2) to be administered roughly 24 hours before a still higher dose (the MTD) of FUra. Such a regimen may be expected to yield even better therapeutic results.

Biochemical modulation with methotrexate (MTX) and FUra

The sequential use of MTX and FUra is based on *in vivo* observations in several murine tumour model systems (Bertino *et al.*, 1977; Heppner and Calabresi, 1977; Martin *et al.*, 1976) and, subsequently, extensive biochemical studies on cells in culture (Benz and Cadman 1981; Benz *et al.*, 1982; Cadman *et al.*, 1979, 1981). MTX is a folate antagonist that inhibits dihydrofolate reductase (DHFR). Since *de novo* purine biosynthesis requires reduced folate-dependent enzymes, glycineamide ribonucleotide transformylase, or GAR TFase, and 5-aminoimidazole-4-carboxamide ribonucleotide transformylase, or AICAR TFase (Figure 2), the resulting depletion of tetrahydrofolates inhibits *de novo* purine synthesis, causing an accumulation of PRPP. PRPP is an important compound for *de novo* purine biosynthesis (Figure 2). *In vitro* work suggests that one reason that a sequenced MTX–FUra combination is synergistic is because MTX increases PRPP in MTX-sensitive cells (Cadman *et al.*, 1979, 1981). Since supplies of PRPP can be rate-limiting for the phosphoribosylation of FUra into its active ribonucleotides (Allegra *et al.*, 1985), the MTX-induced increased intracellular pools of PRPP result in greater intracellular conversion of FUra into nucleotides, increased incorporation of drug into RNA, and therefore greater anti-cancer activity (Cadman *et al.*, 1979, 1981).

There are other reasons for synergism in a sequenced MTX–FUra combination. MTX + 5-FUra sequence-dependent synergy may occur at the level of thymidylate synthetase (TS). Theoretically, reduction of tetrahydrofolates by MTX could antagonize FUra's inhibitory action on TS since FdUMP requires the tetrahydrofolate cofactor, N_5N_{10}-methylene tetrahydrofolate, for a tight binding ternary complex with TS. However, MTX is converted by both susceptible tumours and normal tissues (e.g., bone marrow and intestine) to polyglutamate derivatives (e.g., MTX-PGs), and this occurs in an MTX concentration-dependent and time-dependent pattern; thus, high-dose MTX favours formation of MTX-PGs. MTX-PGs are retained longer in cells, have high affinity for TS and markedly enhance covalant binding of FdUMP to TS. Thus, the enhanced TS block that ensues following MTX-before-FUra treatment may be still another reason for the synergy found with MTX treatment before FUra in tumour-bearing mice (Allegra *et al.*, 1985; Bertino *et al.*, 1983; Koizumi, *et al.*, 1985; Matherly *et al.*, 1983, 1986).

Treatment with MTX before FUra in MTX-sensitive tumour cells that readily form MTX-PGs usually results in effective inhibition of TS by the MTX-PGs themselves (Allegra *et al.*, 1985). Thus high levels of either MTX-PGs, or MTX-PGs + FUra are sufficient for an optimum block of TS. Regardless of the particular mechanism, as a consequence of either the MTX-PG or MTX-PG + 5-FU block on TS, there is a decrease in dTTP pools, and a consequent inhibition of DNA synthesis. Further, there may be an incorporation of dUTP and FdUTP into DNA when dUMP and dUTP and FdUTP levels increase following the TS block, with subsequent excision of the misincorporated uracil entities leading to DNA strand breaks that may also contribute to cytotoxicity (Bertino *et al.*, 1983; Goulian *et al.*, 1980; Sedwick *et al.*, 1981; Cheng, 1984). Whether or not this misincorporation contributes to the cytotoxicity has not been established (Danenberg *et al.*, 1981). The enhanced cytotoxicity induced by the sequenced MTX-FUra combination likely results from increased activation of FUra to FUTP and incorporation into RNA (Allegra *et al.*, 1985).

Synergism between MTX and FUra depends on both the proper sequence (MTX before FUra) and the interval between the two agents (Benz *et al.*, 1982). *In vitro* studies using human carcinoma lines have shown that optimal tumour toxicity has been achieved by 18–24 hours sequencing of these drugs (Benz and Cadman, 1981; Benz *et al.*, 1982).

The initial clinical trials of sequential MTX-before-FUra therapy employed a one hour scheduling interval between agents. This timing was based on the initial preclinical studies (Bertino *et al.*, 1977; Cadman *et al.*, 1979; Martin *et al.*, 1976). However, preclinical timing intervals do not necessarily directly transpose into successful clinical trial, and it is not surprising that most of these one hour interval clinical trials were reported with negative results. In marked contrast, most of the clinical studies with longer scheduling intervals (e.g., four hours or more, and probably better closer to 24 hours) were reported to show enhanced tumour response rates over FUra alone (Benz *et al.*, 1983, 1985; Cannobbio *et al.*, 1986; Drapkin *et al.*, 1983; Glimelius *et al.*, 1986; Herrman *et al.*, 1984; Ignoffo *et al.*, 1984; Kaye *et al.*, 1984; Kemeny *et al.*, 1984; Saks *et al.*, 1985; Weinerman *et al.*, 1982). It is to be noted that, in addition to the varying timing interval between the drugs, the intensity of administration also varied between protocols (e.g., weekly vs. every 2–3 weeks), and there were differences in the doses employed of the two agents. There are all pilot studies, and their clinical findings should be considered as preliminary until appropriately randomized controlled studies are done.

Biochemical modulation with leucovorin (LV) and FUra

A major cytotoxic action of FUra involves the conversion of FUra into FdUMP, which inhibits thymidylate synthetase (TS) and results in the suppression of DNA synthesis by depletion of dTTP (Heidelberger, 1975). FdUMP binds tightly to TS in the presence of the folate cofactor, N_5N_{10}-methylene tetrahydrofolate (5,10-MeTHF) (Cannobbio *et al.*, 1986; Santi *et al.*, 1974). Preclinical biochemical and *in vitro* studies have demonstrated that an excess of intracellular reduced folates is necessary for maximum creation of the ternary complex (FdUMP + TS + 5,10-MeTHF; Figure 4), the result being optimal inhibition of TS and increased cytotoxic efficacy of FUra (Cannobbio *et al.*, 1986; Evans *et al.*, 1981; Glimelius *et al.*, 1986; Hakala *et al.*, 1982; Houghton *et al.*, 1981; Kaye *et al.*, 1984; Ullman *et al.*, 1978; Waxman *et al.*, 1978; Waxman and Bruckner, 1982; Yin *et al.*, 1983). The increased toxic effects are due to the stabilization of the ternary complex, resulting in more prolonged inhibition of TS activity (Kaye *et al.*, 1984). These preclinical findings have suggested that the clinical coadministration of large doses of LV (5-formyltetrahydrofolate) may retard TS recovery from FUra administration and thereby increase FUra's anti-cancer activity. *In vivo*, LV is rapidly converted to 5-methyltetrahydrofolate, and then to the biologically active coenzyme of TS, 5,10-MeTHF.

Pilot clinical trials of this concept have been reported with both encouraging (Machover *et al.*, 1986; Madajewicz *et al.*, 1984) and discouraging (Bertrand, *et al.*, 1986; Byrne *et al.*, 1983; Cunningham *et al.*, 1984) results. These pilot studies are all compared to historical controls treated with FUra as a single agent; however, there is evidence (Diehl and Perry, 1986) that such a comparison may not be valid. Such comparisons may be misleading because prognostic factors, measurements of tumour size (e.g., some protocols use ultrasonographic and/or scintigraphic procedures while others employ measurement by palpation), and patient performance level may vary between current protocols and those of historical controls. The current protocols also vary in certain treatment details, such as different doses of LV and different timings between LV and FUra. These studies should all be considered as only preliminary until appropriately randomized controlled studies are done.

Randomized studies are now in progress comparing FUra alone with FUra and high-dose LV in cancer patients previously unexposed to chemotherapy that should provide the answer as to whether or not LV can improve the therapeutic efficacy of FUra. However, one caveat seems in order. The comparison of the LV + FUra combination should be with a randomized control group receiving the maximum tolerated dose (MTD) of FUra as a single agent in a regimen that is equitoxic and equi-intensive (Hryniuk and Bush, 1984) to that of the LV + FUra combination. It should be noted that there is an increase of FUra toxicity in the presence of excess LV (Bruckner *et al.*, 1981) that usually necessitates a lower dose of FUra in the LV + FUra combination than the MTD of FUra alone. Hence, a study comparing the same lower FUra dose as that employed in the LV + FUra combination is likely to demonstrate a therapeutic advantage for the combination, but perhaps would not to a randomized group at the MTD of FUra as a single agent.

The special clinical needs of "modulatory" combination chemotherapy

It has become apparent that the translation of preclinical results with biochemical modulation to the clinic requires careful attention to specific details. The inclusion of "modulatory" agents in combination chemotherapy does not depend on the ability of the modulating agents to kill tumour cells as single agents; they are given to obtain a desired intracellular biochemical alteration in the tumour cells which will permit greater differential toxicity in the tumour cells by the appropriate "effector" agent(s) in the combination. As explained earlier, parameters of dosage, ratios of agents, and sequence and time interval between administration of agents are much more critical in this approach than in the classical approach in which the independent activity of each agent is the desired effect.

In the PALA + FUra "modulatory" combination chemotherapy example noted previously, an outstanding difference between the preclinical and clinical anti-tumour findings with PALA emerges. In the preclinical laboratory, against experimental tumours, both moderate and high doses of PALA are reported to exert anti-tumour activity, whereas in contrast, in the clinic, even high doses of PALA are considered therapeutically inactive. The apparent major reason for this ostensible difference in therapeutic activity is that entirely different endpoints are utilized for determining therapeutic activity in animal tumour models and in the clinic (Martin *et al.*, 1984, 1986). In the clinic, drugs are defined as clinically active only if the drugs elicit tumour regression ($\geqslant$50% in at least 20% of evaluable patients). In marked contrast, inhibition of tumour growth is the criterion of effectiveness employed to define the same tumour agents as active in the laboratory tumour models.

The fact that different endpoints are being used to identify anti-cancer activity in humans and in animals merits consideration by clinical investigators in the design of clinical trials involving biochemical modulation. In the laboratory tumour model, various degrees of tumour growth inhibition can be discerned and interpreted as evidence for therapeutic gain. For example, both PALA-before-FUra, and MTX-before-FUra, can be clearly shown to be better than the MTD of FUra alone on the basis of tumour growth inhibition measurements, even though only a very low, unimpressive, and statistically insignificant percentage of chemotherapeutically-induced partial tumour regressions is evident (Martin *et al.*, 1983 b). In the clinic, however, tumour growth inhibition criteria cannot be employed, and the therapeutic incremental gains induced by each of these single manipulations of FUra metabolism may not be sufficient (and particularly in the usual small pilot study) to overcome the inherently more extreme tumour cell heterogeneity at the level of statistically significant improvement in the number of tumour regressions. For this reason, it is stressed that preclinical studies have demonstrated *in vivo* that unequivocally improved tumour regression rates of a "modulated" effector agent can be brought out by the concurrent administration of more than one "modulating" agent (Table 3).

Specifically, sequential modulation at several steps in the metabolic activation of FUra has been demonstrated in an experimental solid tumour to effect tumour regressions, whereas manipulation of a single step in the metabolism of FUra only augments FUra's inhibition of tumour growth. Thus, in Table 3, whereas the very small number of partial regressions induced by either double combination (PALA + 5-FUra, 3%, or MTX + FUra, 5%) is not persuasive of therapeutic gain, the combination of all three agents (PALA + MTX + FUra) followed by appropriate rescue is clearly a therapeutic advance in producing 27–32% partial tumour regressions in very advanced murine breast cancers (Martin *et al.*, 1983 b). Of course, the "modulating" agents were administered in appropriate sequence, interval and

Table 3. More than one biochemical modulator of 5-fluorouracil (FUra) is necessary to clearly induce unequivocally improved tumour regression rates.

	Treatment	% of PR†
1.	FUra	0%
2.	PALA → FUra → LV + UR "Rescue"	5%
3.	MTX → FUra → LV + UR "Rescue"	3%
4.	PALA → MTX → FUra → LV + UR "Rescue"	27–32%

Results are pooled data from four murine experiments with advanced CD8F1 breast cancer (Tables 5,6,7 of Martin *et al.*, 1983 a). Methotrexate (MTX) and PALA are administered in *non-therapeutic* but biochemically active regimens. LV = Leucovorin; UR = uridine. FUra is at its MTD in group 1, as are each of the drug combinations in groups 2–4, but the UR "rescue" allows for the safe administration of FUra at higher doses than would be otherwise tolerated.
† PR = partial regressions of ⩾50% of initial tumour size.

dosage ratio. Since both "modulating" agents, PALA and MTX, were administered in *non*-therapeutic (but biochemically active) regimens, and both rescue agents, leucovorin and uridine, were administered well after the effector agent, the conclusion is clear that the markedly improved tumour regression rate was due to the "modulated" heightened efficacy of the effector agent, FUra. The message in these experimental studies is that the concurrent administration of several appropriate modulating agents in biochemically active regimens can enhance the opportunity for discerning clinical success with biochemical modulation of an effector agent.

Conclusions

The past decade has brought major advances in our understanding of the biochemistry of purine and pyrimidine antimetabolites. This chapter has attempted to integrate the old with the new biochemical information with specific reference to cancer chemotherapy. It is clear that the new findings have stimulated great interest in the manipulation of intracellular biochemical events for therapeutic gain, and that these biochemical perturbations have indeed succeeded in improving chemotherapeutic efficacy, but so far, only in the preclinical laboratory.

Why have the clinical attempts to reproduce the preclinical findings of effective biochemical modulation been disappointing? As has been discussed, appropriate ratios of agents, and the sequence and time interval between administration of agents are critical determinants of success in preclinical studies of biochemical modulation but these parameters have not been scientifically incorporated into the design of clinical protocols. Instead, the choice of these parameters has been "admittedly largely arbitrary... [because]... there is little in the way of reliably predictable animal model experimentation to serve as a foundation for rational dosage administration in humans' (Buroker *et al.*, 1985). The implication of this statement that the animal model may be predictable in the sense that preclinical regimens, despite their being scientifically determined, nevertheless may be *roughly* transposable to the clinic, is not warranted. The known quantitative biochemical differences between mouse and man require that *scientific*, and *not arbitrary*, determinations in patients be the basis for setting the details of the treatment plans in clinical protocols evaluating preclinical findings of biochemical modulation.

These quantitative differences indicate that the appropriate dose of an agent, and the appropriate time interval between administration of agents probably will be different in the two species. In order to translate successful preclinical results in biochemical modulation into the the clinical setting it will be necessary to determine in patients (by direct biochemical measurements at the tissue level) the dose and temporal relationship between agents that produces the pertinent biochemical changes in human tumours that were associated with the therapeutic success of that particular drug combination in the murine tumour model.

The cure of some human cancers has been possible through the use of combinations of agents, but the inherent heterogeneity of neoplastic cells has precluded similar success with other cancers. The search for new and better anti-cancer agents will (and should, of course) continue, but all evidence indicates that when found each new drug will still have to be integrated into a therapeutic combination. The possibilities for improvement in combination chemotherapy may well depend not only upon a clearer understanding of how an agent affects intracellular biochemistry, but upon how deliberate further biochemical manipulation by other agents may facilitate therapeutic gain. The potential for clinical benefit may only be realized by determining the details of a clinical treatment plan on a scientific basis by measuring in patients the intracellular biochemical change produced by a particular dose of an agent and the time interval it takes to produce this effect. After all, that is what was required for therapeutic progress in the preclinical murine model. Should the intracellular biochemistry and pharmacology of anti-cancer agents in humans be less complex?

Acknowledgements

The research from the author's laboratory was supported in part by grant POICA25842 from the National Cancer Institute and in part by the Chemotherapy Foundation of New York.

The author wishes to express his appreciation to his colleagues, Drs. R. Sawyer, R. Stolfi, E. Balis, and J. Colofiore for their contributions to the data and their helpful criticisms, and to Mrs. Margaret Petrosino for her excellent secretarial assistance.

References

Ackerman, W. W. and Potter, V. R., 1949, Enzyme inhibition in relation to chemotherapy. *Proc. Soc. Biol. Med.* **72**, 1–9.

Allan, P. W. and Bennett, L. L., Jr., 1971, 6-Methylthioguanylic acid, a metabolite of 6-thioguanine. *Biochem. Pharmacol.*, **20**, 847–852.

Allegra, C. J., Chabner, B., Drake, J. C., Lutz, R., Rodbard, D. and Jolivet, J., 1985, Enhanced inhibition of thymidylate synthase by methotrexate polyglutamates. *J. Biol. Chem.*, **260**, 9720–9726.

Anderson, D. and Brockman, R. W., 1964, Feedback inhibition of uridine kinase by cytidine triphosphate and uridine triphosphate. *Biochim. Biophys. Acta*, **91**, 380–386.

Ardalan, B., Cooney, D. A., Jayaram, H. N., *et al.*, 1980 a, Mechanism of sensitivity and resistance of murine tumors to 5-fluorouracil. *Cancer Res.*, **40**, 1431–1437.

Ardalan, B., Glazer, R., Kensler, T., *et al.*, 1980 b, Biochemical mechanism for the synergism of 5-fluorouracil (5-FU) and phosphonacetyl-L-aspartate (PALA) in human mammary carcinoma cells. *Proc. Am. Assoc. Cancer Res.*, **21**, 8.

Armstrong, R. D., Vera, R., Snyder, P. and Cadman, E., 1982. Enhancement of 6-thioguanine cytotoxic activity with methotrexate. *Biochem. Biophys. Res. Commun.*, **109**, 595–601.

Atkinson, D. E., 1969, Regulation of energy metabolism: Exploitable molecular mechanisms and neoplasia. The University of Texas M. D. Anderson Hospital and Tumor Institute at Houston, 22nd Annual Symposium on Fundamental Cancer Research, 1968 (Baltimore: Williams and Wilkins), pp. 397–413.

Atkinson, D. E. and Fall, L., 1967, Adenosine triphosphate conservation in biosynthetic regulation. *J. Biol. Chem.*, **242**, 3241–3242.

Atkinson, M. R., and Murray, A. W., 1965, Inhibition of purine phosphoribosyltransferases of Ehrlich ascites-tumor cells by 6-mercaptopurine. *Biochem. J.*, **94**, 64–74.

Atkinson, M. R., Eckermann, G., and Stephenson, J., 1965, Formation of 6-thioxanthosine-5′-phosphate from 6-mercaptopurine and from 6-thioxanthine in Ehrlich ascites-tumor cells. *Biochim. Biophys. Acta*, **108**, 320–322.

Atkinson, M. R., Jackson, J. F. and Morton, R. K., 1961, Substrate specific and inhibition of nicotinamide mononucleotide adenyltransferase of liver nuclei: possible mechanism of effect of 6-mercaptopurine on tumor growth. *Nature*, **192**, 946–948.

Atkinson, M. R., Jackson, J. F., Morton, R. K. and Murray, A. W., 1962, Nicotinamide 6-mercaptopurine dinucleotide and related compounds: Potential sources of 6-mercaptopurine nucleotide in chemotherapy. *Nature*, **196**, 35–36.

Atkinson, M. R,, Morton, R. K. and Murray, A. W., 1963, Inhibition of inosine 5′-phosphate dehydrogenase from Ehrlich ascites tumor cells by 6-thioinosine 5′-phosphate. *Biochem. J.*, **89**, 167–172.

Atkinson, M. R., Morton, R. K. and Murray, A. W. 1964, Inhibition of adenylosuccinate synthetase and adenylosuccinate lyase from Ehrlich ascites-tumor cells by 6-thioinosine 5′-phosphate. *Biochem. J.*, **92**, 398–404.

Baylin, S. B., 1982, Clonal selection and heterogeneity of human solid neoplasms. In *Design of Models for Testing Cancer Chemotherapeutic Agents*, edited by I. J. Fidler and R. J. White (New York: Van-Nostrand Reinhold), pp. 50–63.

Bedikian, A. Y., Strochlein, J. R., Karlin, D. A., 1981, Chemotherapy for colorectal cancer with a combination of PALA and 5-FU. *Cancer Treat. Rep.*, **65**, 747–753.

Bennett, L. L., Jr, and Adamson, D. J., 1970, Reversal of the growth inhibitory effects of 6-methyliopurine ribonucleoside. *Biochem. Pharmacol.*, **19**, 2172–2176.

Bennett, L. L., Simpson, L., Golden, J. and Barker, T. L., 1963, The primary site of inhibition by 6-mercaptopurine on the purine biosynthetic pathway in some tumors *in vivo*. *Cancer Res.*, **23**, 1574–1580.

Bennett, L. L., Brockman, R. W., Schnebli, H. P., Chumley, S., Dixon, G. J., Schabel, F. M., Dulmadge, E. A., Skipper, H. E., Montgomery, J. A. and Thomas, H. J., 1965, Activity and mechanism of action of 6-methylthiopurine ribonucleoside in cancer cells resistant to 6-mercaptopurine. *Nature*, **205**, 1276–1279.

Bennett, L. L., Jr., Schnebli, H. P., Vail, M. H., Allan, P. W. and Montgomery, J. A., 1966 Purine ribonucleoside kinase activity and resistance to some analogs of adenosine. *Molec. Pharmacol.*, **2**, 432–443.

Benz, C. and Cadman, E., 1981, Modulation of 5-fluorouracil metabolism and cytotoxicity by antimetabolite pretreatment in human colorectal adenocarcinoma, HCT-8. *Cancer Res.*, **41**, 994–999.

Benz, C., Tillis, T., Tattelman, E. *et al.*, 1982, Optimal scheduling of methotrexate and 5-fluorouracil in human breast cancer. *Cancer Res.*, **42**, 2081–2086.

Benz, C., Silverberg, M. and Cadman, E., 1983, Use of high-dose oral methotrexate sequenced at 24 hours with 5-FU: A clinical toxicity study. *Cancer Treat. Rep.*, **67**, 297–299.

Benz, C., DeGregorio, M., Saks, S., Sambol, G., Holleran, W., Ignoffo, R., Lewis, B. and Cadman, E., 1985, Sequential infusions of methotrexate and 5-fluorouracil in advanced cancer: pharmacology, toxicity, and response. *Cancer Res.*, **45**, 3354–3358.

Berger, N. A. Catino, D. M., and Vietti, T. J., 1982, Synergistic antileukemic effect of 6-aminonicotinamide and 1-3 bis-(2-chloroethyl)-1-nitrosourea on L1210 cells *in vitro* and *in vivo*. *Cancer Res.*, **42**, 4382–4386.

Bertino, J. R., 1979, Toward improved selectivity in cancer chemotherapy: The Richard and Hinda Rosenthal Foundation Award Lecture. *Cancer Res.*, **39**, 293–304.

Bertino, J. R., 1981, Clinical use of methotrexate—with emphasis on use of high doses. *Cancer Treat. Rep.*, **65**, 131–135.

Bertino, J. R., Mini, E. and Fernandes, D. J., 1983, Sequential methotrexate and 5-fluorouracil: mechanisms of synergy. *Seminars in Oncology.*, **10** (No. 2, Suppl. 2) 2–5.

Bertrand, M., Doroshow, J. H., Mulythavf, P., *et al.*, 1986, High-dose continuous infusion folinic acid and bolus 5-fluorouracil in patients with advanced colorectal cancer: a phase II study. *J. Clin. Oncol.*, **4**, 1058–1061.

Bieber, S., Dietrich, L. S., Elion, G. B., Hitchings, G. H. and Martin, D. S., 1961, incorporation of 6-mercaptopurine-S35 into the nucleic acids of sensitive and nonsensitive tranplantable tumors. *Cancer Res.*, **21**, 228–231.

Bloch, A., 1974, Metabolic conditioning and metabolic actuation: Experimental approaches to cancer chemotherapy involving combinations of metabolites and antimetabolites. *Cancer Chemother. Rep.*, **53**, 471–477.

Bresnick, E., 1962, Feedback inhibition of aspartate transcarbamylase in liver and in hepatoma. *Cancer Res.*, **22**, 1246–1251.

Bresnick, E. and Blatchford, K., 1964, Inhibition of dihydroorotase by purines and pyrimidines. *Biochim. Biophys. Acta.*, **81**, 150–151.

Bresnick, E., Thompson, V. B., Morris, H. P. and Liebelt, A. G., 1964, Inhibition of thymidine kinase activity in liver and hepatomas by TTP aned d-CTP. *Biochem. Biophys. Res. Commun.*, **16**, 278–281.

Breter, H. J. and Zahn, R. K., 1979, Quantitation of intracellular metabolites of (^{35}S)-6-mercaptopurine in L5178Y cells grown in time-course incubates *Cancer Res.*, **39**, 3744–3748.

Britell, J. C., Moertel, C. G., Kvols, L. K., O'Connell, J., Rubin, J. and Schutt, A. J., 1981, Phase II trial of i.v. 6-thioguanine in advanced colorectal carcinoma. *Cancer Treat. Rep.*, **65**, 909–910.

Brockman, R. W., 1963, Mechanism of resistance to anticancer agents. *Adv. Cancer Res.*, **7**, 129–234

Brockman, R. W., 1964, Biochemical aspects of mercaptopurine inhibition and resistance. Cancer Res., **23**, 1191–1201.

Bruckner, H. W., Storch, J. A. and Holland, J. F., 1981, Leucovorin increases the toxicity of 5-fluorouracil: Phase I clinical pharmacological trials. *Proc. Am. Assoc. Cancer Res.* **22**, 192.

Burchenal, J. H., Murphy, M. L., Ellison, R. R., Sykes, M. P., Tan, T. C., Leone, L. A., Karnofsky, D. A., Craver, L. F., Dargeon, H. W. and Rhoads, C. P., 1953, Clinical evaluation of a new antimetabolite, 6-mercaptopurine, in the treatment of leukemia and allied diseases. *Blood*, **8**, 965–999.

Buroker, T. R., Moertel, C. G., Fleming, T. R., *et al.*, 1985, A controlled evaluation of recent approaches to biochemical modulation or enhancement of 5-fluorouracil therapy in colorectal carcinoma. *J. Clin. Oncol.*, **3**, 1624–1631.

Byrne, P., Smith, F., Treat, J., *et al.*, 1983, 5-Fluorouracil and higher dose folinic acid treatment of colorectal carcinoma patients. *Proc. Am. Soc. Clin. Oncol.*, **2**, 121.

Cadman, E., Davis, L. and Heimer, R., 1979, Enhanced 5-fluorouracil nucleotide formation after methotrexate administration: explanation for drug synergism. *Science*, **205**, 1135–1137.

Cadman, E., Heimer, R. and Benz, C., 1981, The influence of methotrexate pretreatment on 5-fluorouracil metabolism in L1210 cells. *J. Biol. Chem.*, **256**, 1695–1704.

Calabresi, P. and Parks, R. E., 1985, Chemotherapy of neoplastic diseases. In *The Pharmacological Basis of Therapeutics*, 7th ed., edited by L. S. Goodman and A. G. Gilman (New York: Macmillan), p. 1276.

Caldwell, I. C., Henderson, J. F. and Paterson, A. R. F., 1966, The enzymic formation of 6-(methylmercapto)purine ribonucleoside 5′-phosphate. *Can. J. Biochem.*, **44**, 229–245.

Cannobbio, L., Nobile, M., Ardizzoni, A., Tatarek, R. and Rosso, R., 1986, Phase II study of sequential methotrexate and 5-FU combination in the treatment of advanced colorectal cancer. *Cancer Treat. Rep.*, **70**, 419–420.

Carrico, C. K. and Sartorelli, A. C., 1977, Effects of 6-thioguanine on macromolecular events in regenerating rat liver. *Cancer Res.*, **37**, 1868–1875.

Carroll, D. S., Gralla, R. J. and Kemeny, N. E., 1980, Phase II evaluation of N-(phosphonacetyl)-L-aspartic acid (PALA) in patients with advanced colorectal carcinoma. *Cancer Treat. Rep.*, **64**, 339–342.

Caskey, C. T., Ashton, P. N. and Wyngarden, J. B., 1964, The enzymology of feedback inhibition of glutamine phosphoribosylpyrophosphate amidotransferase by purine ribonucleotides. *J. Biol. Chem.*, **239**., 2570–2579.

Casper, E. S., Vale, K., Williams, L. J., Martin, D. S. and Young, C. W. 1983, Phase I and clinical pharmacological evaluation of biochemical modulation of 5-fluorouracil with N-(phosphonacetyl)-L-aspartic acid. *Cancer Res.*, **43**, 2324–2326

Chabner, B. A., Fine, R. L., Allegra, C. J., Yeh, G. W and Curt, G. A., 1984, Cancer chemotherapy. Progress and expectations, 1984. *Cancer*, **54**, 2599–2608.

Cheng, Y. C., 1984, The preclinical rationale for 5-fluorouracil–leucovorin combination. Correlation with clinical response. *Adv. Cancer Chemother.*, November 1984, p. 46.

Cheng, Y. C. and Nakayama, K., 1983, Effects of 5-fluoro-2′-deoxyuridine on DNA metabolism in Hela cells. *Mol. Pharmacol.*, **23**, 171–174.

Christie, N. T., Drake, S., Meyn, R. E. and Nelson, J. A., 1984, 6-Thioguanine-induced DNA damage as a determinant of cytotoxicity in cultured Chinese Hamster ovary cells. *Cancer Res.*, **44**, 3664–3671.

Coffey, J. J., White, C. A., Lesk, A. B., Rogers, W. I. and Serpick, A. A., 1972, Effect of allopurinol on the pharmacokinetics of 6-mercaptopurine (NSC 755) in cancer patients. *Cancer Res.*, **32**, 1283–1289.

Cohen, M. B. and Sadie, W., 1983, Contributions of the depletions of guanine and adenine nucleotides to the toxicity of purine starvation in the mouse T lymphoma cell line. *Cancer Res.*, **43**, 1587–1591.

Collins, K. D. and Stark, G. R., 1971, Aspartate transcarbamylase, interaction with the transition state analogue N-(phosphonacetyl)-L-aspartate. *J. Biol. Chem.*, **246**, 6599–6605.

Cory, J. G. and Chiba, P., 1985, Combination chemotherapy directed at the components of nucleoside diphosphate reductase. *Pharmac. Ther.*, **29**, 111–127.

Crabtree, G. W. and Henderson, J. F., 1971, Rate-limiting steps in the interconversion of purine ribonucleotides in Ehrlich ascites tumor cells *in vitro.*, *Cancer Res.*, **31**, 985–991.

Cunningham, J., Bukowski, R., Budd, G., *et al.*, 1984, 5-Fluorouracil and folinic acid: A phase I–II trial in gastrointestinal malignancy. *Invest. New Drugs.*, **2**, 391–395.

Danenberg, P. V., Heidelberger, C., Mulkins, M. A. and Peterson, A. R., 1981, The incorporation of 5-fluoro-2′-deoxyuridine into DNA of mammalian tumor cells. *Biochem. Biophys. Res. Commun.*, **102**, 654–658.

Davidson, J. D. and Winter, T. S., 1964, Purine nucleotide pyrophosphorylases in 6-mercaptopurine-sensitive and -resistant human leukemias. *Cancer Res.*, **24**, 261–267.

Diehl, L. F. and Perry, D. J., 1986, A comparison of randomized concurrent control groups with matched historical groups: Are historical controls valid? *J. Clin. Oncol.*, **4**, 114–1120.

Dietrich, L. S., 1975, Cytotoxic analogs of pyridine nucleotide coenzymes. In *Antineoplastic and Immunosuppressive agents.*, edited by A. C. Sartorelli and D. G. Johns (New York: Springer-Verlag), pp. 539–542.

Dietrich, L. S., Kaplan, L. and Friedland, I. M., 1958 a, Pyridine nucleotide metabolism: Mechanism of action of the niacin antagonist, 6-aminonicotinamide. *J. Biol. Chem.*, **233**, 964–968

Dietrich, L. S., Kaplan, L. A., Friedland, I. M. and Martin, D. S., 1958 b, Quantitative differences between tumor and host tissue. VI. 6-aminonicotinamide antagonism of DPN-dependent enzymatic systems. *Cancer Res.*, **18**, 1272–1280.

Dolnick, B. J. and Pink, J. J., 1985, Effects of 5-fluorouracil on dihydrofolate reductase and dihydrofolate reductase in RNA from methotrexate-resistant KB cells. *J. Biol. Chem.*, **260**, 3006–3014.

Drake, S., Burns, R. L. and Nelson, J. A., 1982, Metabolism and mechanisms of action of 9-(tetrahydro-2-furyl)-6-mercaptopurine in Chinese hamster ovary cells. *Chem.-Biol. Interact.*, **41**, 105–115.

Drapkin, R., McAloon, E. and Lyman, G., 1983, Sequential methotrexate (MTX) and 5-fluorouracil in advanced measurable colorectal cancer. *Proc. Am. Soc. Clin. Oncol.*, **2**, 118.

Elion, G. B., 1967, Biochemistry and pharmacology of purine analogs. *Fred. Proc.*, **26**, 898–903.

Elion, G. B. 1975, Interaction of anticancer drugs with enzymes. In *Pharmacological Basis of Cancer Chemotherapy* (A collection of papers presented at the Twenty-Seventh Annual Symposium on Fundamental Cancer Research, 1974, at the University of Texas M. D. Anderson Hospital and Tumor Institute at Houston). (Baltimore: Williams and Wilkins), pp. 547–564.

Elion, G. B., 1985, Selectivity-key to chemotherapy: Presidential address. *Cancer Res.*, **45**, 2943–2950.

Elion, G. B., Burgi, E. and Hitchings, G. H., 1952, Studies on condensed pyrimidine systems. IX. The synthesis of some 6-substituted purines. *J. Am. Chem. Soc.*, **74**, 411–414.

Elion, G. B., Callahan, S., Nathan, H., Bieber, S., Rundles, R. W. and Hitchings, G. H., 1963, Potentiation by inhibition of drug degradation: 6-substituted purines and xanthine oxidase. *Biochem. Pharmacol*, **12**, 85–93.

Erlichman, C., Donhower, R. C., Speyer, J. L., *et al.*, 1982, Phase I–II trial of *N*-phosphonacetyl-L-aspartic acid given by intravenous infusion and 5-fluorouracil given by bolus injection. *J. Natl Cancer Inst.*, **68**, 227–231.

Esterhay, R. J., Aisner, J., Levi, J. A. and Wiernik, P. H., 1978, High-dose 6-mercaptopurine in advanced refractory cancer. *Cancer Treat. Rep.*, **62**, 1229–1231.

Evans, R. M., Laskin, J. D. and Hakala, M. T., 1980, Assessment of growth limiting events caused by 5-fluorouracil. *Cancer Res.*, **40**, 4113–4122.

Evans, R. M., Laskin, J. D. and Hakala, M. T., 1981, Effect of excess folates and deoxyinosine on the activity and site of action of 5-fluorouracil. *Cancer Res.*, **41** 3288–3295.
Fox, I. H. and Kelly, W. N., 1971, Phosphoribosylpyrophosphate in man: biochemical and clinical significance. *Ann. Intern. Med.*, **74**, 424–433.
Glock, G. E. and McLean, P., 1957, Levels of oxidized and reduced diphosphopyridine nucleotide and triphosphopyridine nucleotide in tumors. *Biochem. J.*, **65**, 413–416.
Goldie, J. H., 1983, Relevance of drug resistance in cancer treatment strategy. In *Cancer Chemotherapy*, edited by I. F. M. Muggia (Boston: Martinus Nijhoff), pp. 1–30.
Goulian, M., Bleile, B. and Tseng, B., 1980, Methotrexate-induced misincorporation of uracil into DNA. *Proc. Natl. Acad. Sci. USA*, **77**, 1956–1960.
Grassetti, D. R., 1986, The antimetastatic and tumor growth retarding effects of sulfur containing analogs of nicotinamide. *Cancer Lett.*, **31**, 187–195.
Green, H. and Chan, T. S., 1973, Pyrimidine starvation induced by adenosine in fibroblasts and lymphoid cells: Role of adenosine deaminase. *Science*, **182**, 836–837.
Grindey, G. B., Lowe, J. K., Divekar, A. Y. and Hakala, M. T., 1976, Potentiation by guanine nucleosides of the growth-inhibitory effects of adenosine analogs on L1210 and Sarcoma 180 cells in culture. *Cancer Res*, **36**, 379–383.
Gusella, J. G. and Housman, D., 1976, Induction of erythroid differentiation *in vitro* by purines and purine analogues. *Cell*, **8**, 263–269.
Hakala, M. T., Yin, M.-B. and Zakrzewski, S. F., 1982, Role of the composition of tetrahydrofolate pools in response to 5-fluorouracil. *Fed. Proc.*, **41**, 1476.
Heidelberger, C., 1975, Fluorinated pyrimidines. *Prog. Nucleic Acid. Mol. Biol.*, **4**, 1–50.
Heidelberger, C., Danenberg, P. V. and Moran, R. G., 1983, Fluorinated pyrimidines and their nucleosides. *Adv. Enzymol.*, **4**, 58–119.
Henderson, J. F.and Khoo, M. K. Y., 1965, On the mechanism of feedback inhibition of purine biosynthesis de novo in Ehrlich ascites tumor cells in vitro. *J. Biol. Chem*, **240**, 3104–3109.
Henderson, J. F., Caldwell, I. C, and Paterson, A. R. P., 1967, Decreased feedback inhibition in a 6-(methylmercapto) purine ribonucleoside-resistant tumor. *Cancer Res.*, 27, 1773–1778.
Henderson, J.F., Bagnara, A. S., Crabtree, G. W., Lomax, C. A., Shantz, G. D. and Snyder, F. F., 1975, Regulation of enzymes of purine metabolism in intact tumor cells. *Adv. Enzyme Regul.*, **13**, 37–64.
Heppner, G. H., 1984, Tumor heterogeneity. *Cancer Res.*, **44**, 2259–2265.
Heppner, G. and Calabresi, P. C., 1977, Prolonged survival in mammary tumor-bearing mice treated with a regimen of methotrexate, leucovorin and 5-fluorouracil (Abstract). *Clin. Res.*, **25**, 407.
Herrman, R., Spehn, J., Beyer, J. H., von Franque, V., Schmieder, A., Holzman, K., and Abel, V. 1984, Sequential methotrexate and 5-fluorouracil: improved response rate in metastatic colon cancer. *J. Clin. Oncol.*, **2**, 591–594.
Hershfield, M. S. and Seegmiller, J. E., 1977, Coordinate regulation of the proximal and distal steps of the pathway of purine synthesis *de novo* in W1-L_2 lymphoblasts. *Adv. Exp. Med. Biol.*, **76**A, 19–29.
Hershko, A., Rozin, T., Shoshani, T. and Mager, J., 1969, Regulation of the synthesis of 5-phosphoribosyl-1-pyrophosphate in intact red blood cells and in cell-free preparation. *Biochim. Biophys. Acta*, **184**, 64–76.
Hewlett, J. S., 1979, Combination 6-mercaptopurine and 6-methylmercaptopurine

riboside in the treatment of adult acute leukemia: A Southwest Oncology Group Study. *Cancer Treat. Rep.*, **63**, 156–157.

Hill, D. L. and Bennett, L. L. Jr., 1969, Purification and properties of 5-phosphoribosylpyrophosphate amidotransferase from adenocarcinoma 755 cells. *Biochemistry*, **8**, 122–130.

Hitchings, G. H. and Elion, G. B., 1972, Mechanisms of action of purine and pyrimidine analogues. In *Cancer Chemotherapy II*, the Twenty-Second Hahnemann Symposium, edited by I. Brodsky, S. B. Kahn and J. H. Moyer (New York: Grune and Stratton), pp. 26–36.

Houghton, J. A., Maroda, S. J., Phillips, J. O. and Houghton, P. J., 1981, Biochemical determinants of responsiveness to 5-fluorouracil and its derivatives in xenografts of human colorectal adenocarcinoma in mice. *Cancer Res.*, **41** 144–149.

Hryniuk, W. M., 1986, Is More Better? *J. Clin. Oncol.*, **4**, 621–422

Hryniuk, W. M. and Bush, H., 1984, The importance of dose intensity in chemotherapy of metastatic breast cancer. *J. Clin. Oncol.*, **2** 1281–1288.

Hugles, S. M., 1984, Are guanine nucleotide binding proteins a distinct class of regulatory proteins? *FEBS Lett.*, **164**, 1–8.

Hunting, D., Gowans, B. and Henderson, J. F., 1985, Effects of 6-aminonicotinamide on cell growth. Poly (ADP)ribose synthesis and nucleotide metabolism. *Biochem. Pharmacol*, **34**, 3999–4003.

Ignoffo, R. J., Friedman, M. A., Gribble, M., Hannigan, J., Reynolds, R., Yu, K. P., Schiff, S. and Congdon, J. E., 1984, Phase II study of sequential methotrexate and 5-FU plus mitomycin and leucovorin in patients with disseminated large bowel cancer. A Northern California Oncology Group Study. *Cancer Treat. Rep.*, **68**, 983–988.

Ishiguro, K. and Sartorelli, A. C., 1984, Altered 5-phosphoribosyl 1-pyrophosphate amidotransferase activity in 6-thioguanine-resistant HL-60 human acute promyelocytic leukemia cells. *Cancer Res.*, **44**, 3679–3685.

Ishiguro, K. and Sartorelli, A. C., 1985, Enhancement of the differentiation-inducing properties of 6-thioguanine by hypoxanthine and its nucleosides in HL-60 promyelocytic leukemic cells. *Cancer Res.*, **45**, 91–95.

Ishiguro, K., Schwartz, E. L. and Sartorelli, A. C., 1984, Characterization of the metabolic forms of 6-thioguanine responsible for cytoxicity and induction of differentiation of HL-60 acute promyelocytic leukemic cells. *J. Cell Physiol.*, **121**, 383–390.

Ishii, K. and Green, H., 1973, Lethality of adenosine for cultured mammalian cells by interference with pyrimidine biosynthesis. *J. Cell Sci.*, **13**, 429–439.

Jackson, R. C., Ross, D. A., Harkrader, R. J. and Epstein, J., 1980, Biochemical approaches to enhancement of antitumor drug selectivity: selective protection of cells from 6-thioguanine and 6-mercaptopurine by adenosine. *Cancer Treat. Rep.*, **64**, 1347–1353.

Jediken, L. A. and Weinhouse, S., 1955, Metabolism of neoplastic tissue. VI. Assay of oxidized and reduce diphosphopyridine nucleotide in normal and neoplastic tissues. *J. Biol. Chem.*, **213**, 271–280.

Johnson, W. J. and McColl, J. D., 1955, 6-Aminonicotinamide—a potent nicotinamide antagonist. *Science.*, **122**, 834.

Johnson, R. K., Clement, J. J. and Howard, W. S., 1980, Treatment of murine tumors with 5-fluorouracil in combination with *de novo* pyrimidine synthesis inhibitors PALA or pyrazofurin. *Proc. Am. Assoc. Cancer Res.*, **21** 292.

Kawahata, R. T., Chuang, L. F., Holmberg, C. A., Osburn, B. I. and Chuang, R. Y., 1983, Inhibition of human lymphoma DNA-dependent RNA polymerase activity by 6-mercaptopurine ribonucleoside triphosphate. *Cancer Res.*, **43**, 3655–3659.

Kaye, S. B., Sangster, G., Hutcheon, A., *et al.*, 1984, Sequential methotrexate plus 5-FU in advanced breast and colorectal cancers: A Phase II study. *Cancer Treat. Rep.*, **68**, 547–548.

Kemeny, N., Ahmed, T., Michaelson, R., Harper, H., and Yip, L., 1984, Activity of sequential low-dose methotrexate and fluorouracil in advanced colorectal carcinoma: attempt at correlation with tissue and blood levels of phosphoribosylpyrophosphate. *J. Clin. Oncol.*, **2**, 311–315.

Keppler, D., Rudiger, J., Bischoff, E. and Decker, K., 1970, The trapping of uridine phosphates by D-galactosamine, D-glucosamine, 2-deoxy-D-galactose. A study on the mechanism of galactosamine hepatitis. *Eur. J. Biochem.*, **17**, 246–253.

Klubes, P. and Cerna, I., 1983, Use of uridine rescue to enhance the antitumor selectivity of 5-fluorouracil. *Cancer Res.*, **43**, 3182–3186.

Klubes, P., Cerna, I. and Meldon, M., 1982, Uridine rescue from the lethal toxicity of 5-fluorouracil in mice. *Cancer Chemother. Pharmacol.*, **8**, 17–21.

Koizumi, S., Curt, G., Fine, R., Griffen, J. and Chabner, B., 1985, Formation of methotrexate polyglutamates in purified myeloid precursor cells from normal human bone marrow. *J. Clin. Invest.*, **75**, 1008–1014.

Konits, P. H., Egorin, M. J., Van Echo, D. A., Aisner, J., Andrews, P. A., May, M. E., Bachur, N. R. and Wiernik, P. H., 1982, Phase II evaluation and plasma pharmacokinetics of high-dose intravenous 6-thioguanine in patients with colorectal carcinoma. *Cancer Chemother. Pharmacol.*, **8**, 199–203.

Krakoff, I. H. and Balis, M. E., 1959, Studies of the uricogenic effect of 2-substituted thiadiazoles in man. *J. Clin. Invest.*, **38**, 904–915.

Kufe, D. W. and Egan, E. M., 1981, Enhancement of 5-fluorouracil incorporation into human lymphoblast ribonucleic acid. *Biochem. Pharmacol.*, **30**, 129–133.

Kufe, D. W., and Major, P. P., 1981, 5-Fluorouracil incorporation into human breast carcinoma RNA correlates with cytoxicity. *J. Biol. Chem.*, **256**, 9803–9805.

Kufe, D. W., Major, P. P., Egan, E. M. and Loh, E., 1981, 5-Fluoro-2′-deoxyuridine incorporation in L1210 DNA. *J. Biol. Chem.*, **256**, 8885–8888.

Kwan, S-W., Kwan, S-P. and Mandel, H. G., 1973, The incorporation of 6-thioguanine into RNA fractions and its effect on RNA and protein biosynthesis in mouse sarcoma 180 cells. *Cancer Res.*, **3**, 950—955.

Laskin, J. D., Evans, R. M., Slocum, H. K., *et al.*, 1979, Basis for natural variation in sensitivity to 5-fluorouracil in mouse and human cells in culture. *Cancer Res.*, **39**, 383–390.

Lazo, J. S., Hwang, K. M. and Sartorelli, A. C., 1977, Inhibition of L-fucose incorporation into glycoprotein of sarcoma 180 cells by 6-thioguanine. *Cancer Res.*, **37**, 4250–4255.

Lazo, J. S., Shansky, C. W. and Sartorelli, A. C., 1979, Reduction in cell surface concanavalin A binding and mannose incorporation into glycoproteins of sarcoma 180 by 6-thioguanine. *Biochem. Pharmacol.*, **28**, 583–588.

Lee, M. Y. W. T., Byrnes, J. J., Downey, K. M. and So, A. G., 1980, Mechanisms of inhibition of deoxyribonucleic acid synthesis by 1-β-D-arabinofuranosyladenosine triphosphate and its potentiation by 6-mercaptopurine ribonucleoside 5′-monophosphate. *Biochemistry*, **19**, 215–219.

Lee, S. H. and Sartorelli, A. C., 1981 a, The effects of inhibitors of DNA biosynthesis on the cytotoxicity of 6-thioguanine. *Cancer Biochem. Biophys.*, **5**, 189–194.

Lee, S. H. and Sartorelli, A. C., 1981 b, Conversion of 6-thioguanine to the nucleoside level by purine nucleoside phosphorylase of Sarcoma 180 and Sarcoma 180 ITG ascites cells. *Cancer Res.*, **41**, 1086–1090.

Lee, S. H., Huang, Y-M. and Sartorelli, A. C., 1978, Alkaline phosphatase activities of 6-thiopurine-sensitive and -resistant sublines of sarcoma 180. *Cancer Res.*, **38**, 2413–2418.

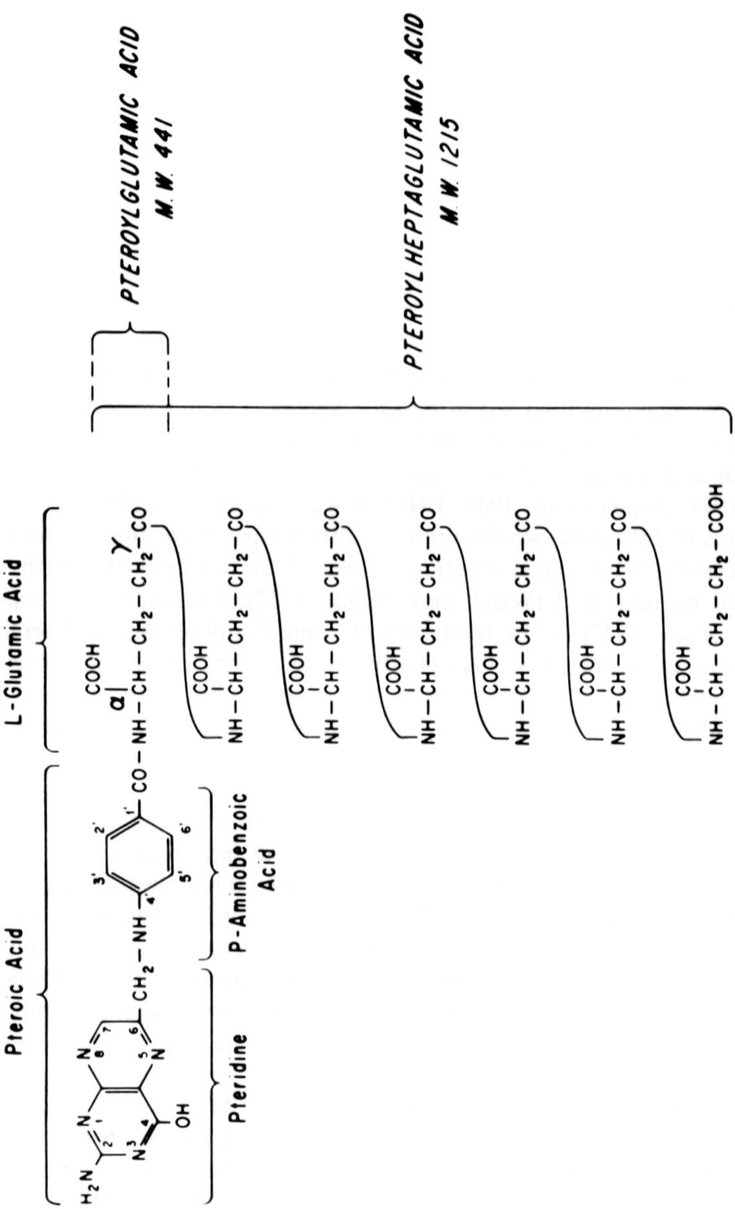

Figure 1. The structure of folic acid (pteroylglutamine) and its heptaglutamate derivative is shown. By convention, folic acid is the monoglutamate. Therefore, the heptaglutamate is folate plus six additional glutamate residues.

heroic feat. Readers needing more data are encouraged to seek additional information from these more specialized, detailed texts (for example, see texts of Hutchison and Schmid, 1984; Winick *et al.*, 1985; Blakely, 1984).

Clinical use of MTX

The spectrum of clinical activity of MTX is extensive. It is a mainstay in the treatment of acute lymphoblastic leukaemia (ALL) of childhood, both for systemic and central nervous system (CNS) components of the disease. MTX is also a commonly used agent in the treatment of lymphomas, osteogenic sarcoma and in squamous cell carcinoma of the head and neck. In combination therapy or as a single agent with other agents it is also used in the treatment of breast cancer, brain tumours and malignant carcinomatosis. It is given orally, intramuscularly, intravenously, subcutaneously and as already noted it is one of the few agents that can be given intrathecally. Use of a biochemical antidote, 5-formyltetrahydrofolate (leucovorin, citrovorum factor) has also allowed dose escalations from 0·5 mg to >30 g/m^2. The rationale and basis for leucovorin rescue will be discussed below and has been reported elsewhere (Goldman and Matherly, 1985).

Acute lymphoblastic leukaemia

Aminopterin was initially used in the 1940s, but due to more predictable dose-related toxicities, MTX has become the anti-fol of choice for the treatment of ALL. Although it causes a clinical remission in 20–30% of cases treated (Acute Leukemia Group B, 1961), MTX is primarily used in the continuation phase of therapy (Acute Leukemia Group B, 1965, 1969; Frei, 1984). It is usually administered in doses ranging from 20–40 mg/m^2 weekly in combination with 6-mercaptopurine. Results of more recent studies allow the suggestion that periodic pulses of moderate doses (1000 mg/m^2) may lower the incidence of testicular leukaemia and bone marrow relapse (Moe *et al.*, 1981); however it has not lowered the incidence of CNS leukaemia in the typical child with ALL (Freeman *et al.*, 1983; Haas *et al.*, 1983). High-dose MTX during induction therapy has also proven too toxic when given with other agents (Rivera *et al.*, 1985). In addition to systemic administration, MTX is also given intrathecally, either alone or in combination with hydrocortisone and cytosine arabinoside to treat and prevent the occurrence of CNS leukaemia. Routine prophylactic therapy of the CNS has decreased the incidence of CNS disease from approximately 80 to 5% (Frei, 1984). Current studies are evaluating different combinations of chemo- and radiotherapy in order to maintain the successful prevention of CNS disease but with less toxicity (see below).

Lymphoma

As the efficacy of MTX in the treatment of leukaemia evolved, its activity in lymphoma was also established (Levitt *et al.*, 1972). Recent studies with high-dose MTX (HDMTX) and with moderate- and high-dose MTX in combination chemotherapy regimens also support the use of MTX in the treatment of lymphomas of all histological types (Fisher *et al.*, 1983; Cabanillas *et al.*, 1982; Skarin *et al.*, 1983). The treatment of patients with CNS lymphoma with intrathecal or intraventricular MTX has also been shown to be effective (Abelson *et al.*, 1981). Current clinical trials have been designed to test HDMTX vs. standard or moderate-dose MTX in combination with other known effective lymphoma agents. So far, there is no strong evidence to support the superiority of HDMTX compared to more standard or conventional doses (Ginsberg *et al.*, 1985; Shipp *et al.*, 1985; Vogler *et al.*, 1979).

Osteogenic sarcoma

Soon after the introduction of HDMTX by Djerassi *et al.*, in 1972, the successful treatment of a few patients with metastatic osteogenic sarcoma was reported (Jaffe, 1972). Since then a series of studies from Memorial Sloan-Kettering by Rosen and associates have reported the successful treatment of osteogenic sarcoma using HDMTX (10–20 g/m^2) in combination with other agents, primarily anthracyclines, platinum, bleomycin, cyclophosphamide and actinomycin D (Pratt, 1981; Rosen *et al.*, 1982). The apparent therapeutic efficacy of combination chemotherapy in an adjuvant setting has been reported by the Pediatric Oncology Group (Link *et al.*, 1986) and other cooperative groups (Winkler *et al.*, 1984). However, despite its widespread use in this relatively uncommon malignancy, there is little dose–response data and only a very limited analysis of tumour MTX content following HDMTX (Samuels *et al.*, 1984). This latter point is important when one considers the morbidity and expense of HDMTX. Since other clinical trials in breast cancer, squamous cell carcinoma of the head and neck and lymphoma have failed to show the superiority of HDMTX over more standard doses (Taylor *et al.*, 1984; Vogler *et al.*, 1979; Shipp *et al.*, 1985) and laboratory studies revealed little dose response with respect to MTX tissue content in both animals and clinical samples (Winick *et al.*, 1985), a trial of conventional, perhaps even orally administered MTX vs. HDMTX should be considered.

Head and neck squamous cell carcinoma

This is clearly a drug-sensitive tumour. Responses to antimetabolites, natural products and alkylating agents have been documented. Combination chemotherapy and chemotherapy regimens with radiation and surgery are used in curative attempts. MTX and platinum are two of the most active drugs. As in the treatment of other malignancies, the optimal schedule and dose have not yet been determined. Clinical trials during the 1980s have not shown the superiority of HDMTX with leucovorin rescue over more conventional, lower doses of MTX (Kirkwood *et al.*, 1981; Taylor *et al.*, 1984, Coleman *et al.*, 1981).

Breast cancer

MTX has been shown to have activity against breast cancer (Carter 1974). Objective responses in 30–35% of patients treated with weekly doses of 25–50 mg/m^2 are not significantly improved with escalation to the "high-dose" range (HDMTX), but the response rate seen is still among the highest of any single agent tested. Recent studies have been designed to evaluate the effectiveness of different doses and schedules in combination with other agents (Hortobagyi *et al.*, 1983). The combination of MTX with hormonal treatment (which may synchronize cells) has been promising, but more clinical trials are needed (Allegra, 1983). MTX has also been used intraventricularly or intrathecally for the treatment of meningeal carcinomatosis (Abelson *et al.*, 1981; Yap *et al.*, 1982).

Gestational trophoblastic neoplasms (GTN)

This group of malignancies, which includes hydatidiform moles, invasive moles and choriocarcinoma, has been a model disease which is cured with single-agent chemotherapy (Li *et al.*, 1956). The production of a tumour marker, chorionic gonadotrophin, long-term follow-up for toxicity (so far nearly three decades) and the high percentage of complete remissions with single-agent therapy are some of the reasons why this group of tumours has been a model for chemotherapy (Ross *et al.*, 1965, Hammond *et al.*, 1967). Current trials of combination chemotherapy for advanced stage disease (metastatic) include MTX and appear to be promising, but additional follow-up time is needed in order to more completely assess the efficacy of these newer regimens (Begent and Bagshawe, 1982; Newlands, 1982).

The initial therapy of GTN was based upon data suggesting that folic acid was required for normal embryonic development and that MTX inhibited the oestrogen-induced growth of the chick oviduct (Hertz and Tullner, 1949). The initial success in the treatment of patients with metastatic disease was followed by additional single-agent studies and combination therapy with MTX and actinomycin D (Ross *et al.*, 1965). Studies of MTX doses and schedule are in progress (Smith *et al.*, 1982). To date, repetitive low-dose (15–25 mg daily for five days without leucovorin rescue is a commonly used schedule for MTX and has become the gold standard for treatment.

Brain tumours

MTX can be safely administered intrathecally and intraventricularly. It was initially used for the treatment of CNS leukaemia (Whiteside *et al.*, 1958), but has also been used for meningeal carcinomatosis (Yap *et al.*, 1982) and in the treatment of primary brain tumours (Rosen *et al.*, 1977; Mooney *et al.*, 1983). Since MTX does not significantly cross the blood–brain barrier (about 1–2% of the concomitant plasma concentration), most investigators have used HDMTX or agents such as mannitol to "open" the blood–brain barrier for short periods of time with the simultaneous administration of intracarotid MTX (Neuwelt *et al.*, 1981, 1982). The efficacy of this regimen has yet to be proven. In light of recent data showing a saturable, specific transport system for folate and MTX which is functional in the nanomolar range, the utility of HDMTX and/or intracarotid infusion should be carefully evaluated (Kamen, 1986). This is especially true since a review of the clinical literature reveals significant neurological sequelae in patients who received MTX with or without irradiation (Allen *et al.*, 1980; Abelson, 1978).

Non-malignant disorders

MTX was used in the early 1950s for the treatment of psoriatic arthritis (Gubner *et al.*, 1951). During the past three decades it has become accepted therapy in psoriasis (Stern *et al.*, 1982) and more recently has achieved more general use in the treatment of patients with arthritis who have failed conventional steroidal and non-steroidal anti-inflammatory therapy (Anderson *et al.*, 1984; Ward, 1984; Weinstein and Frost, 1971; Willkens and Watson, 1982). The exact mechanism of action of MTX in these disorders is not yet fully understood. The drug is acting as an anti-flammatory agent, not necessarily as an immuno-suppressive agent. Recent clinical trials of MTX in arthritis have been published and the reader is referred to them for more specific information (Weinblatt *et al.*, 1985; Kremer, 1985).

Toxicity

As with other anti-proliferative (anti-neoplastic agents), MTX exerts its toxicity primarily on growing, self-renewing tissues. The primary toxicity is to the bone marrow and gastrointestinal system, in particular mucositis. In addition to these obvious toxicities, MTX is also associated with hepatic (Parker *et al.*, 1980; Lawrence *et al.*, 1983; Harb *et al.*, 1983; Custer *et al.*, 1977; Nyfors and Poulsen, 1977), pulmonary (Sostman *et al.*, 1976; see Clinical-Pathological Conference, *New England Journal of Medicine*, **312**, 359–369, 1985) and CNS toxicity (Fritsch and Urban, 1984; Allen *et al.*, 1980; Abelson, 1978). These problems may or may not be related to anti-proliferative effects of MTX and are often not dose-related. In particular the long-term CNS toxicity of MTX seen in patients, especially children with acute lymphoblastic leukaemia, may be related to the effect of MTX on folate metabolism in specific cells in the CNS or some as yet undefined parameter. The subject of neurotoxicity of the brain and in the inter-relationships of MTX and folate have been reviewed (Abelson, 1978; Kamen, 1986). MTX with or without cranial irradiation has been associated with a devastating leukoencephalopathy and mineralizing microangiopathy (Bleyer, 1981). In the spinal cord, it has also been implicated in the development of a leukomyelopathy, a pathological lesion similar to the encephalopathy seen in the white matter of the brain. Recent studies of the folate and MTX content of tissues obtained from animals and patients treated with repetitive low-dose MTX for periods of more than one year have shown a significant folate deficiency in several tissues, including the brain (Kamen *et al.*, 1981, 1984 a). Accumulation of MTX polyglutamates has also been shown (Krakower and Kamen, 1983). The mechanism for the folate loss is not fully understood, but may be related to MTX accumulation and alterations in the normal homeostatic mechanisms for folate. The biochemical interactions between folate(s) and MTX are presented in more detail below.

Biochemical features

Introduction

The prototypic anti-fol is a 4-amino-substituted pterin compound (figure 2 and compare figure 1). The substitution of the 4-hydroxyl with an amino moiety results in a folate analogue which has a several thousand-fold increase in affinity for the main intracellular target, dihydrofolate reductase (DHFR). The K_m for the natural substrate, dihydrofolate, is generally in the micromolar range while the K_i for MTX is below 10^{-10} M. It is this remarkable increase in affinity compared to the natural substrate that resulted in MTX being considered a "stoichiometric inhibitor" of DHFR.

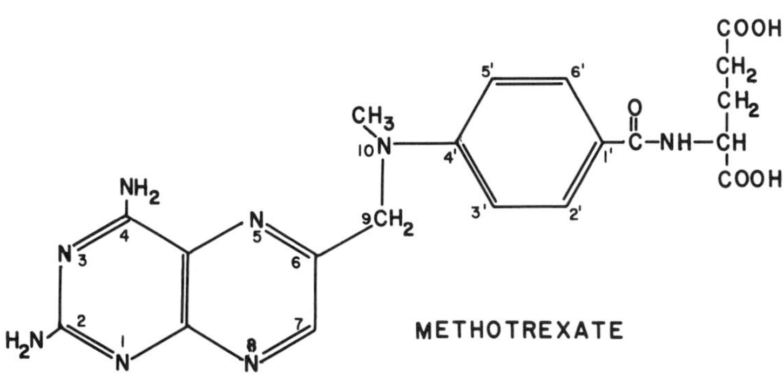

Figure 2. The structure of methotrexate is shown. Compare to figure 1. The N-10 methyl group is the difference between methotrexate and aminopterin.

In regard to MTX metabolism, until the mid 1970s little besides MTX transport and the MTX–DHFR interaction was studied. However, with the recognition that MTX was a substrate for folate polyglutamate synthetase (Baugh *et al.*, 1973) an additional, new field was opened. MTX polyglutamates have an extended intracellular half-life compared to MTX and are inhibitors of enzymatic reactions other than DHFR reduction of folate (see below). Combining the techniques of HPLC and radio-ligand binding assay, also developed and refined during the past decade, allows the assay of MTX and derivatives in human tissue biopsy samples containing as little as 20–30 pmol of MTX (Kamen and Winick, 1986). This facilitates an analysis of human pharmacodynamics of MTX *in situ* and has resulted in a reappraisal and refinement of MTX dose and scheduling.

The number of studies of the hydroxylation reaction to form 7-hydroxymethotrexate increased during the 1970s as this metabolite was found in plasma after the administration of HDMTX. Although this metabolite is not a potent inhibitor of DHFR, it has a very long plasma half-life compared to MTX (Breithaupt and Kuenzlen, 1982). It is found intracellularly but its effects on normal folate homeostasis are not fully understood. However, several studies have shown that 7OHMTX can be polyglutamated. Further, the mono- and polyglutamate compounds can interfere with both folate and MTX metabolism and transport (Fabre *et al.*, 1983; Gaukroger and Wilson, 1984; McGuire *et al.*, 1984).

Transport of MTX is via the same pathway cells used for the reduced folate co-factors (serum folate is 5-methyltetrahydrofolate). The membrane receptor for folate has been characterized (Kamen and Capdevila 1986, McHugh and Cheng, 1979; Antony *et al.*, 1985) but the precise mechanism of folate transport across the membrane is not yet known. Similarly, the control mechanism(s) of folate accumulation is not yet defined.

Selected recent advances in our understanding of DHFR, MTX and folate transport and polyglutamation, and additional target enzymes are detailed below. If a more thorough, historically complete overview is needed, previously noted texts and symposia should be reviewed (see texts of Hutchison *et al.*, 1984 and Winick *et al.*, 1985). The material discussed here is predominantly work done during this decade.

Dihydrofolate reductase

DHFR has been purified, cloned and sequenced (Bolin *et al.*,1982; Pan *et al.*, 1983). The identification and selection of human cell lines containing large quantities of DHFR have facilitated the study of the human enzyme (Domin *et al.*, 1981; Delcamp *et al.*, 1983; Morandi and Attardi, 1981). This has been important because, as opposed to animal tissues and cell lines *in vitro*, human tissue obtained by biopsy contains little DHFR (Kamen *et al.*, 1985). The reasons are not fully known. There is a great deal of similarity among the several enzymes that have been purified and sequenced. A typical DHFR is a single polypeptide of approximately 20–21 kilodalton, making DHFR one of the smallest enzymes requiring a reduced pyridine nucleotide co-factor. The preferred substrate is dihydrofolate as opposed to the fully oxidized folic acid. The turnover number for dihydrofolate by human enzyme is 850–1000 per minute. This compares to a value of 1–2 for folic acid per minute (Capdevila and Kamen, 1985). Studies with X-ray crystallography are revealing more information about the mechanism of drug binding and the interaction of the reduced pyridine co-factor in the formation of a ternary rather than a simple binary enzyme–MTX complex. The presence of NADPH has been shown to increase the affinity of the enzyme for MTX (and in studies of bacterial enzymes, trimethoprim) by several orders of magnitude (see Blakely, 1984). In fact, in the absence of adequate amounts of NADPH, MTX is a competitive but reversible inhibitor of DHFR (Kamen *et al.*, 1983).

A great number of structure–activity studies of anti-fols with DHFR have clearly shown the requirement for the 4-amino substitution. Alterations of the N10 position, quinazoline compounds (5,8-dideaza-pteridine structure) or alterations of the glutamic acid moiety have also been shown to have effects on the enzyme–drug complex. This work has been reviewed in detail (Blakely, 1984). The results of the computer–X-ray studies may assist in the development of better anti-fols based upon the structure–activity requirements for tight binding of the drug and enzyme.

Folate and methotrexate transport

It is important to understand folate and MTX transport and accumulation by normal and neoplastic cells, because the drug exerts its cytotoxic effects in the cell, not the plasma or tissue culture media. MTX is transported into cells via the carrier system present for the naturally occurring reduced folates (reviewed by Sirotnak, 1985). Folic acid is generally considered not to share this system (see below). The carrier-mediated transport of MTX and folate is unusual in several respects with regard to energy requirements. Specifically, certain metabolic poisons such as dinitrophenol will actually increase the accumulation of MTX intracellularly by inhibiting the efflux carrier but not the influx system (Fry *et al.*, 1980). Thus, the currently accepted model for folate and MTX transport consists of two parallel systems, one for influx and the other for efflux. In general, the K_m for influx of reduced folates and MTX is approximately μM in many different cell lines studied *in vitro* (Sirotnak, 1985).

The identification of both membrane-bound and soluble high-affinity folate binding factors (K_m of $<$ nM) has resulted in a re-evaluation of folate and MTX accumulation *in vitro*. Three laboratories (Kamen and Capdevila, 1986, McHugh and Cheng, 1979; Antony *et al.*, 1985) have shown that the high-affinity folate binder present on the membrane of both human KB cells and monkey kidney epithelial cells binds reduced and oxidized folates and MTX at physiological plasma folate concentrations (10–20 nM). Moreover, it was shown that at these concentrations the cells were capable of transporting and accumulating folate such that the intracellular concentration of folate exceeded that in the medium by several hundred-fold after four hours of uptake at 37°C (Kamen and Capdevila, 1986). Interestingly, folic acid had the greatest affinity for the receptor (K_d of 0·4 nM) but the slowest rate of accumulation. This apparent paradox is explained by knowing that the folic acid was not released intracellularly because the affinity for the receptor is great, relative to the reduced folates. This may explain why previous studies failed to recognize that folic acid shared the transport system with reduced folates and MTX. It also explains why low (but physiological) concentrations of folic acid cannot support the growth of cells *in vitro* as well as reduced folates. Since most prior studies of folate and anti-fol transport analysed folate and MTX uptake in folate-replete cells often grown in a large excess of a non-physiological folate (folic acid), the observed K_m values may be high compared to plasma folate (0·01 μM). This is because the receptor is either saturated or down-regulated by the high folate content of medium and cells (Kamen and Capdevila, 1986). The failure of the cells to significantly concentrate folate from the medium can also be explained by knowing the cells are already folate-replete. The "accumulation" of the radiolabelled folate could simply represent exchange with an internal pool of folate polyglutamates.

Folate polyglutamate synthetase

As early as the 1940s it was known that folate growth factors were most likely in a more complex polypeptide structure. The early nomenclature referred to this growth factor as vitamin Bc conjugate. Incubation of tissue extracts at 37°C converted the inactive complex to an active growth factor (microbiological assay). The complex was shown to contain folate with extra glutamic acid residues added via the gamma carboxyl of the terminal glutamate residue (Figure 1). The report of McBurney and Whitemore in 1974 clearly established the importance of folate polyglutamates for normal cellular growth. Intracellular folates are primarily in this form, with 5–7 extra glutamyl residues predominating (Covey, 1980). Studies of folate-requiring enzymes (e.g., methylene tetrahydrofolate reductase, *de novo* purine synthesis (see below)) have shown that these folate polyglutamate derivatives are not merely storage forms of the vitamin but are actually the preferred substrates. As the glutamyl chain length increases, there is often an increase in the V_{max} and decrease in the K_m until a certain number of glutamates have been added. Thereafter, there is little increase in enzyme activity (Mathews, 1980).

Despite the studies of folate polyglutamates, it was not until 1973 that MTX was shown to be a substrate for folate polyglutamate synthetase by rat liver (Baugh *et al.*, 1973). Several years later MTX was found in a polygamma-glutamyl form in human liver (Jacobs *et al.*, 1977; see also metabolic studies below). MTX polyglutamates have a long intracellular half-life compared to MTX, inhibit enzymes other than DHFR (see next section) and may inhibit folate accumulation at the level of membrane transport and polyglutamation.

The study of purified folate polyglutamate synthetase (FPGS) from mammalian liver (McGuire *et al.*, 1980, 1983; Moran and Colman, 1984; Schoo *et al.*, 1985) has revealed a stringent requirement for the terminal glutamate and confirmed the requirement for a purine nucleoside triphosphate (ATP or dATP) as an energy source. FPGS has a molecular size of approximately 60–70 kilodalton and a pH optimum in the alkaline range. The reaction is a highly ordered Ter Ter mechanism. The nucleotide binds first, followed by the folate and then the glutamate. Tetrahydrofolate is the preferred substrate but substituted folates and oxidized folates are also substrates. In regard to specific inhibitors of FPGS, several groups have synthesized folate congeners in attempts to inhibit FPGS and/or DHFR (Rosowsky *et al.*, 1984; McGuire and Coward, 1985; Galivan *et al.*, 1985). Since folate polyglutamates are required for cellular proliferation, it is clearly a worthwhile target for anti-neoplastic agents. Whether or not the therapeutic index will be sufficient to warrant clinical trials remains to be seen.

Purine synthesis

De novo purine synthesis (carbon atoms at positions 2 and 8) requires two steps dependent on folate cofactors. The enzymes, 5-aminoimidazole-4-carboxamide ribotide (AICAR) transformylase and glycinamide ribonucleotide (GAR) transformylase utilize 10-formyltetrahydrofolate as a substrate. Studies of these two enzymes has revealed that folate polyglutamates are the preferred substrates. For example, the K_m and V_{max} for the pentaglutamate are approximately 8-fold lower and 1·3-fold higher respectively than the monoglutamate when partially purified AICAR transformylase from MCF-7 breast cancer cells was analysed (Allegra *et al.*, 1985 a). Inhibition by MTX polyglutamates is greater than that seen with the monoglutamate. Inhibition is competitive in nature and AICAR tranformylase is more affected by the glutamyl chain length than the GAR transformylase enzyme. In addition to the direct inhibition of these enzymes by MTX metabolites, the formation of oxidized folates, generated by MTX inhibition of DHFR, may also ihibit *de novo* purine synthesis as well as other enzymes such as thymidylate synthase (Baggott *et al.*, 1986).

Pharmacology

Human pharmacology of MTX has been extensively studied. The disposition of radiolabelled MTX administered to animals has been detailed elsewhere (Zaharko *et al.*, 1971). Current pharmacokinetic studies are done using radio-ligand binding assays (Myers *et al.*, 1975; Kamen *et al.*, 1976; Buice *et al.*, 1980) or if less sensitivity is required and time is important, EMIT assays are used. The former methods are generally sensitive to 0·5 nM and the latter to 100 nM. During the last decade many pharmacokinetic studies of intravenously and enterally administered MTX have been done. Thorough reviews have been published (Bleyer, 1978; Schornagel and McVie, 1983).

MTX equilibrates in total body water, including "third spaces" such as pleural effusions and ascites. The drug exits these spaces more slowly and therefore toxicity can develop in patients with significant effusions. MTX enters the CNS compartment slowly. The blood–brain barrier limits the penetration of MTX into the cerebrospinal fluid to about 2% of the concomitant plasma concentration. Age of the patient, duration of therapy and other drugs may also influence MTX pharmacokinetics (Lokiec *et al.*, 1982).

In low-dose regimens (<50 mg/m^2), MTX undergoes little metabolism. Most of the drug detectable in the urine is unmetabolized. At doses up to approximately 25–30 mg/m^2 oral MTX is nearly completely absorbed. However, there is a great deal of inter-patient variability as to the peak concentration achieved as well as the time of the peak plasma concentration (Pinkerton *et al.*, 1980 a, b). This has been most completely documented in children with ALL taking MTX on a weekly schedule as part of a continuation phase of therapy. The absorption is also affected by the particular preparation used (Mahoney *et al.*, 1984).

The importance of monitoring plasma MTX during HDMTX therapy (Bertino, 1981) cannot be overstated. There is clearly a threshold plasma concentration above which MTX is toxic. Based upon empirical clinical experience, studies of MTX cell kill *in vitro* and the analysis of receptor-mediated folate and MTX transport noted above, a plasma MTX greater than 0.1 μM would be expected to be cytotoxic. Since plasma folate concentration is approximately 0·01 μM, this value is not surprising. Administering HDMTX also results in the formation of 7OHMTX, primarily via hepatic aldehyde oxidase. This metabolite of MTX has a longer half-life than MTX (23·8 vs. 2·1 hours; Breithaupt and Kuenzlen, 1982) and is actually five times less soluble than MTX at acid pH. Evans and colleagues (1983) also noted the rapid appearance and prolonged half-life of 7OHMTX during the following 24 h infusions of MTX (1000 mg/m^2) for the treatment of leukaemia in children. Despite the higher, more prolonged plasma concentration of 7OHMTX compared to MTX, no metabolite was found in the spinal fluid.

The effects of protein binding on the elimination of MTX and 7OHMTX have also been studied. Paxton (1982) noted that approximately half of plasma MTX is bound. Binding was measured by ultrafiltration dialysis. The percentage bound was independent of the plasma concentration in the range of 100 μM to 1 nM. This implies that there is a high-capacity, essentially unsaturable, low-affinity binding of MTX by serum proteins. Serum binding of

7OHMTX was reported by Lopez *et al.* (1986). As compared to MTX, there are two binding sites for 7OHMTX on human serum albumin (free of fatty acid contaminants) based upon Scatchard analysis. One site is at least partially competitive with MTX, the second was not and considered to be unique for 7OHMTX compared to MTX due to the presence of the OH group. A total of 65% of the 7OHMTX was bound when the initial conditions were set up to mimic the peak plasma concentration of 7OHMTX (560 μM) after a six-hour infusion of HDMTX. This is somewhat higher than the 40–50% of MTX bound to serum proteins. At a concentration of 10 μM, which is the plasma concentration of 7OHMTX 60 hours after an HDMTX infusion, 93% of the 7OHMTX was bound. This value agrees well with the value of 95% reported by Breithaupt and Kuenzlen (1982). The clinical significance of these findings is not yet clear. Sixty hours after an HDMTX infusion, the concentration of MTX would be significantly less than 10 μM and will generally be in the non-toxic range. The clinical significance of 7OHMTX must await further knowledge of the intracellular interaction of MTX, folate and this metabolite. However, it is reasonable to assume that an elevated plasma concentration of 7OHMTX could cause renal damage by direct precipitation in the tubules. Since 7OHMTX has such a long half-life and its concentration will exceed that of MTX by several hundred-fold, this could be a source of the major renal damage associated with HDMTX regimens. This point may assume more significance in light of reports of unexplained but significant morbidity and mortality associated with the administration of HDMTX following treatment with platinum, a renal toxic anti-neoplastic (Haim *et al.*, 1984 and see chapter 6).

Biological activity and metabolism

As briefly reviewed above and presented in greater detail elsewhere (Goldman and Matherly, 1985; Matherly *et al.*, 1983, 1984, 1986), there is a distinct relationship between the cytotoxic action and the metabolism of MTX. In the early years, the main site of action, and the cause/effect relationship of the drug's activity was considered to be the inhibition of DHFR. This inhibition would indirectly cause a thymine-less and in some cases eventually a purine-less death. This presumed mechanism of action also led to several hypotheses to explain cellular resistance and the rationale for the development of HDMTX therapy. Mechanisms of resistance include an altered or increased concentration of DHFR or decreased transport of the drug (Bertino *et al.*, 1981). The identification of the now well recognized phenomena of gene amplification and homogeneously staining regions of chromosomes containing the DHFR gene was an early example of mechanism for drug resistance (Schimke, 1986). These models defined or selected for *in vitro* have not yet been found to be clinically significant. However, the availability of a biochemical antidote (5-formyltetrahydrofolate, leucovorin) and the laboratory data to support the efficacy of HDMTX with leucovorin rescue (Goldin *et al.*, 1953) has led to the continued use of HDMTX. As noted earlier, few studies support the superiority of HDMTX over more conventional doses. This may be explained by more recent observations concerning the inter-relationship of folate and MTX transport and accumulation. The time of exposure to the drug is clearly a more important parameter than the concentration in the medium (or plasma) once a certain critical concentration has been reached (Keefe *et al.*, 1982). That is, intracellular metabolism rather than transport may be a more critical factor of cytotoxicity and the rate-limiting step. The accumulation of MTX by select tissues *in situ* seems to bear this point out. Specifically, there was little dose response over a 1000-fold increase in dose when tissue MTX was determined 3–24 hours after a single injection of MTX was given to rats (Winick *et al.*, 1985). In other words, once the plasma (or extracellular) concentration of drug exceeds the K_m for transport (e.g., at a V_{max} concentration), increasing the concentration further may add little to the observed cytotoxicity and in fact may contribute to acute toxicity, *in vivo*, if the drug or metabolite was to precipitate in the renal tubules (see pharmacology section).

The current studies showing the metabolism of MTX to polyglutamates and the inhibition of other folate-mediated reactions noted above by these MTX metabolites or even oxidized folate polyglutamates (Allegra *et al.*, 1985 a, b; Baggott *et al.*, 1986) are assuming a more prominent role in our understanding the possible mechanism(s) of action of MTX. These additional sites of action are also potential targets for the development of new anti-fols having enzymes other than DHFR as a prime target.

The metabolism of MTX to polyglutamates and the subsequent development of a tissue folate deficiency may be important factors with regard to long-term administration and potential toxicity (Kamen, 1986). The exact mechanism of the MTX-induced folate deficiency is not yet fully known, but it is probably related to MTX metabolism to polyglutamates and either the inhibition of folate accumulation or the resultant accumulation and then loss of partially oxidized folates from tissues. Since inborn errors of folate metabolism are associated with neurological and other developmental abnormalities, it is not unreasonable to assume that the drug-induced folate deficiency could be at least partially responsible for some of the long-term sequelae of repetitive therapy with MTX, especially seen in the CNS of young children treated for leukaemia.

In summary, as an anti-fol anti-metabolite, MTX interferes with folate homeostasis at many different sites. During the three decades of its use, a more detailed and complete understanding of the importance of folate metabolism and folate-mediated reactions has been acquired. Thus MTX has been both a successfully used anti-neoplastic agent and a probe to aid in our understanding of normal and neoplastic cell growth and multiplication.

Future prospects

As may be implied from the summary, a more complete understanding of enzyme reactions requiring folate co-factors and the relationship of MTX and folate metabolism may lead to a better understanding of one-carbon metabolism and its critical role in cell processes. As a corollary, this knowledge could lead to the development of second- and third-generation anti-fols with more specific or select targets. The new quinazoline anti-fols such as trimetrexate (Elslager *et al.*, 1983; Kamen *et al.*, 1984) or BW301U (Iland *et al.*, 1985) designed to overcome resistance to MTX defined *in vitro* represent such a class of compounds. In addition, MTX analogues and pyrimidine analogues have also been synthesized (Sirotnak *et al.*, 1982; Currie *et al.*, 1980) in efforts to improve efficacy or overcome resistance. Whether or not folate polyglutamate synthetase, thymidylate synthase, purine synthetic enzymes or the folate receptor can be successfully exploited as targets for anti-metabolite therapy remains to be seen. If folate homeostasis is critically related to or regulated by events in the cell cycle, then perhaps a more thorough understanding of these events in normal and neoplastic cells may result in drugs with a higher therapeutic index than those currently in use. The selected use of novel anti-fols with selected targets may be useful both as biochemical tools to further study cell metabolism and as anti-neoplastic agents.

References

Abelson, H. T., 1978, Methotrexate and central nervous system toxicity. *Cancer Treat. Rep.*, **62**, 1999.

Abelson, H. T., Kufe, D. W., Skarin, A. T., Major, P., Ensminger, W., Beardsley, G. P. and Canellos, G. P., 1981. Treatment of central nervous system tumors with methotrexate. *Cancer Treat. Rep.*, **65**, (Suppl), 137–140.

Acute Leukemia Group B, 1961, Studies of sequential and combination anti-metabolite therapy in acute leukemia: 6-mercaptopurine and methotrexate. *Blood*, **18**, 431.

Acute Leukemia Group B, 1965, New treatment schedule with improved survival in childhood leukemia. *J. Am. Med. Ass.*, **194**, 187–193.

Acute Leukemia Group B, 1969, Acute lymphocytic leukemia in children; maintenance therapy with methotrexate administered intermittently. *J. Am. Med. Ass.*, **207**, 923.

Allegra, C. J., 1983, Methotrexate and 5-fluorouracil following tamoxifen and Premarin in advanced breast cancer. *Seminars in Oncology*, **10**, (2, Suppl 2) 23–28.

Allegra, C. J., Chabner, B. A., Drake, J. C., Lutz, R., Rodband, D. and Jolivet, J., 1974, Enhanced inhibition of thymidylate synthase by methotrexate polyglutamates. *J. Bio. Chem.*, **249**, 4100–4103.

Allegra, C. J., Chabner, B. C., Drake, J. C., Lutz, R., Rodbard, D. and Jolivet, J., 1985 a, Enhanced inhibition of thymidylate synthase by methotrexate polyglutamates. *J. Bio. Chem.*, **260**, 9720–9726.

Allegra, C. J., Drake, J. C., Jolivet, J. and Chabner, B. A., 1985 b, Inhibition of phosphoribosyl aminoimidazolecarboxamide transformylase by methotrexate and dihydrofolic acid polyglutamates. *Proc. Nat. Acad. Sci. USA*, **82**, 4881–4885.

Allen, J. C., Rosen, G., Mehta, B. M. and Horten, B. 1980, Leukoencephalopathy following high-dose IV methotrexate chemotherapy with leucovorin rescue. *Cancer Treat. Rep.*, **64**, 1261.

Anderson, P. A., West, S. G. and Claypool, R. C., 1984, Pulse methotrexate therapy for rheumatoid arthritis: a double-blind crossover study. *Arth. Rheum.*, **27**, 4(Supplement): S25, 60.

Angier, R. B., Boothe, J. H. and Hutchings, B. L., 1945, Synthesis of a compound identical with the *L. casei* factor isolated from liver. *Science*, **102**, 227–228.

Angier, R. B., Boothe, J. H., Hutchings, B. L., 1946, The structure and synthesis of the liver *L. casei* factor. *Science*, **103**, 667–669.

Antony, A. C., Kane, M. A., Portillo, R. M., Elwood, P. C. and Kolhouse, J. F., 1985, Studies of the role of a particulate folate-binding protein in the uptake of 5-methyltetrahydrofolate by cultured human KB cells. *J. Bio. Chem.*, **260**, 14911–14917.

Baggott, J. E., Vaughn. W. H. and Hudson, B. B., 1986, Inhibition of 5-aminoimidazole-4-carboxamide ribotide transformylase, adenosine deaminase and 5′-adenylate deaminase by polyglutamates of methotrexate and oxidized folates and by 5-aminoimidazole-4-carboxamide riboside and ribotide. *Biochemical J.*, **236**, 192–300.

Baugh, C. M., Krumdieck, C. L. and Nair, M. G. 1973, Polygammaglutamyl metabolites of methotrexate. *Biochem. Biophys. Res. Commun.*, **52**, 27.

Begent, R. H. J. and Bagshawe, K. D., 1982, The management of high risk choriocarcinoma. *Seminars in Oncology*, **9**, 198.

Bertino, J. R., 1981, Clinical use of methotrexate—with emphasis on use of hish doses. *Cancer Treat. Rep.*, **65**, 131–135.

Bertino, J. R., Dolnick, B. J., Berenson, R. J., Scheer, D. I. and Kamen, B. A., 1981, Cellular mechanisms of resistance to methotrexate. In *Molecular Actions and Targets for Cancer Chemotherapeutic Agents.*, edited by A. C. Sartorelli, J. S. Lazo and J. R. Bertino (New York: Academic Press), pp. 385–400.

Blakely, R. L., 1984, *Dihydrofolate Reductase in Folates and Pterins*, edited by R. L. Blakely and S. J. Benkovic (New York: John Wiley), Vol. 1, pp. 191–254.

Bleyer, W. A., 1978, The clinical pharmacology of methotrexate: new application of an old drug. *Cancer*, **41**, 36–51.

Bleyer, W. A., 1981, Neurologic sequelae of methotrexate and ionizing radiation: a new classification. *Cancer Treat Rep.*, **65**, 89.

Bolin, J. T., Filman, D. J., Matthews, D. A., Hamlin, R. C. and Kraut, J., 1982, Crystal structures of *Escherichia coli* and *Lactobacillus casei* dihydrofolate reductase defined at 1.7 Å resolution. *J. Biol. Chem.*, **257**, 13650–13662.

Breithaupt, H. and Kuenzlen, E., 1982, Pharmacokinetics of methotrexate and 7-hydroxymethotrexate following infusions of high-dose methotrexate. *Cancer Treat. Rep.*, **66**, 1733–1741.

Buice, R. G., Evans, W. E., Karas, J., Nicholas, C. A., Paramjeet, S., Straughn, A. B., Meyer, M. C. and Crom, W. R., 1980, Evaluation of enzyme immunoassay, radioassay, and radioimmunoassay of serum methotrexate, as compared with liquid chromatography. *Clin. Chem.*, **26**, 1902–1904.

Cabanillas, F., Hagemeister, F. B., Bodey, G. P and Freirech E. J., 1982, IMVP-16: an effective regimen for patients with lymphoma who have relapsed after initial combination chemotherapy. *Blood*, **60**, 693–697.

Capdevila, A. and Kamen, B., 1985, Binding and substrate specificity of human dihydrofolate reductase purified from hepatoma *in vivo*. *Proc. Am. Ass. Cancer Res.*, **26**, 232.

Carter, S. K., 1974, The chemical therapy of breast cancer. *Seminars in Oncology*, **1**, 131–144.

Coleman, C. N., Cohen, J. R., Burke, J. S. and Rosenberg, S. A., 1981, Lymphoblastic lymphoma in adults: results of a pilot protocol. *Blood*, **57**, 679–684.

Covey, J. M., 1980, Polyglutamate derivatives of folic acid coenzymes and methotrexate. *Life Sciences.*, **26**, 665–678.

Currie, V. W., Kempin, S. J. and Young, C. W., 1980, Phase I trial of metoprine in patients with advanced cancer. *Cancer Treat. Rep.*, **64**, 951–956.

Custer, R. P., Freeman-Narrod, M. and Narrod, S. A., 1977, Hepatotoxicity in Wistar rats following chronic methotrexate administration: a model of human reaction. *J. Nat. Cancer Inst.*, **58**, 1011–1017.

Delcamp, T. J., Susten, S. S., Blankenship, D. T. and Freisheim, J. H., 1983, Purification and characterization of dihydrofolate reductase from methotrexate-resistant human lymphoblastoid cells. *Biochemistry* **22**, 633.

Djerassi, I., Rominger, C. J., Kim, J. S., Turchi, J., Suvansri, V. and Hughes, D., 1972, Phase I study of high doses of methotrexate with citrovorum factor in patients with lung cancer. *Cancer*, **30**, 22–29.

Domin, B. A., Cheng, Y-C. and and Hakala, M. T., 1981, Properties of dihydrofolate reductase from a methotrexate-resistant subline of human KB cells and comparison with enzyme from KB parent cells and mouse S180 AT/3000 cells. *Mol. Pharmacol.*, **21**, 231–238.

Elslager, E. F., Johnson, J. L. and Werbel, L. M., 1983, Folate antagonists. 20. Synthesis and antitumor and antimalarial properties of trimetrexate and related 6-((phenylamine)methyl)-2, 4-quinazolinediamines. *J. Med. Chem.*, **26**, 1753–1760.

Evans, W. E., Hutson, P. R., Stewart, C. F., Cairnes, D. A., Bowman, W. P., Rivera, G. and Crom, W. R., 1983, Methotrexate cerebrospinal fluid and serum concentrations after intermediate-dose methotrexate infusion. *Clin. Pharmacol. Ther.*, **33**, 301–307.

Farber, S., Diamond, L. K., Mercer, R. D., *et al.*, 1948, Temporary remissions in acute leukemia in children produced by folic acid antagonist, 4-aminopteroyl-glutamic acid (aminopterin). *New England J. Med.*, **238**, 787–793.

Fabre, G., Matherly, L. H., Favre, R., Catalin, J. and Cano, J. P., 1983, *In vitro* formation of polyglutamyl derivatives of methotrexate and 7-hydroxymethotrexate in human lymphoblastic leukemia cells. *Cancer Res.*, **43**, 4648–4652.

Fisher, R. I., DeVita, V. T., Hubbard, S. M., Longo, D. Z., Wesley, R., Chabner, B. A. and Young, R. C., 1983, Diffuse aggressive lymphomas: increased survival after alternative flexible sequences of ProMACE and MOPP chemotherapy. *Ann. Int. Med.*, **98**, 304–309.

Franklin, A. L., Belt, M., Stokstad, E. L. R. and Jukes, T. H., 1949, Biological studies with 4-amino-10-methylpteroylglutamic acid. *J. Biol. Chem.*, **177**, 621–629.

Freeman, A. I., Weinberg, V., Brecher, M. L., *et al.*, 1983, Comparison of the intermediate-dose methotrexate with cranial irradiation for the post-induction treatment of acute lymphocytic leukemia in children. *New England J. Med.*, **308**, 477–484.

Frei, E., 1984, Acute leukemia in children. *Cancer*, **53**, 2013–2025.

Fritsch, G. and Urban, C., 1984, Transient encephalopathy during the late course of treatment with high-dose methotrexate. *Cancer*, **53**, 1849.

Galivan, J., Inglese, J., McGuire, J. J., Nimec, Z. and Coward, J. K., 1985, γ-Fluoromethotrexate: synthesis and biological activity of a potent inhibitor of dihydrofolate reductase with greatly diminished ability to form poly-γ-glutamates. *Proc. Natl. Acad. Sci. USA*, **82**, 2598–2602.

Gaukroger, J. M. and Wilson, L., 1984, Protection of cells from methotrexate toxicity by 7-hydroxymethotrexate. *Brit. J. Cancer.*, **50**, 327–333.

Ginsberg, S., Anderson, J., Bloomfield, C., Norton, L., Barcos, M., Gottlieb, A. J. and Holland, J., 1985, Therapy of advanced, intermediate grade lymphoma with cyclophosphamide, adriamycin, vincristine and prednisone with or without bleomycin (CAVPB vs. CAVP) follwed by high dose methotrexate or standard dose methotrexate (HMTX vs. LMTX): a randomized trial. *Proc. Am. Soc. Clin. Oncol.*, **4**, 202.

Goldin, A., Mantel, N., Greenhouse, S. W., Venditti, J. M., and Humphreys, S. R., 1953, Effect of delayed administration of citrovorum factor on the antileukemic effectiveness of aminopterin in mice. *Cancer Res.*, 43–48.

Goldman, I. D., and Matherly, L. H., 1985, The cellular pharmacology of methotrexate. *Pharmacol. Ther.*, **28**, 77–102.

Gubner, R., August, S. and Ginsberg, V., 1951, Therapeutic suppression of tissue reactivity; effect of aminopterin in rheumatoid arthritis and psoriasis *Am. J. Med. Sci.*, **221**, 176–182.

Haas, R. J., Janka, G., Gaedicke, G., *et al.*, 1983, Therapy of acute lymphocytic leukemia of childhood with intermediate dose methotrexate and CNS irradiation. A report of the ALL 77-02 study group. *Blut*, 321–331.

Haim, N., Kedar, A. and Robinson, E., 1984, Methotrexate-related deaths in patients previously treated with cis-diamminodichloride platinum. *Cancer Chemother. Pharmacol.*, **13**, 223–225.

Hammond, C. B., Hertz, R., Ross, G. T., Lipsett, M. B. and Odell, W. D., 1967, Primary chemotherapy for non-metastatic gestational trophoblastic neoplasms. *Am. J. Obs. Gyne.*, **98**, 71.

Harb, J. M., Werlin, S. L., Camitta, B. M., Oechler, H., Kamen, B. A. and Blank, E. L., 1983, Hepatic ultrastructure in leukemic children treated with methotrexate and 6-mercaptopurine. *Am. J. Pediat. Hemat./Oncol.*, **5**, 323–331.

Hertz, R. and Tullner, W. W., 1949, Quantitative interference with estrogen-induced tissue growth by folic acid antagonists. *Endocrinology*, **44**, 278.

Hortobagyi, G. N., Yap, H. Y., Blumenschein G. R., Buzdar, A. U., Barnes, B. C., Legha, S. S. and Wiseman, C. L., 1983, Phase II evaluation of vinblastine, methotrexate, and calcium leukovorin rescue in patients with refractory metastatic breast cancer. *Cancer*, **51**, 769–772.

Hutchinson, D. J. and Schmid, F. A., 1984, *Experimental Cancer Chemotherapy with Folate Antagonists in Folate Antagonists as Therapeutic Agents.*, edited by F. M. Sirotnak, J. J. Burchall, W. B. Ensminger and J. A. Montgomery (New York: Academic Press), Vol. 2, pp. 1–22.

Iland, H. J., Laszlo, J. and Sedwick, W. D., 1985, Paradoxical effect of BW 301U, a lipophilic antifolate, on methotrexate-inhibitable deoxyuridine incorporation by human hematopoietic cells. *Cancer Res.*, **45**, 3962–3968.

Jackson, R. C., 1984, Biological effects of folic acid antagonists with antineoplastic activity. *Pharmacol. Ther.*, **25**, 61–82.

Jacobs, S. A., Derr, C. J. and Johns, D. G., 1977, Accumulation of methotrexate diglutamate in human liver during methotrexate therapy. *Biochem Pharmacol.*, **26**, 2310–2313.

Jaffe, N., 1972, Recent advances in the chemotherapy of metastatic osteogenic sarcoma. *Cancer*, **30**, 1627–1631.

Kamen, B. A., 1986, Folate, MTX and the brain. *J. Neurotoxicol.*, **7**, 209–216.

Kamen, B. A. and Capdevila, A., 1986, Receptor mediated folate and methotrexate transport is regulated by the intracellular folate pool. *Proc. Natl. Acad. Sci.*, **83**, 5983–5987.

Kamen, B. A. and Winick, N. J., 1986, Analysis of methotrexate polyglutamate derivatives *in vivo*. In *Methods in Enzymology*, edited by F. Chytil and D. B. McCormick (Orlando: Academic Press), Vol. 122, pp. 339–346.

Kamen, B. A., Nylen, P. A., Camitta, B. M. and Bertino, J. R., 1981, Methotrexate accumulation in cells as a possible mechanism of chronic toxicity to the drug. *Brit. J. Haematol.*, **49**, 355.

Kamen, B. A., Bauer, W. W. and Bertino, J. R., 1983, A mechanism of resistance to NADPH but not NADH stimulates methotrexate binding to a dihydrofolate reductase *Biochem. Pharmacol.*, **32**, 1837–1844.

Kamen, B. A., Moulder, J. E., Kun, L. E., *et al.*, 1984 a, Effects of single dose and fractionated cranial irradiation on rat brain accumulation of methotrexate. *Cancer Res.*, **44**, 5092–5094.

Kamen, B. A., Holcenberg, J. S., Turo, K. and Whitehead, V. M., 1984 b, Methotrexate and folate content of erythrocytes in patients receiving oral vs. intramuscular therapy with methotrexate. *J. Pediat.*, **104**, 131–133.

Kamen, B. A., Eibl, B., Cashmore A. and Bertino, J. R., 1984 c, Uptake and efficacy of trimetrexate (TMQ, 2,4-diamino-5-methyl-6-[3,4,5-trimethoxyanilinomethyl]-quinazoline) a non-classical antifolate in MTX resistant leukemia cells *in vitro*. *Biochem. Pharmacol.*, **33**, 1697–1699.

Kamen, B. A., Nylen, P. A., Whitehead, V. M., Abelson, H. T., Dolnick, B, J. and Peterson, D. W., 1985, Lack of dihydrofolate reductase in human tumor and leukemia cells *in vivo*. *Cancer Drug Delivery*, **2**, 133–138.

Keefe, D. A., Capizzi, R. L. and Rudnick, S. A., 1982, Methotrexate cytotoxicity for L5178Y/Asn lymphoblasts: relationship of dose and duration of exposure to tumor cell viability. *Cancer Res.*, **42**, 1641–1645.

Krakower, G. R. and Kamen, B. A. 1983, *In situ* methotrexate polyglutamate formation in rat tissues. *J. Pharmacol. Exp. Ther.*, **227**, 633–638.

Kremer, J. M., 1985, Longterm methotrexate therapy in rheumatoid arthritis: a review. *J. Rheumatol.*, **12**, 25–28.

Lawrence, C. M., Strange, R. C. and Summerly, R., 1983, Assessment of liver function using fasting bile salt concentrations in psoriasis prior to and during methotrexate therapy. *Clin. Chim. Acta*, **129**, 341–351.

Levitt, M. D., Marsh, J. C., DeConti, R. C., Mitchell, M. S., Skeel, R. T., Farner, L. R. and Bertino, J. R., 1972, Combination sequential chemotherapy in advanced reticulum cell sarcoma. *Cancer*, **29**, 630–636.

Li, M. C., Hertz, R. and Spencer, D. B., 1956, Effect of methotrexate therapy upon choriocarcinoma and chorioadenoma. *Proc. Soc. Exp. Biol. Med.*, **93**, 361.

Link, M. P., Goorin, A. M., Miser, A. W., Green, A. A., Pratt, C. B., Belasco, J. B., Pritchard, J., Malpas, J. S., Baker, A. R, Kirkpatrick, J. A., Ayala, A. G., Shuster, J. J., Abelson, H. T., Simone, J. V. and Vietti, T. J., 1986, The effect of adjuvant chemotherapy on relapse-free survival in patients with osteosarcoma of the extremity. *New England J. Med.*, **314**(25), 1600–1606.

Lokiec, F., Poirier, O., Gisselbrecht, C., Marty, M., Boiron, M. and Najean, Y., 1982, Effect of combination chemotherapy, duration of methotrexate administration, and patient's age on methotrexate pharmacokinetics. *Cancer Chemother. Pharmacol.*, **9**, 165–168.

Lopez, C., Bourdeaux, M., Chauvet, M., Gilli, R. and Briand, C., 1986, Binding of 7-hydroxy-methotrexate to human serum albumin. *Biochem. Pharmacol.*, **35**, 2834–2836.

Mahoney, M. J., Murphy, M. S., Wadsworth, J. and Mott, M. G., 1984, Modification of oral methotrexate absorption in children with leukemia. *Cancer Chemother. Pharmacol.*, **12**, 131–133.

Matherly, L. H., Fry, D. W. and Goldman, I. D., 1983, Role of methotrexate polyglutamylation and cellular energy metabolism in inhibition of methotrexate binding to dihydrofolate reductase by 5-formyltetrahydrofolate in Ehrlich ascites tumor cells *in vitro*. *Cancer Res.*, **43**, 2694–2699.

Matherly, L. H., Anderson, L. A. and Goldman, I. D., 1984, Role of the cellular oxidation–reduction rate in methotrexate binding to dihydrofolate reductase and dissociation induced by reduced folates. *Cancer Res.*, **44**, 2325–2330.

Matherly, L. H., Barlowe, C. K. and Goldman, I. D., 1986, Antifolate polyglutamylation and competitive drug displacement at dihydrofolate reductase as important elements in leucovorin rescue in L1210 cells. *Cancer Res.*, **46**, 588–593.

Mathews, R. G. and Baugh, C. M., 1980, Interactions of pig liver methylenetetrahydrofolate reductase with methylenetetrahydropteroylpolyglutamate substrates and with dihydropteroylpolyglutamate inhibitors. *Biochemistry*, **19**, 2040–2045.

McBurney, M. W. and Whitemore G. F., 1974, Isolation and biochemical characterization of folate deficient mutants of chinese hamster cells. *Cell* **2**, 173–182.

McGuire, J. J., Hsieh, P., Coward, J. K. and Bertino, J. R., 1980, Enzymatic synthesis of folylpolyglutamates: characterization of the reaction and its products. *J. Biol. Chem.*, **255**, 5776–5788.

McGuire, J. J., Hsieh, P., Coward, J. K. and Bertino, J. R., 1983, In vitro methotrexate polyglutamate synthesis by rat liver folylpolyglutamate synthetase and inhibition by bromosulfophthalein. *Adv. Exp. Med. Biol.*, **163**, 199–214.

McGuire, J. J., Hsieh, P. and Bertino, J. R., 1984, Enzymatic synthesis of polyglutamate derivatives of 7-hydroxymethotrexate. *Biochem. Pharmacol.*, **33**, 1355–1361.

McGuire, J. J. and Coward, J. K., 1985, DL-threo-4-fluoroglutamic acid: a chain-terminating inhibitor of folylpolyglutamate synthesis. *J. Biol. Chem.*, **260**, 6747–6754.

McHugh, M. and Cheng, Y-C., 1979, Demonstration of a high affinity folate binder in human cell membranes and its characterization in cultured human KB cells. *J. Biol. Chem.*, **254**, 11312–11318.

Mitchell, H. K., Snell, E. E. and Williams, R. J., 1941, The concentration of "folic acid". *J. Am. Chem. Soc.*, **62**, 2284.

Moe, P. J., Seip, M. and Finne, P. H., 1981, Intermediate dose methotrexate (IDM) in childhood acute lymphocytic leukemia in Norway. Preliminary results of a national treatment program. *Acta Paediat. Scand.*, **70**, 73–79.

Mooney, C., Souhami, R. and Pritchard, J., 1983, Recurrent medulloblastoma. Lack of response to a high-dose methotrexate. *Cancer Chemother. Pharmacol.*, **10**, 135–136.

Morandi, C. and Attardi, G., 1981, Isolation and characterization of dihydrofolic acid reductase from methotrexate-sensitive and -resistant human cell lines. *J. Biol. Chem.*, **256**, 10169–10175.

Nelson, M. M. and Evans, H. M., 1949, Pteroylglutamic acid and reproduction in the rat. *J. Nut.*, **38**, 11.

Neuwelt, E. A., Diehl, J. T., Vu L. H., Hill, S. A., Michael, A. J. and Frenkel, E. P., 1981, Monitoring of methotrexate delivery in patients with malignant brain tumors after osmotic blood–brain barrier disruption. *Ann. Int. Med.*, **94**, 449–454.

Neuwelt, E. A., Barnett, P. A., Bigner, D. D. and Frenkel, E. P., 1982, Effects of adrenal cortical steroids and osmotic blood–brain barrier opening on methotrexate delivery to gliomas in the rodent: the factor of the blood–brain barrier. *Proc. Natl. Acad. Sci. USA.*, **79**, 4420–4423.

Newlands, E. S., 1982, New chemotherapeutic agents in the management of gestational trophoblastic disease. *Seminars in Oncology*, **9**, 239.

Nyfors, A. and Poulsen, H., 1977, Morphogenesis of fibrosis and cirrhosis in methotrexate-treated patients with psoriasis. *Am. J. Surg. Path.*, **1**, 235–243.

Pan, Y-CE., Domin, B. A., Li, SS-L. and Cheng, Y. C., 1983, Studies of amino-acid sequence in dihydrofolate reductase from a human methotrexate-resistant cell line KB/6b. *Eur. J. Biochem.*, **132**, 351–359.

Parker, D., Bate, C. M., Craft, A. W., Graham-Pole, J., Malpas, J. S. and Stansfeld, A. G., 1980, Liver damage in children with acute leukaemia and non-Hodgkin's lymphoma on oral maintenance chemotherapy. *Cancer Chemother. Pharmacol.*, **4**, 121–127.

Paxton, J. M., 1982, The protein binding and elimination of methotrexate after intravenous infusions in cancer patients. *Clin. Exp. Pharmacol. Physiol.*, **9**, 225–234.

Pinkerton, C. R., Glasgow, J. F. T., Welshman, S. G. and Bridges, J. M., 1980, Can food influence the absorption of methotrexate in children with acute lymphoblastic leukaemia? *Lancet*, **1**, 944.

Pinkerton, C. R., Welshman, S. G., Dempsey, S. I., Bridges, J. M. and Glasgow, J. F. T., 1980, Absorption of methotrexate under standardized conditions in children with acute lymphoblastic leukaemia. *Brit. J. Cancer*, **42**, 613–615.

Pratt, C. B., 1981, Selected applications of methotrexate alone and in combination in osteosarcoma. *Cancer Treat. Rep.*, **65**, (Suppl 1), 107–111.

Rivera, G. K., Evans, W. E., Kalwinsky, D. K., *et al.*, 1985, Unexpectedly severe toxicity from intensive early treatment of childhood lymphoblastic leukemia. *J. Clin. Oncol.*, **3**, 201–206.

Rosen, G., Fereshteh, G., Nirenberg, A., Mosende, C. and Mehta, B. M., 1977, High-dose methotrexate with citrovorum factor rescue for the treatment of central nervous system tumors in children. *Cancer Treat. Rep.*, **61**, 681–690.

Rosen, G., Caparros, B., Huvos, A. G., Kosloff, C., Nirenberg, A., Cacavio, A., Marcove, R. C., Lane, J. M., Mehta, B. and Urban C., 1982, Preoperative chemotherapy for osteogenic sarcoma: selection of postoperative adjuvant chemotherapy based on the response of the primary tumor to preoperative chemotherapy. *Cancer.*, **49**, 1221–1230.

Rosowsky, A., Moran, R. G., Forsch, R., Colman, P., Uren, J. and Wick, M., 1984, Methotrexate analogues—XVII. Antitumor activity of 4-amino-4-deoxy-N^{10}-methylpteroyl-D,L-homocysteic acid and its dual inhibition of dihydrofolate reductase and folyl polyglutamate synthetase. *Biochem. Pharmacol.*, **33**, 155–161.

Ross, T. G., Goldstein, D. P., Hertz, R., Lipsett, M. B. and Odell, W. D., 1965, Sequential use of methotrexate and actinomycin D in the treatment of metastic choriocarcinoma and related trophoblastic diseases in women. *Am. J. Obst. Gynec.*, **93**, 223.

Sakami, W. and Welch, A. D., 1950, Synthesis of labile methyl groups *in vitro*. *J. Biol. Chem.*, **18**, 379–384.

Samuels, L. L., Feinberg, A., Moccio, D. M., Sirotnak, F. M. and Rosen, G., 1984, Detection by high performance liquid chromatography of methotrexate and its metabolites in tumor tissue from osteosarcoma patients treated with high-dose methotrexate/leucovorin rescue. *Biochem. Pharmacol.*, **33**, 2711–2714.

Schalhorn, A., Sauer, H., Wilmanns, W. and Stupp-Poutot, G., 1982, Pharmacokinetics of erythrocyte methotrexate after high-dose methotrexate. *Cancer Chemother. Pharmacol.*, **9**, 65–69.

Schimke, R. T., 1986, Methotrexate resistance and gene amplification. *Cancer*, **57**, 1912–1917.

Schornagel, J. H. and McVie, J. G., 1983, The clinical pharmacology of methotrexate. *Cancer Treat Rev.*, **10**, 53–75.

Seeger, D. R., Smith, J. M., Jr and Hultquist, M. E., 1947, Antagonist for pteroylglutamic acid. *J. Am. Chem. Soc.*, **69**, 567.

Shipp, M., Klatt, M., Harrington, D., Pinkus, G., Jochelson, M., Rosenthal, D., Skarin, A. and Canellos, G., 1985, M-BACOD and m-BACOD in the treatment of unfavourable prognosis lymphoma: analysis of prognostic variables. *Proc. Am Soc. Clin. Oncol.*, **4**, 205.

Sirotnak, F. M., DeGraw, J. I., Chello, P. L., Moccio, D. M. and Dorick, D. M., 1982, Biochemical and pharmacologic properties of a new folate analog, 10-deaza-aminopterin, in mice. *Cancer Treat. Rep.*, **66**, 351–358.

Sirotnak, F. M., 1985, Obligate genetic expression in tumor cells of a fetal membrane property mediating "folate" transport: biological significance and implications for improved therapy of human cancer. *Cancer Res.*, **45**, 3992–4000.

Skarin, A. T., Canellos, G. P., Rosenthal, D. S., Case, D. C., Jr., MacIntyre, J. M., Pinkus, G. S., Moloney, W. C. and Frei, E., III, 1983, Improved prognosis of diffuse histiocytic and undifferentiated lymphomas by use of high-dose methotrexate alternating with standard agents (M-BACOD). *J. Clin. Oncol.*, **1**, 91–98.

Smith, E. B., Weed, J. C., Tyrey, L. and Hammond, C. B., 1982, Treatment of nonmetastatic gestational trophoblastic disease: Results of methotrexate alone versus methotrexate-folinic acid. *Am. J. Obs. Gynec.*, **144**, 88.

Stern, R. S., Zierler, S. and Parrish, J. A., 1982, Methotrexate used for psoriasis and the risk of noncutaneous or cutaneous malignancy. *Cancer*, **50**, 869–872.

Taylor, S. G., McGuire, W. P., Hauck, W. W., Showel, J. L. and Lad, T. E., 1984, A randomized comparison of high-dose infusion methotrexate versus standard-dose weekly therapy in head and neck squamous cancer. *J. Clin. Oncol.*, **2**, 1006–1011.

Ward, J. R., 1984, A prospective randomized controlled trial of low dose pulse methotrexate (MTX) in rheumatoid arthritis (RA). *Arthr. Rheum.*, **27**, 4(Supplement): S40 (150).

Weinblatt, M. E., Coblyn, J. S., Fox, D. A., Fraser, P. A., Holdsworth, D. E., Glass, D. N. and Trentham, D. E., 1985, Efficacy of low dose methotrexate in rheumatoid arthritis. *New England J. Med.*, **312**, 818–822.

Weinstein, G. D. and Frost, P., 1971, Methotrexate for psoriasis. *Arch. Dermatol.*, 103, 33–38.

Welch, A. D. and Nichol, C. A. 1952, Water-soluble vitamins concerned with one and two carbon intermediates. *Ann. Rev. Biochem*, **21**, 633–686.

Whiteside, J. A., Philips, F. S., Dargeon, H. W. and Burchenal, J. H., 1958, Intrathecal amethopterin and neurological manifestations of leukemia. *AMA Arch. Int. Med.*, **101**, 279–285.

Wilkens, R. F., and Watson, M. A., 1982, Methotrexate: a perspective of its use in the treatment of rheumatic diseases. *J. Lab. Clin. Med.*, **100**, 314.

Winick, N. J., Krakower, G. R. and Kamen, B. A., 1985, Metabolism of MTX to polyglutamyl derivatives and the relationship to folate pools *in vivo.*, In *Proceedings of the Second Workshop on Folyl and Antifolyl Polyglutamates*, edited by I. D., Goldman (Westport, CN: Praeger), pp. 297–307.

Winkler, K., Beron, G., Kotz, R., Salzer-Kuntschik, M., Beck, J., Beck, W., Brandeis, W., Ebell, W., Erttmann, R., Gobel, U., Havers, W., Henze, G., Hinderfeld, L., Hocker, P., Jobke, A., Jurgens, H., Kabisch, H., Presser, P., Prindull, G., Ramach, W., Ritter, J., Sekera, J., Treuner, J., Wust, G. and Landbeck, G., 1984, Neoadjuvant chemotherapy for osteogenic sarcoma: results of a cooperative German/Austrian study. *J. Clin. Oncol.* **2**(6), 617–624.

Yap, H-Y., Yap, B. S., Rasmussen, S., Levens, M. E., Hortobagyi, G. N. and Blumenschein, G. R., 1982, Treatment of meningeal carcinomatosis in breast cancer. *Cancer.*, **50**, 219–222.

Zaharko, D.S., Dedrick, R. L. and Bischoff, I. C. B., 1971, Methotrexate tissue distribution: prediction by a mathematical model. *J. Nat. Cancer Inst.*, **46**, 775–784.

6. The platinum anti-tumour drugs

Richard F. Borch

Introduction

cis-Diamminedichloroplatinum(II), known to chemists as Peyrone's chloride and now also to biomedical scientists as cisplatin, is a neutral square planar coordination complex first synthesized in 1845 and structurally characterized in 1893. Interest in this compound was markedly stimulated in 1965 following Rosenberg's report that platinum electrolysis products inhibited bacterial cell growth (Rosenberg *et al.*, 1965). Cisplatin was subsequently shown to possess potent anti-tumour activity *in vivo* (Rosenberg *et al.*, 1969), and phase I clinical trials were initiated in 1971. Recent reviews of the clinical experience with cisplatin attest to the remarkable contribution of this drug to the oncologist's armamentarium (Prestayko *et al.*, 1980; Hacker *et al.*, 1984; Loehrer and Einhorn, 1984). During the 1970s a large number of cisplatin analogues were synthesized and evaluated, in the hope that appropriate modification of the amine ligands and/or the labile leaving groups might provide a second-generation drug lacking the nephrotoxicity associated with cisplatin. Several of these analogues are now in clinical trials and appear to have both anti-tumour and toxicity profiles somewhat different from cisplatin. Mechanistic elucidation of both anti-tumour and host cytotoxicity has attracted the recent attention of numerous investigators. The history, chemistry, cytotoxicity and clinical applications of cisplatin have been the subjects of recent reviews (Rosenberg, 1985; Lippard, 1982, 1983; Douple, 1984; Prestayko *et al.*, 1980; Hacker *et al.*, 1984; Loehrer and Einhorn, 1984). Therefore this review will not attempt to be comprehensive but will focus on recent studies of platinum drug metabolism and its relationship to host and tumour cytotoxicity.

Cisplatin is clearly one of the most important anti-tumour agents to enter the clinic in the last 20 years. It has become an integral part of multi-drug regimens for treating a wide variety of solid tumours. Its use in combination with vinblastine and bleomycin revolutionized the treatment of non-seminomatous testicular cancer; even in the presence of disseminated disease, five-year disease-free survivals approach 90% (Drasga *et al.*, 1982; Ozols *et al.*, 1983; Loehrer and Einhorn, 1984). Cisplatin has also been an important addition to several drug combinations in the treatment of bladder cancer (Yagoda, 1983). It is among the most active agents in the treatment of ovarian cancer, producing response rates of 60–80% in combination with other drugs, compared with 40% for other single agents (Ozols and Young, 1984). The use of cisplatin with sytemic thiosulphate (Pfeifle *et al.*, 1985) and with hypertonic saline (Ozols and Young, 1985) have provided strategies for administration of very high cisplatin doses with acceptable toxicity, giving improved responses in patients refractory to other treatments. The major dose-limiting side-effect in these high-dose regimens is neurotoxicity, which currently limits treatment to a maximum of four cycles at 200 mg/m^2. Carboplatin is a new cisplatin analogue with minimal nephrotoxicity and neurotoxicity; its dose-limiting toxicity is myelosuppression. Carboplatin has activity similar to cisplatin in ovarian cancer and also appears to be effective in heavily pretreated patients (Evans *et al.*, 1983; Ozols and Young, 1985).

Cisplatin has also become an important drug in the treatment of lung cancer. Although not a first-line drug in the treatment of small cell lung cancer, the combination of etoposide and cisplatin may be the most active therapy currently for refractory disease (Greco *et al.*, 1985). A recent report also suggests that carboplatin is highly active against this tumour (Smith *et al.*, 1985). In non-small cell lung cancer, cisplatin in combination with either etoposide or vindesine can achieve a response rate of 30–40% compared to 5% with previous regimens (Klastersky and Sculier, 1985). Unfortunately, improvement in overall survival has been less impressive, increasing only from 4 to 8 months. Cisplatin-containing regimens are also useful in the treatment of cervical cancer, but their use is limited to patients with adequate renal function because of cisplatin's nephrotoxicity (Guthrie, 1985). Finally, combined modality treatment of squamous cell carcinoma of the head and neck, in which induction chemotherapy containing cisplatin is used, is beginning to have an impact on this disease. Combinations of cisplatin with bleomycin–vincristine, bleomycin–methotrexate, and 5-fluorouracil (5-FU) have been used successfully (Ervin *et al.*, 1985); one study reported a 54% complete response rate with 62% 18-month disease-free survival using cisplatin and 5-FU induction therapy (Rooney *et al.*, 1985).

The toxicity of cisplatin and its analogues has been well documented (Von Hoff *et al.*, 1979; Harrap *et al.*, 1980; Rose *et al.*, 1982). Nephrotoxicity is dose-limiting for cisplatin when standard regimens are used; the major site of toxicity in animals is the P3 segment of the proximal tubule, and in man it is characterized by decreased creatinine clearance and magnesium wasting (Blachley and Hill, 1981). Development of nephrotoxicity appears to correlate with elevated plasma platinum levels during infusion (Campbell *et al.*, 1983). Forced diuresis reduces the degree of nephrotoxicity (Hayes *et al.*, 1977), and recently introduced regimens using high-dose cisplatin and hypertonic saline (Ozols *et al.*, 1984) have largely alleviated this problem. Cisplatin is also highly emetogenic, and a variety of anti-emetic regimens have had only limited success. Myelosuppression is minimal with conventional cisplatin doses and becomes acutely severe but without cumulative effects using high-dose regimens (Ozols and Young, 1985). Ototoxicity is manifested by high-frequency hearing loss and is cumulative. Neurotoxicity is emerging as the dose-limiting toxicity in the high-dose cisplatin regimens and appears as a progressive peripheral neuropathy with increasing cumulative dose (Ozols and Young, 1985). Preliminary evidence suggest that the toxicity involves axonopathic changes with secondary demyelination (Gastaut and Pellissier, 1985).

Identification of active compounds that lack the severe toxicities of cisplatin has been the major goal of analogue development. Carboplatin (Evans *et al.*, 1983) and iproplatin (Creaven *et al.*, 1983) are currently the most promising second-generation drugs in clinical trials. Both drugs are essentially devoid of nephrotoxicity, but myelotoxicity is now dose-limiting. Carboplatin is less neurotoxic than cisplatin and causes significantly less emesis (Evans *et al.*, 1983; Ozols and Young, 1985). Preliminary clinical evidence suggests that these analogues may be active in patients heavily pretreated with and refractory to cisplatin.

Chemistry

There is currently no evidence that enzymes participate in the metabolism of the platinum drugs; presumably their biotransformations result from ligand displacement reactions with various biological nucleophiles. The chemistry of cisplatin has been reviewed extensively (Lippard, 1982, 1983; Pinto and Lippard, 1985 a); this section will focus on those reactions that are important to the metabolism of cisplatin and its analogues.

Platinum complexes are characterized by slow rates of ligand substitution reactions compared to other metal complexes. Therefore both kinetic and thermodynamic factors will be important in metabolic reactions. Cisplatin is a square planar complex in which the metal and liganded atoms retain their geometry and lie in a common plane (Figure 1). When cisplatin is dissolved in water, the more labile chloride ligands are displaced in a stepwise fashion (Figure 2). Although the rate of aquation of cisplatin is independent of chloride ion concentration, the equilibrium composition of the resulting substitution products is highly dependent on chloride levels (Tables 1–3). This is an important factor for cisplatin metabolism; in plasma, where $[Cl^-] =$ 100 mM, cisplatin would be expected to exist predominantly as the neutral dichloro complex. Intracellular chloride ion concentrations are very low however, and the aquated species should predominate in this environment (Table 3). Two important properties of the aquated complexes should be noted. First, the oxygen-bound protons become acidic when water is bound to platinum. Second, the water ligands (but not the hydroxide ligands of the

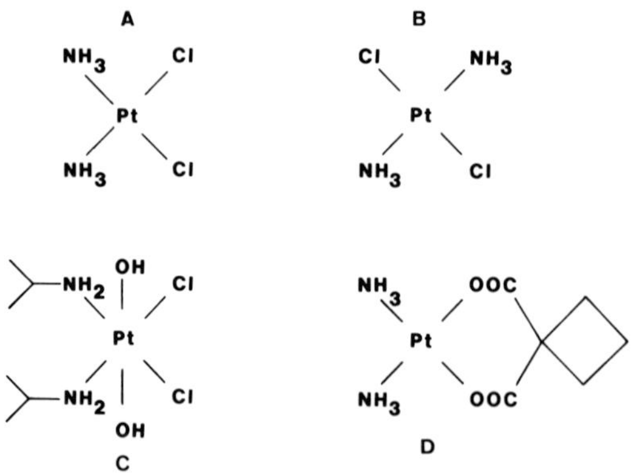

Figure 1. Structures of the major platinum complexes. A, *cis*-Diamminedichloroplatinum(II) (cisplatin); B, *trans*-Diamminedichloroplatinum(II) (trans-platinum); C, *cis*-Dichloro-*trans*-dihydroxy bis-isopropylamine platinum(IV) (iproplatin); D, *cis*-Diammine 1,1-cyclobutane-dicarboxylato platinum(II) (carboplatin).

neutral complexes) are far more reactive than the chloride ligands and are readily replaced by a variety of biological nucleophiles. It has been suggested that the neutral cisplatin enters the cell and is trapped there by rapid aquation to give a cationic complex. It should be noted, however, that the aquation reaction has a half-life of almost two hours at 37°C, and half of the mono-aquo product exists as a neutral hydroxo-liganded species. It is convenient to consider the ligand exchange reactions of cisplatin metabolites in two groups:

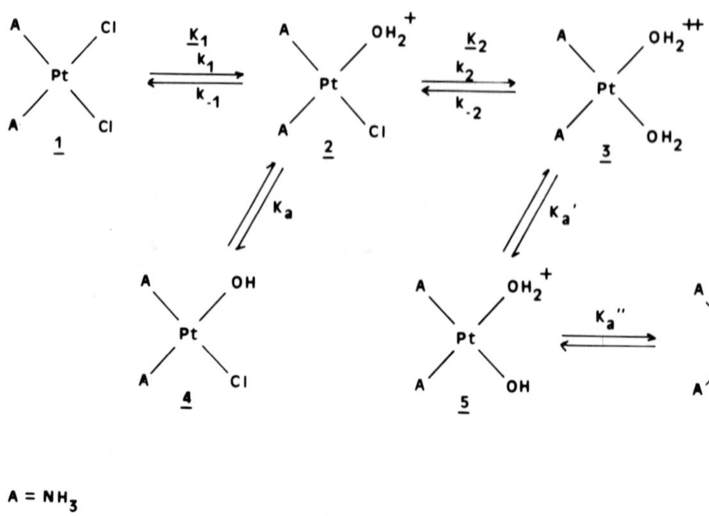

Figure 2. Aquation reactions of cisplatin.

Table 1. Rate and equilibrium constants for reactions of cisplatin and its hydrolysis products

Constant	Value	Source
k_1	$1 \cdot 1 \times 10^{-4}\,s^{-1}$ (37°)	Bodenner *et al.* (1986 a)
k_2	$4 \cdot 2 \times 10^{-5}\,s^{-1}$ (37°)	Segal and LePecq (1986)
k_{-1}	$2 \cdot 5 \times 10^{-2}\,M^{-1}\,s^{-1}$ (37°)	From k_1/K_1
k'_2	$2 \cdot 2 \times 10^{-1}\,M^{-1}\,s^{-1}$ (37°)	From k_2/K_2
K_1	$4 \cdot 37 \times 10^{-3}$ M (35°)	Lee and Martin (1976)
K_2	$1 \cdot 88 \times 10^{-4}$ M (35°)	Lee and Martin (1976)
pK_a	7·4 (estimate)	Lippard (1982)
pK_a'	5·56 (20°)	Jensen (1939)
pK_a''	7·32 (20°)	Jensen (1939)

Table 2. Estimated half-lives for interconversion of cisplatin and its hydrolysis products (for structures 1–3, see Figure 2)

	Interconversion half-life (min)			
$[Cl^-]$ (mM)	1 → 2	2 → 1	2 → 3	3 → 2
100	105	4·6	275	0·5
4	105	115	275	13·1

Table 3. Estimated cisplatin hydrolysis product composition (%) at plasma and intracellular chloride ion concentrations at pH 7·4 (for structures 1–6, see Figure 2).

	Product percentage					
$[Cl^-]$ (mM)	1	2	3	4	5	6
100	90·9	4·0	<0·1	4·0	0·5	0·6
4	9·1	9·9	0·5	9·9	32·1	38·5

those with nucleophiles of low reactivity, which require activation by prior aquation, and those with nucleophiles of high reactivity where reaction can occur with either the chloro or aquo complexes. Nitrogen and oxygen-based ligands are in the former category and sulphur ligands in the latter.

Cisplatin reactions with DNA

Persuasive evidence exists to support the hypothesis that cisplatin's anti-tumour effect is mediated by reaction with DNA and inhibition of its replication. The reader is referred to recent reviews (Douple, 1984; Pinto and Lippard, 1985 a) for thorough coverage of this subject. The order of reactivity for mononucleotides is GMP > AMP > CMP ≫ TMP (Mansy *et al.*, 1978), and the N-7 position of guanine appears to be most reactive in DNA as well. This nitrogen is relatively unreactive, however, and aquation of cisplatin appears to be rate-limiting for platination of DNA (Johnson *et al.*, 1980; Ushay *et al.*, 1981). Because *trans*-diamminedichloroplatinum(II) (trans-DDP) and monofunctional platinum complexes are orders of magnitude less effective than cisplatin as anti-tumour agents, it has been assumed that the cytotoxic lesion is a platinum cross-link formed between two bases in DNA. Cisplatin, its *trans* isomer and the monochloro analogue $Pt(dien)Cl^+$ inhibited DNA synthesis in L1210 cells *in vitro*, but the IC_{50} values were 2·3, 67 and 271 μM, respectively, after two-hour drug exposure. 50% inhibition of DNA replication occurred at a platinum/nucleotide ratio of 1/5000 (Salles *et al.*, 1983). Recently it was shown that cisplatin and its *trans* isomer generate different cytotoxic lesions in SV40 chromosomes. Fourteen-fold higher doses of *trans*-platinum are needed to provide equal inhibition of DNA replication (50%) and equal binding of platinum to DNA (1/2500 nucleotides). The kinetics of adduct formation are also very different; during continuous drug exposure the *trans*-platinum lesion peaks at 6 hours and is rapidly repaired, but the cisplatin lesion continues to increase over 48 hours (Ciccarelli *et al.*, 1985).

In a formal sense the replacement of two chlorides by DNA bases in cisplatin is analogous to the well-known reactions of bis(chloroethylamine) anti-tumour alkylating agents, and by analogy an inter-strand cross-link was assumed to be the major one formed by cisplatin. Inter-strand cross-links account for <1% of platinum–DNA adducts (Roberts and Friedlos, 1982; Eastman, 1985), however, and in a series of cisplatin-resistant L1210 sublines there was no correlation between inter-strand cross-links and cytotoxicity (Strandberg *et al.*, 1982). The geometry of cisplatin is unique in allowing it to form an intra-strand cross-link: numerous investigators have now demonstrated that the intra-strand cross-link between adjacent guanine residues is the major product from reaction of cisplatin with DNA (Eastman, 1983, 1986; Rahn, 1984; Fichtinger-Schepman *et al.*, 1985), and the X-ray structure of the cisplatin–d(pGpG) adduct has been determined (Sherman *et al.*, 1985). The approximate intra-strand adduct composition is: GpG, 50–65%; GpNpG, 5–10%; and ApG, 25%; the G–A adduct was not observed (Fichtinger-Schepman *et al.*, 1985; Eastman, 1986). The kinetics of the platinum–DNA reaction are of interest and may be of significance with respect to selective toxicity. Inter-strand cross-linking in cultured cells reaches a peak in 6–12 hours followed by a decline attributed to repair processes. The delay in cross-link formation was proposed to be the result of rapid mono-adduct formation followed by a slow step involving inter-strand adduct formation (Zwelling *et al.*, 1979). A "pre-cross-link" platinum–DNA lesion with an inter-strand cross-linking half-life of 3·5 hours has been described that provides supporting evidence for a fast mono-adduct–slow cross-link time course (Knox *et al.*, 1986). In contrast, the mono-adduct with an adjacent guanine or adenine residue reacts rapidly to form the intra-strand cross-link (Johnson *et al.*, 1985). Examination of cisplatin–DNA adducts after brief reaction times showed that the intra-strand GpG adduct represented 40% (Eastman, 1986) and 60% (Fichtinger-Schepman *et al.*, 1985) of bound platinum at 15 and 30 minutes, respectively; the guanosine mono-adduct comprised 40% and 15% of total platinum, respectively, at these times. The quantity of GpG adduct was also much higher than predicted if all guanines in DNA were equally reactive, suggesting that a kinetic preference exists between the reactive platinum species and d(GpG) sequences (Fichtinger-Schepman *et al.*, 1985). Thus reaction of cisplatin with DNA occurs via initial formation of a mono-adduct at the N-7 position of guanine. Rapid intra-strand cross-linking of this mono-adduct predominates; a minor fraction of the mono-adduct presumably lacks an appropriately positioned intra-strand base and undergoes slow inter-strand cross-linking to a nearest-neighbour guanine.

Which lesion is responsible for cisplatin's cytotoxicity? The frequency of DNA lesions argues in favour of the intra-strand cross-link. Recent studies of second-strand DNA synthesis using cisplatin-treated template DNA showed that inhibition occurred at all $(dG)_n$ sequences in the strand where $n > 1$. *Trans*-platinum also formed adducts that inhibited DNA synthesis, but these adducts occurred with much lower specificity. $Pt(dien)Cl^+$ mono-adducts did not inhibit DNA synthesis. Therefore d(GpG) sequences represent the major binding sites for both single-strand and double-strand DNA, and these represent the template sites where DNA synthesis is blocked (Pinto and Lippard, 1985 b).

We recently described results that, taken together with the data presented above, provide additional support for the intra-strand cross-link as the cytotoxic lesion. Diethyldithiocarbamate (DDTC) rapidly reacts with and removes platinum from mono-guanine adducts but is completely unreactive toward the cisplatin–bis-guanine adducts (Bodenner *et al.*, 1986 a). When L1210 cells were treated with cisplatin *in vitro*, washed, and immediately treated with DDTC, inter-strand cross-linking was reduced by approximately 50%, but clonogenicity was unaffected (Figure 3). Inter-strand cross-link reversal is not surprising considering DDTC's reactivity toward mono-adducts and the long half-life reported for the "inter-strand mono-adduct" (Knox *et al.*, 1986). The absence of effect on L1210 cell clonogenicity suggests that the cytotoxic bis-adducts were already formed when the cells were treated with DDTC. These data implicate the rapidly formed intra-strand cross-link as the cytotoxic lesion.

The reaction of cisplatin analogues with DNA has not been studied extensively. Carboplatin is assumed to form the same platinum–DNA adducts based upon the structural identity of the intermediates after replacement of the cyclobutanedicarboxylate ligand vs. the two chloride ligands in cisplatin. Equivalent cytotoxicity and DNA inter-strand cross-linking requires 45-fold

nucleophiles also react with aquated platinum metabolites at rates too fast to measure; thus these compounds may transform platinum metabolites in the plasma by rapid reaction with the aquated species.

The role of cysteine and methione in cisplatin metabolism and toxicity is not well defined. Cysteine was reported both to have no effect on (Nechay and Neldon, 1984) and to completely block (Daley-Yates and McBrien, 1982 b) cisplatin inhibition of renal ATPase. Both groups found that methionine increased cisplatin-induced enzyme inhibition. Methione was also administered two hours before cisplatin in the rat; in contrast to the protective effects expected, pretreatment with the methionine actually increased cisplatin-induced nephrotoxicity (Alden and Repta, 1984). The 1:1 cisplatin–methionine adduct was not nephrotoxic, however, when administered to rats (Daley-Yates and McBrien, 1984). These results suggest that cisplatin forms adducts with these amino acids but the adducts may be more reactive and/or toxic than the parent drug.

Reactions with proteins

Abundant evidence exists to show that cisplatin binds to plasma proteins both *in vitro* and *in vivo*. Reported half-times for protein binding are 60 (Robins, 1982; Daley-Yates and McBrien, 1985 a) and 90 minutes (Repta and Long, 1980). Binding was non-specific among protein classes; although cisplatin binding did not affect the biological activity of the immunoglobulins (Robins, 1982), α_2-macroglobulin was cross-linked and inactivated by cisplatin (Gonias *et al.*, 1984). The reaction of cisplatin with albumin has been studied in more detail; approximately one mole of platinum was bound per mole of protein, and reaction of the single sulphydryl residue with a sulphydryl reagent abolished cisplatin binding. Dialysis experiments showed that the albumin–cisplatin complex did not dissociate to a significant extent (Gonias and Pizzo, 1983), in agreement with the findings of Repta and Long (1980). Recent equilibrium dialysis experiments, however, indicate that the platinum drugs are reversibly bound to plasma protein; 65%, 26% and 7% of platinum was irreversibly protein-bound for cisplatin, carboplatin and iproplatin respectively. Reversal of the labile platinum complex was generally complete within three hours (Daley-Yates and McBrien, 1985 a). The basis for these contradictory observations is not clear. Protein-bound cisplatin is devoid of cytotoxic activity (Patton *et al.*, 1978).

It has been proposed by numerous investigators that cisplatin may exert its toxic effects by inhibition of critical enzymes; these inhibitory effects have now been documented for a number of enzymes *in vitro* (Aull *et al.*, 1979), including ATPase (Daley-Yates and McBrien, 1982 b), γ-glutamyl transpeptidase (Bodenner *et al.*, 1986 a), and α_2-macroglobulin (Gonias *et al.*, 1984). The non-nephrotoxic analogues carboplatin and iproplatin minimally inhibited ATPase at concentrations 8-fold higher than maximally inhibiting levels of cisplatin (Dedon *et al.*, 1986; Dedon and Borch, 1987), and the chemoprotector diethyldithiocarbamate was shown to reverse inhibition of both macroglobulin (Gonias *et al.*, 1984) and γ-glutamyl transpeptidase (Bodenner *et al.*, 1986 a). However, there is no evidence of significant enzyme inhibition *in vivo* following administration of cisplatin to the rat (Litterst, 1984; Dedon *et al.*, 1986; Dedon and Borch, 1987). There appears to be a correlation between inhibition and restoration of certain enzyme activities and platinum drug nephrotoxicity, but a causative role for enzyme inhibition has not been established.

Glutathione and cisplatin metabolism

There has been considerable interest in the role of glutathione on both the nephrotoxicity and the anti-tumour effects of cisplatin. Glutathione is the most abundant intracellular non-protein thiol (0·5–10 mM; Kosower and Kosower, (1978), and reaction of this thiol with platinum species may inhibit subsequent cytotoxic reactions. It has been reported that cisplatin does not react directly with sulphydryl groups (Levi *et al.*, 1980). In fact, cisplatin reacts with both cysteine and glutathione in a second-order reaction with half-times of approximately 1 and 3 hours respectively at 5 mM thiol and 37° C. The reaction between glutathione and aquated cisplatin, however, is essentially instantaneous (Dedon and Borch, 1987). This suggests that direct participation of glutathione in reducing cytotoxicity occurs via reaction with metabolites rather than with cisplatin itself.

Cisplatin treatment alters renal glutathione levels in a time-dependent manner. Total renal glutathione levels in the rat were increased 50% 20 minutes after cisplatin administration but returned to normal levels within an hour: there was no evidence of glutathione depletion over 4 hours (Leyland-Jones *et al.*, 1983). Total glutathione levels increased significantly beyond 5 days (3- and 5-fold at 8 and 12 days respectively); reduced glutathione was unchanged over this period (Litterst *et al.*, 1982). Pretreatment with glutathione was reported to cause a dose-dependent reduction in cisplatin-induced lethality, weight loss and blood urea nitrogen (BUN) elevation in the mouse and rat without altering the anti-tumour effect (Zunino *et al.*, 1983; Litterst and Uozumi, 1986). Renal glutathione levels were increased 40% by pretreatment, and cytosolic platinum concentrations increased 25–50% compared with a 30% decrease in microsomal platinum. Depletion of renal glutathione by pretreatment with buthione sulphoximin (BSO) or diethyl maleate enhanced lethality, BUN elevation, and weight loss. BSO also increased cytosolic platinum concentration but caused little change in other cell fractions (Litterst and Uozumi, 1986). 30% of cytosol platinum was associated with glutathione and <5% was protein-bound in cisplatin-treated rats (Litterst *et al.*, 1982). BSO pretreatment markedly enhanced cisplatin but not carboplatin lethality in nude mice (Hamilton *et al.*, 1986). These data suggest that alteration of renal glutathione levels can modify nephrotoxicity, but the changes in toxicity presumably result from differences in metabolite structure rather than intracellular distribution of platinum.

Glutathione is an important determinant in the sensitivity of many tumour lines to nitrogen mustards (Arrick and Nathan, 1984). Glutathione depletion has been shown to potentiate melphalan cytotoxicity in human ovarian cancer cell lines (Green *et al.*, 1984; Andrews *et al.*, 1985). The effect of glutathione depletion on the response of both cisplatin-sensitive and -resistant cell lines to cisplatin *in vitro* appears to depend on both the duration and extent of glutathione depletion. Andrews *et al.* showed that 24-hour pretreatment of COLO 316 and 2008 human ovarian tumour cells depleted glutathione to about 10% of control levels but did not potentiate the cytotoxicity of cisplatin or its analogues carboplatin and iproplatin. Baseline glutathione levels were very high and identical in both sensitive and resistant lines; levels after BSO depletion were in the range 1·5–6 ng/10^6 cells (Andrews *et al.*, 1985). It is interesting to note that BSO pretreatment significantly potentiated the cytotoxicity of trans-DDP; this is consistent with the observation that trans-DDP reacts with glutathione approximately 300 times faster than cisplatin, and the half-life for trans-DDP in the presence of 1 mM glutathione at 37° C is 3 minutes (Dedon and Borch, 1987).

Ozols *et al.* carried out similar experiments with sensitive and resistant lines of A2780 human ovarian carcinoma cells, except that the cells were exposed to BSO for 48 hours before and also during cisplatin treatment. Potentiation of cytotoxicity occurred with both cell lines; dose modification factors were 4·3 and 3·2 respectively. Glutathione levels were three times higher in the resistant cells (6·1 vs. 1·9 ng/10^6 cells), but the depleted levels were essentially identical in the two lines (0·7 vs. 0·6 ng/10^6 cells). There are two possible explanations for the different responses to glutathione depletion observed by these two groups. First, removal of BSO during cisplatin treatment may allow glutathione levels to recover sufficiently to negate the effect of prior depletion. Second, the depleted glutathione levels observed in the COLO 366 cells are similar to the control levels seen in A2780 cells. It is possible that glutathione must be depleted below 1 ng/10^6 cells before potentiation can occur.

The role of glutathione in the development of resistance to cisplatin is not clear. Glutathione levels were identical in both sensitive and resistant lines of COLO 316 and 2008 cells. Although resistance to cisplatin in A2780 cells was associated with a threefold elevation in glutathione levels, depletion of glutathione to identical levels in both sensitive and resistant lines did not abolish resistance. In fact, when the dose modification factors are taken into account, the relative resistance actually increased in the presence of BSO compared to control (19 × vs. 14 ×). We have shown that glutathione inhibition of cisplatin binding to DNA is concentration dependent; 5 mM glutathione decreases the rate of cisplatin binding to DNA 4·4-fold, but 0·5 mM glutathione has minimal inhibitory effect (P. C. Dedon and R. F. Borch, unpublished results). This concentration difference approximates that which can be achieved intracellularly by BSO treatment, and the rate differences for cisplatin–DNA binding approximate the dose modification factors observed by Ozols *et al.* in both sensitive and resistant cells. A recent report indicates that glutathione depletion by BSO reverses the marked cross-resistance of these ovarian cell lines to carboplatin (Hamilton *et al.*, 1986). It is unlikely that this resistance is mediated by direct reaction of glutathione with carboplatin, since the half-life for this reaction exceeds 40 hours at 5 mM glutathione concentration (Dedon and Borch, 1987). These data suggest that intracellular glutathione may be an important determinant for both nephrotoxicity and tumour cell cytotoxicity. The mechanistic basis for glutathione's effect, however, has not been established.

Metallothionein and cisplatin metabolism

Metallothioneins are cytosolic proteins of molecular weight 6000–7000 that contain 20 cysteine residues, all of which are present in the reduced state and configured to provide seven tetrahedral metal binding sites. Because of the unusually high cysteine content of metallothionein, numerous investigators have studied the role of these proteins in cisplatin cytotoxicity. Two factors should be kept in mind when considering the interactions between platinum complexes and metallothionein. First, metallothionein binds with extremely high affinity to those metals (zinc and cadmium, for example) that have tetrahedral geometry. Platinum (II) complexes possess square planar geometry and should be incapable of forming a tetracoordinate complex with metallothionein. Second, the cysteine residues of metallothionein do not exist as free sulphydryl groups; they are tightly associated with divalent metals, usually zinc. Reaction of metallothionein with a platinum complex therefore requires prior dissociation of a high-affinity metal from the protein and preferential reaction of the dissociated complex with platinum. On this basis one would predict that reactions of cisplatin and metallothionein should be very slow. Although the reaction between aquated cisplatin and cysteine or glutathione is essentially instantaneous, reaction of aquated cisplatin and Zn-metallothionein (Pt : Zn ratio = 12·5) for 1 hour led to incorporation of only two platinum atoms and retention of approximately 60% of bound zinc (Kraker *et al.*, 1985).

Several investigators have reported that cisplatin binds to metallothionein or to a "metallothionein-like" protein; identification was based primarily on platinum analysis of peaks collected from Sephadex chromatography. Analysis of rat kidney 24 hours after cisplatin administration showed that approximately 25%, 25% and 50% of total platinum eluted in a high molecular weight fraction, a "metallothionein" fraction, and a low molecular weight (perhaps glutathione) fraction respectively (Sharma and Edwards, 1983). A similar analysis 8 hours after cisplatin showed a much smaller peak in the metallothionein elution volume. Pretreatment with cisplatin gave identical results; however, pretreatment with cadmium chloride, a potent inducer of metallothionein, significantly increased the amount of platinum in the metallothionein fraction (Litterst, 1984). A third study examined platinum binding in rat kidney fractions 15 minutes and 24 hours after cisplatin. After 15 minutes most of the platinum was in the low molecular weight fraction; no platinum was found in the metallothionein fraction. By 24 hours the low molecular weight platinum peak was markedly reduced and was replaced by a broad heterogeneous peak in the metallothionein region. Pretreatment with cadmium chloride induced metallothionein synthesis but did not increase the quantity of platinum associated with the metallothionein peak. Cisplatin did not induce metallothionein. These authors concluded that metallothionein does not have a significant role in the renal metabolism of cisplatin in the rat (Mason *et al.*, 1984). A fourth report also provided evidence for increased platinum in the metallothionein fraction after cadmium chloride pretreatment. Platinum appeared to replace zinc in the (Zn–Cd)metallothionein, and radioimmunoassay showed that the platinum-metallothioneins were cross-reactive with the native metallothionein. The reaction of excess cisplatin with (Zn–Cd)metallothionein was also examined *in vitro*. After 2 hours, less than 10% of the platinum eluted in the metallothionein fraction. Equilibrium was finally reached after 72 hours, when approximately 40% of the platinum was bound to metallothionein (Zelazowski *et al.*, 1984). These data confirm that cisplatin or a metabolite binds to a metallothionein-like protein via displacement of zinc, but that the rate of binding is very slow. Although pretreatment with metallothionein-inducing metals has been shown to reduce the lethal toxicity of cisplatin in mice, there was no correlation between renal metallothionein levels and degree of protection (Naganuma *et al.*, 1985). If one assumes that the toxic lesion in the kidney is formed within minutes after cisplatin administration, it is difficult to postulate a role for metallothionein in the renal metabolism of this drug.

The contribution of metallothionein to resistance against cisplatin is ambiguous. Human epithelial and mouse fibroblast cell lines containing trace amounts of metallothionein were made resistant to cadmium chloride; the resistant lines contained very high levels of metallothionein with a metal content >95% cadmium. Growth curves showed that the cadmium-resistant cells were also resistant to cisplatin; clonogenic assay indicated a cisplatin resistance factor of 1·6 ($LC_{99} = 50\ \mu M$ vs. $30\ \mu M$). 70% of the cytosolic platinum was bound to metallothionein in the cadmium-resistant cells, but these measurements were made after four days of cisplatin treatment (Bakka *et al.*, 1981). Evaluation of the sensitive and resistant mouse fibroblast cell lines *in vivo* showed that both lines were equally responsive to cisplatin at a dose of 8 mg/kg, but only the parent cell line responded to a 4 mg/kg dose (Endreson *et al.*, 1984). Two cadmium-resistant sublines of human ovarian cells were 2- and 3-fold resistant to cisplatin but were also resistant to melphalan. The corresponding cisplatin-resistant lines, however, were not cross-resistant to cadmium (Murphy *et al.*, 1985). Ehrlich cells are highly sensitive to cisplatin, although they have substantial levels of cytosolic metallothionein. Under conditions where cisplatin is cytotoxic, 30% of cytosolic platinum is bound to the metallothionein fraction after 25 hours (Kraker *et al.*, 1985). It is apparent that cadmium pretreatment can induce cross-resistance to cisplatin, and that platinum is associated with metallothionein after many hours. However, there is no evidence that metallothionein contributes to resistance developed against cisplatin. We have shown that treatment of L1210 cells with a powerful platinum chelator 30–60 minutes after cisplatin exposure has no effect on cytotoxicity (Bodenner *et al.*, 1986a). The highly unfavourable kinetics of the cisplatin–metallothionein reaction imply that metallothionein is unlikely to alter cisplatin cytotoxicity by a mechanism involving direct coordination of the metal.

Pharmacokinetics

The pharmacokinetics and distribution of cisplatin have been studied extensively in animal models and in man. The pharmacokinetic data must be interpreted with caution, however, because the results are highly dependent upon whether total platinum or non-protein bound platinum was measured. Distribution studies using radiolabelled platinum indicate that cisplatin was rapidly distributed to all organs after i.v. administration, with relatively high retention in kidney, liver, skin, and spleen in the dog (Lagasse *et al.*, 1981) and rat (Harrison *et al.*, 1983). In the rat, plasma clearance of free platinum was biphasic with α and β half-lives of 2 and 10 minutes respectively; renal clearance of free platinum exceeded inulin clearance, indicating net tubular secretion. 54% of plasma platinum was protein-bound after one hour, and 40–50% of the platinum dose was excreted in the urine in the first 72 hours (Siddik *et al.*, 1986; Daley-Yates and McBrien, 1985 a). Free platinum clearance after carboplatin administration in the rat had half-lives of 3 and 26 minutes, with 17% of total plasma platinum bound to protein at 1 hour and 80–90% of the dose excreted in the urine within 72 hours. Conflicting data were obtained for the fractional renal clearance of carboplatin; Siddik *et al.* found that renal clearance of carboplatin was identical to that of inulin. However, Daley-Yates and McBrien observed increased and equivalent fractional renal clearances for cisplatin, carboplatin and iproplatin, indicating net tubular secretion for all three drugs. The pharmacokinetics of iproplatin in the dog showed rapid renal excretion of the parent drug with a half-life of 20–30 minutes; plasma clearance of total platinum was biphasic with half-lives of 35 minutes and 34 hours (Pendyala *et al.*, 1982). Although these values are similar to those for cisplatin in the dog (12 minutes and 54 hours; Lagasse *et al.*, 1981), irreversible protein binding is a major factor for cisplatin but is essentially non-existent for iproplatin (Pendyala *et al.*, 1982; Daley-Yates and McBrien, 1985 a).

Total plasma platinum pharmacokinetics after cisplatin administration in patients was biphasic, with α and β half-lives in the range of 20–50 minutes and 20–80 hours respectively. 30–70% of the platinum dose is excreted in the urine, most in the first 6 hours (Thatcher *et al.*, 1982 and references therein). The pharmacokinetics of free platinum in patients after bolus injection was also biphasic, but the β phase half-life was 48 minutes, suggesting that the very slow terminal phase of total platinum was associated with removal of protein-bound drug. Clearance also depended on rate of drug administration; with a 15-minute infusion the terminal half-life was 48 minutes, and 40% of the dose was excreted in the urine. Following a 6-hour infusion, the early rapid clearance phase was obscured and a single exponential clearance with a half-life of 26 minutes was observed; 75% of the dose was excreted in the urine with this longer infusion (Belt *et al.*, 1979). Free platinum half-lives of 30 minutes have also been reported for bolus (Himmelstein *et al.*, 1981) and infusion routes (Reece *et al.*, 1985). An interesting but unexplained effect on free platinum clearance comparing 30-minute infusions of conventional-dose cisplatin and high-dose cisplatin with hypertonic saline has been reported; clearance half-lives increased from 19 minutes for conventional dose therapy to 31 minutes using high dose with hypertonic saline. No significant increase in half-life was noted when the first and fifth courses of a five-day infusion were compared (Corden *et al.*, 1985). Fractional renal clearance of cisplatin exceeds unity in patients, indicating that net tubular secretion occurs (Jacobs, 1986). The non-linear clearance of ultrafilterable platinum recently reported in patients was interpreted as net tubular secretion coexisting with a saturable reabsorption process (Reece *et al.*, 1985).

The clinical pharmacokinetics of carboplatin and iproplatin have been less extensively studied. Carboplatin is cleared almost exclusively by glomerular filtration, with most of the dose excreted in the urine within 24 hours after administration. Binding of drug to plasma protein is very slow (Calvert *et al.*, 1982; Harland *et al.*, 1984). Ultrafilterable platinum clearance was biphasic with half-lives of 87 and 354 minutes after a 1-hour infusion (Harland *et al.*, 1984) but was mono-exponential with a half-life of 170 minutes after a 24-hour infusion (Curt *et al.*, 1983). Free platinum clearance values of 106 and 123 ml/min have been reported, confirming the importance of glomerular filtration and the apparent absence of tubular secretion for this drug in man (Curt *et al.*, 1983; Harland *et al.*, 1984). A recent study in patients with compromised renal function showed excellent correlation between total body clearance of ultrafilterable platinum and creatinine clearance (Egorin *et al.*, 1984).

The pharmacokinetics of iproplatin appear to be dose-dependent. Total platinum clearance was biphasic when tracer doses (1–2 mg) of drug were used; half-lives were 17 minutes and 78 hours, and 60% of the drug dose was excreted in the urine (Thatcher *et al.*, 1982). Administration of therapeutic doses (20–350 mg/m^2) resulted in total platinum clearance half-lives of 1 and 64 hours. Plasma clearance of filterable platinum was mono-exponential at low doses ($t_{1/2} = 1{\cdot}75$ h) but biexponential at high doses ($t_{1/2} = 1{\cdot}1$ and 32 h). Iproplatin does not bind to plasma proteins, so the long terminal half-life at high doses presumably results from protein binding of drug metabolites. Clearance of unchanged iproplatin was mono-exponential with a half-life of 55 minutes. Urinary excretion varied widely for this drug (15–60% of total dose at therapeutic levels) (Pendyala *et al.*, 1983). The importance of renal function to the clearance of iproplatin has also been studied in patients with subnormal creatinine clearance. Plasma clearance of iproplatin was biphasic, with half-lives of 25 minutes and 3·2 hours. Total body clearance was 120–330 ml/min (mean 240) and correlated with creatinine clearance (Pendyala *et al.*, 1985). It is interesting to note that the toxicity of both carboplatin and iproplatin measured by reduction in platelet count correlated with the AUC of free drug in the plasma (Egorin *et al.*, 1984; Pendyala *et al.*, 1985).

Renal handling of cisplatin

The kidney is the critical organ involved in cisplatin metabolism; it is the predominant excretory organ (Litterst *et al.*, 1977; Wolf and Manaka, 1976), it is the major site of platinum accumulation and retention, and it represents the target for dose-limiting toxicity. The relationships between nephrotoxicity and renal uptake and excretion are not well understood. Free cisplatin is cleared from plasma with an initial half-life of approximately 30 minutes, predominantly by renal excretion and binding to plasma protein ($t_{1/2}$ approx. 60 minutes) (Daley-Yates and McBrien, 1984). Cisplatin is freely filtered at the glomerulus, and the parent drug represents the predominant form of free platinum in both plasma and urine (Safirstein *et al.*, 1983). The role of tubular secretion and reabsorption has been studied extensively because of its potential importance in drug clearance and as a mechanism for platinum entrance to tubule cells. The clearance ratio (CR) of free (i.e., non-protein bound) platinum may be dependent upon both species and measurement protocol; published results are summarized in table 5. The data obtained via infusion in man indicate net tubular secretion of free platinum which is inhibited by administration of probenecid (Jacobs *et al.*, 1980, 1984). A recent report indicates that ultrafilterable platinum clearance in man is non-linear, with a rapid initial clearance followed by a subsequent decline. The authors suggest that cisplatin is both secreted and reabsorbed, and that reabsorption is a saturable process (Reece *et al.*, 1985). The CR measured via infusion in the

Table 5. Fractional renal platinum clearance following platinum drug administration

Species (Route)	Drug (Metab)†	Other treatment	Clearance ratio	Reference
Perfused rat kidney	CP (UF)		1·25	Daley-Yates and McBrien (1982 a)
		Probenecid	1·95	
		Furosemide	1·24	
Anaesthetized rat (i.p. bolus)	CP (UF)		2·4	Daley-Yates and McBrien (1983)
	CP (CP)		3·5	
Anaesthetized rat (i.v. infusion)	CP (UF)		1·15	Osman and Litterst (1983)
		Probenecid	1·69	
		NMN	0·95	
Conscious rat (i.p. bolus)	CP (UF)		3·08	Daley-Yates and McBrien (1985 a)
		Probenecid	5·05	
		Furosemide	2·07	
		Triethanolamine	4·69	
		Choline	3·89	
	TP (UF)		3·28	
	CB (UF)		3·35	
	IP (UF)		4·04	
Mouse (s.c. bolus)	CP (DER)		0·83	Nelson *et al.* (1984)
		Cimetidine	0·41	
Man (24 h infusion)	CP (UF)		2·7	Jacobs *et al.* (1984)
		Probenecid	1·6	
Man (1 h infusion)	CB (UF)		0·7–0·9	Harland *et al.* (1984)

†Parentheses show the platinum species actually measured. UF = ultrafilterable platinum; DER = derivatized free platinum; CP = cisplatin; TP = trans-platinum; CB = carboplatin; IP = iproplatin.

anaesthetized rat, however, is essentially unity and increases following probenecid but is unaffected by *N*-methylnicotinamide (NMN) administration. The authors suggest that both tubular secretion and reabsorption may be operating and that probenecid may be inhibiting reabsorption (Osman and Litterst, 1983). Studies with the isolated perfused rat kidney show similar results, with CRs of 1·25 and 1·95 respectively in the absence and presence of probenecid (Daley-Yates and McBrien, 1982 a). The CR after i.p. bolus administration in the conscious rat was 3·08 and increased to 5·05 and 4·69 respectively after administration of probenecid and triethanolamine (Daley-Yates and McBrien, 1985 a). In the mouse, the CRs were 0·83 and 0·41 respectively in the absence and presence of cimetidine (Nelson *et al.*, 1984). These data suggest that tubular secretion contributes to platinum clearance *in vivo*, but the effects of both cation (NMN, triethanolamine and cimetidine) and anion (probenecid) transport inhibitors on platinum clearance are not consistent.

Daley-Yates and McBrien have investigated in the rat the pharmacokinetics and toxicity of cisplatin metabolites separable by HPLC. The CR of free platinum (all metabolites) was 2·4; cisplatin and two metabolites showed net secretion (CR 3·5, 4·2 and 2·1), and two metabolites showed net reabsorption (CR 0·35 and 0·55) (Daley-Yates and McBrien, 1983). Although the structures of these metabolites are unknown, two additional metabolites having CR near unity had retention volumes identical to adducts produced by reaction of cisplatin with methionine. The metabolite having CR 2·1 (metabolite "F") had a retention volume identical to the diammine diaquo complex; this metabolite was a minor component during the first hour after cisplatin administration but increased to 40% of plasma metabolites after two hours (Daley-Yates and McBrien, 1984). This metabolite is unlikely to be the aquated species given the high chloride concentration in the plasma and the rapid reaction that occurs between the aquated species and chloride ion ($t_{1/2} < 5$ minutes at 100 mM chloride). Metabolite "F" is unique, however, in that hypertonic saline administration reduces its urinary excretion in the rat (Daley-Yates and McBrien, 1985 b). Administration of the mixture of metabolites to rats and to tumour-bearing mice demonstrated that the mixed metabolites had minimal anti-tumour activity but were more nephrotoxic than a comparable dose of cisplatin (Daley-Yates and McBrien, 1984).

The relationship between cisplatin uptake and cation or anion transport has been examined in several other systems. The Sperber chicken preparation provides a means to evaluate peritubular effects of nephrotoxic drugs. Cisplatin administration preferentially inhibited both cation (tetraethylammonium = TEA) and anion (PAH) transport, and this inhibition was completely blocked by prior administration of the cations quinine and cyanine (Bird *et al.*, 1984). Cisplatin had no effect on either brush border or basolateral PAH transport in the rat tubular membrane vesicle preparation. Transport of the cations TEA and NMN were inhibited by cisplatin treatment for both brush border and basolateral membranes. In the latter case, inhibition was competitive, with $K_i = 0 \cdot 12$ mM (Williams and Hottendorf, 1985). It is unlikely that cisplatin metabolites are responsible for inhibition in these two systems; a 5-minute infusion was used in the Sperber preparation, and the membrane vesicles were incubated for 30 seconds with metabolite-free drug. Cisplatin inhibited both PAH and TEA uptake in mouse kidney slices, and inhibition could be reversed by addition of excess PAH or TEA (Nelson *et al.*, 1984).

Factors affecting platinum uptake in rat kidney cortical slices have also been studied using (^{14}C-en)$PtCl_2$ to facilitate uptake measurements (Safirstein *et al.*, 1984). Drug uptake was both oxygen- and temperature-dependent, with slice/medium ratios (S/M) of 2·5–3·5. PAH and most other organic anions had no effect; probenecid uniquely inhibited uptake 50%. Organic cations inhibited uptake 25–50%, and uncouplers of oxidative phosphorylation inhibited 30–40%. The authors suggest that probenecid may be acting at a site other than that for anion transport. Unbound intracellular platinum analysed after cisplatin exposure was different in both chromatographic mobility and mutagenicity compared to administered or excreted cisplatin. The structure of this intracellular metabolite is unknown; its similar but earlier elution volume using a strong cation exchange column suggests that this substitution product is also neutral.

The relationship between platinum transport and toxicity in the kidney is still controversial. Probenecid was reported to reduce cisplatin nephrotoxicity in the F344 rat, although serum creatinine values still exceeded 3 mg/dl in rats receiving both cisplatin and probenecid (Ross and Gale, 1979). In contrast, probenecid increased cisplatin-induced nephrotoxicity in Wistar rats (Daley-Yates and McBrien, 1985 a). In man, probenecid administration was accompanied by decreases in platinum clearance and nephrotoxicity (Jacobs, 1986). Administration of organic cations inhibited nephrotoxicity in the chicken (quinine and cyanine) (Bird *et al.*, 1984) and in the rat (choline chloride) (Daley-Yates and McBrien, 1985 a). Renal tubular transport of cisplatin or a metabolite may be a necessary but not sufficient condition for nephrotoxicity; fractional clearances of cisplatin, trans-DDP, carboplatin, and iproplatin in the rat are not significantly different, although cisplatin is highly nephrotoxic while the analogues are non-nephrotoxic.

A number of strategies has been developed to inhibit the severe dose-limiting nephrotoxicity of cisplatin. These studies are important because of their potential clinical significance and for the clues they may provide to understand the mechanism of renal tubule toxicity. Hydration–diuresis regimens are now used routinely in cisplatin therapy; they have been discussed extensively in previous reviews (Prestayko *et al.*, 1980; Loehrer and Einhorn, 1984) and will not be considered further. A highly promising variant involves the use of hypertonic saline as the vehicle for cisplatin administration. Litterst has demonstrated significant reductions in nephrotoxicity and platinum concentrations in tissues (particularly kidney) when cisplatin was prepared in 4·5% sodium chloride solution. Coadministration of hypertonic saline with cisplatin prepared in distilled water was not protective, indicating the importance of high salt concentrations in the vehicle itself. Potassium, ammonium and calcium chlorides were also protective; sodium iodide demonstrated the highest degree of protection. The anti-tumour efficacy of cisplatin against intraperitoneal P388 murine leukaemia was not affected (Litterst, 1981), but hypertonic saline has been shown to inhibit anti-tumour effect against intravenous P388 and several other tumour lines (Aamdal *et al.*, 1984). Renal protection correlated best with urinary chloride concentration; sodium and ammonium chloride afforded equivalent protection. Sodium chloride did not protect when given 3 hours after cisplatin (Daley-Yates and McBrien, 1985 b). High-dose cisplatin in hypertonic saline has been used successfully in the clinic

(Corden *et al.*, 1985; Ozols *et al.*, 1984). Although nephrotoxicity was minimal with this dose schedule (40 mg/m^2 in 3% NaCl daily for five days, with continuous saline hydration), systemic side-effects were not diminished.

The mechanistic basis for this protection is not clear. High concentrations of sodium chloride in the vehicle presumably suppress formation of toxic metabolites prior to drug infusion. Plasma chloride concentrations are not changed, however, so it is unlikely that the beneficial effect involves modification of plasma metabolites. The high lumenal chloride concentration and dilute urine should decrease the toxicity of metabolites entering the cell from the lumenal side; however, one study suggests that toxicity is based upon peritubular drug entry (Bird *et al.*, 1984). Reduction of one urinary metabolite has been observed in the rat with sodium chloride pretreatment, but this metabolite constitutes only 3% of the total platinum excreted over five hours (Daley-Yates and McBrien, 1985 b).

Two agents have proved to be effective inhibitors of cisplatin-induced nephrotoxicity when administered just before or concurrent with cisplatin and are currently in clinical trials (Figure 4). The radioprotector WR-2721 blocked toxicity without inhibiting anti-tumour effects in the rat (Yuhas and Culo, 1980), presumably via hydrolysis of the thiophosphate to give a substituted aminoethanethiol (WR-1065) that is capable of chelating platinum. This aminoethanethiol metabolite has been shown to inhibit cisplatin-induced cytotoxicity in V79 cells, with dose modification factors of 2·9, 1·4 and 1·4 when cells were treated with the thiol 30 minutes before, concurrent with, and 30 minutes after cisplatin, respectively (Nagy *et al.*, 1986). Protection against both kidney and systemic toxicity has been observed in the clinic (Glover *et al.*, 1984). Sodium thiosulphate also blocked nephrotoxicity when administered between one hour before and 30 minutes after cisplatin; it was ineffective outside this time period. Renal protection was accompanied by significant inhibition of anti-tumour effect against L1210 leukaemia (Aamdal *et al.*, 1986; Howell and Taetle, 1980). Thiosulphate also inhibited the uptake of platinum by both bacterial and tumour cells exposed to cisplatin but did not significantly

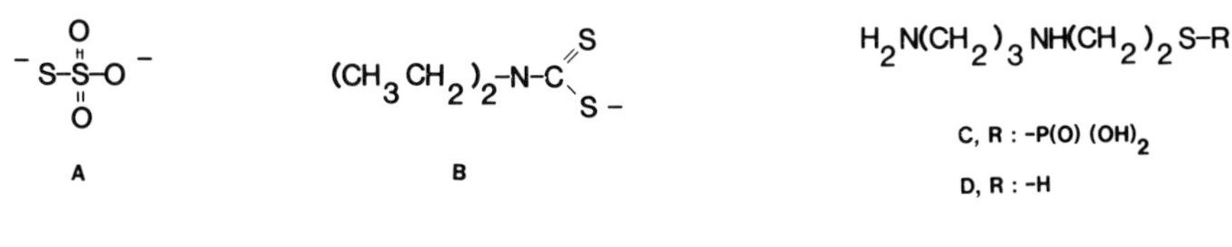

Figure 4. Structures of cisplatin chemoprotectors. A: Thiosulphate; B: Diethyldithiocarbamate; C: WR-2721; D: WR-1065.

alter plasma or renal tissue distribution (Uozumi and Litterst, 1986; Uozumi *et al.*, 1984). The combination of intraperitoneal cisplatin with systemic thiosulphate neutralization is effective for the treatment of intraperitoneal tumour; systemic thiosulphate inhibits nephrotoxicity but not systemic toxicity at high cisplatin doses (Pfeifle *et al.*, 1985; Howell *et al.*, 1983). Presumably WR-2721 and thiosulphate act by reacting with and inactivating highly reactive and toxic platinum metabolites produced shortly alter drug administration.

Sodium diethyldithiocarbamate (DDTC) is also an effective heavy metal chelating agent, but it exhibits selectivity that is unique among cisplatin chemoprotectors. DDTC reacts with and essentially removes platinum from cisplatin adducts *except* for those in which the chloride ligands have been replaced by two guanine residues (Bodenner *et al.*, 1986 a). Thus DDTC acts as a "rescue" agent to remove platinum from all sites except those involving DNA cross-links. Restoration of cisplatin-inhibited α_2-macroglobulin activity (Gonias *et al.*, 1984) and γ-glutamyl transpeptidase activity (Bodenner *et al.*, 1986 a) have been reported. DDTC inhibited cisplatin-induced toxicity to the kidney, bone marrow, and GI tract when administered 2 hours after cisplatin. Inhibition of anti-tumour effect was not observed *in vitro* or *in vivo* (Borch *et al.*, 1980; Bodenner *et al.*, 1986 b). DDTC did not inhibit nephrotoxicity when given concomitantly with cisplatin, suggesting that its protective effects depend upon prior formation of toxic complexes reversible by DDTC. Inhibition of toxicity requires that these complexes be reversed within hours, since protection by DDTC decreases in a time-dependent manner when DDTC is delayed more than 2–3 hours (Borch and Pleasants, 1979; Dedon and Borch, 1986).

Although the exact mechanism of cisplatin-induced nephrotoxicity remains obscure, several aspects merit comment. First, the Sperber chicken and tissue slice studies suggest that parent drug rather than a metabolite enters the tubule cell, probably from the peritubular side. Second, the toxic event is probably initiated by intracellular formation of an unbound metabolite that can be neutralized by thiosulphate. Third, the formation of subsequent reactions of this metabolite may be prevented by agents such as acetazolamide or hypertonic sodium chloride which block toxicity when given 30 minutes before or concurrently with cisplatin but are ineffective 30 minutes later (Heidemann *et al.*, 1985). Fourth, the metabolite presumably binds to an intracelluar target to produce toxicity to the tubule cell. This target may be an enzyme, although the inhibition of γ-glutamyl transpeptidase and ATPase reported with cisplatin *in vitro* is not observed after cisplatin treatment *in vivo* (Dedon and Borch, 1987; Uozumi and Litterst, 1985). DNA is also a possible target, but DNA cross-linking does not correlate with toxicity in normal tissues (Murray *et al.*, 1985), and the ability of DDTC to reverse platinum–DNA cross-links in kidney but not in tumour cells would be difficult to explain. Fifth, toxicity can be prevented by DDTC-induced reversal of platinum binding to the target site within 1–2 hours. Finally, a major dilemma remains in that the toxic lesion presumably forms within minutes and must be reversed within 1–2 hours, but the earliest physiological changes do not occur until 48–72 hours after cisplatin treatment (Winston and Safirstein, 1985).

Future directions

Notwithstanding the tremendous progress of platinum drug research in recent years, several major questions remain to be answered. What is the basis for differential sensitivity to cisplatin and its analogues, with respect to both normal vs. tumour cells and sensitive vs. resistant tumour cells? Does DNA repair play a significant role in differential response? Is the intra-strand DNA cross-link the major determinant of cytotoxicity and, if so, what is the role of the inter-strand cross-link? Do the existing platinum analogues form structurally similar DNA lesions? The recent development of an antibody to the Pt-(GpG) intra-strand complex by Porier and co-workers represents a major advance and should provide a method evaluate the formation and repair of these cross-links under a variety of conditions. What is the mechanistic basis for cisplatin-induced nephrotoxicity? To what extent is drug metabolism a determinant of this toxicity? Cisplatin and carboplatin undergo substitution reactions to form identical products but at significantly different rates. Is this kinetic difference the determining factor in carboplatin's increased bone marrow toxicity and decreased kidney and neurotoxicity? Answers to these questions will be important both to guide the design and synthesis of new analogues and to improve the clinical efficacy of currently used drugs. Cisplatin continues to be a widely used and important drug, and the newer high-dose protocols should extend its therapeutic response in a variety of malignancies. The profound neurotoxicity that has emerged after multiple high doses is currently dose-limiting, and it remains to be seen whether the chemoprotectors currently under investigation will ameliorate this effect. Carboplatin appears to be relatively free of cisplatin's major toxicities, but severe bone marrow suppression currently limits the use of this drug. Recent work in our laboratory has shown that diethyldithiocarbamate protects pluripotent stem cells from carboplatin-induced cytotoxicity; inasmuch as carboplatin's only clinically significant toxicity is to the bone marrow, the combination of carboplatin with DDTC appears worthy of clinical investigation.

The platinum anti-cancer drugs will continue to be an important and fruitful area for basic and clinical research. The continued synthesis and development of new analogues, and continuing efforts to use currently approved drugs more effectively, assure that these drugs will make a major contribution to the future treatment of cancer.

References

Aamdal, S., Fodstad, O., Kaalhus, O. and Pihl, A., 1984, Reduced antineoplastic activity in mice of cisplatin administered with high salt concentration in the vehicle. *J. Natl. Cancer Inst.*, **73**, 743–752.

Aamdal, S., Fodstad, O., Storeng, R. and Pihl, A., 1986, Reduced antitumor activity of cisplatin after concurrent intravenous administration of thiosulfate. *Proc. Am. Ass. Cancer Res.*, **27**, 292.

Abbott, W. A., Bridges, R. J. and Meister, A., 1984, Extracellular metabolism of glutathione accounts for its disappearance from the basolateral circulation of the kidney. *J. Biol. Chem.*, **259**, 15393–15400.

Alden, W. W. and Repta, A. J., 1984, Exacerbation of cisplatin-induced nephrotoxicity by methionine. *Chem. Biol. Interact.* **48**, 121–124.

Andrews, P. A., Murphy, M. P. and Howell, S. B., 1985, Differential potentiation of alkylating and platinating agent cytotoxicity in human ovarian carcinoma cells by glutathione depletion. *Cancer Res.* **45**, 6250–6253.

Arrick, B. A. and Nathan, C. F., 1984, Glutathione metabolism as a determinant of therapeutic efficacy: a review. *Cancer Res.*, **44**, 4224–4232.

Aull, J. L., Allen, R. L., Bapat, A. R., Daron, H. H., Friedman, M. E. and Wilson, J. F., 1979, The effects of platinum complexes on seven enzymes. *Biochim. Biophys. Acta*, **571**, 352–358.

Bakka, A., Endresen, L., Johnsen, A. B. S., Edminson, P. D. and Rugstad, H. E., 1981, Resistance against cis-dichlorodiammineplatinum in cultured cells with a high content of metallothionein. *Toxic. Appl. Pharmacol.* **61**, 215–226.

Belt, R. J., Himmelstein, K. J., Patton, T. F., Bannister, S. J., Sternson, L. A. and Repta, A. J., 1979, Pharmacokinetics of non-protein-bound platinum species following administration of cis-dichlorodiammineplatinum(II). *Cancer Treat. Rep.*, **63**, 1515–1521.

Bird, J. E., Walser, M. M. and Quebbemann, A. J., 1984, Protective effect of organic cation transport inhibitors on Cis-diamminedichloroplatinum-induced nephrotoxicity. *J. Pharmac. Exp. Ther.*, **231**, 752–758.

Blachley, J. D. and Hill, J. B., 1981, Renal and electrolyte disturbances associated with cisplatin. *Ann. Int. Med.*, **95**, 628–632.

Bodenner, D. L., Dedon, P. C., Keng, P. C. and Borch, R. F., 1986 a, Effect of diethyldithiocarbamate on cis-diamminedichloroplatinum(II)-induced cytotoxicity, DNA cross-linking, and γ-glutamyltranspeptidase inhibition. *Cancer Res.*, **46**, 2745–2750.

Bodenner, D. L., Dedon, P. C., Keng, P. C., Katz, J. C. and Borch, R. F., 1986 b, Selective protection against cis-diamminedichloroplatinum(II)-induced toxicity in kidney, gut, and bone marrow by diethyldithiocarbamate rescue. *Cancer Res.*, **46**, 2751–2756.

Borch, R. F. and Pleasants, M. E., 1979, Inhibition of cis-platinum nephrotoxicity by diethyldithiocarbamate rescue in a rat model. *Proc. Natl. Acad. Sci. USA*, **76**, 6611–6614.

Borch, R. F., Katz, J. C., Lieder, P. H. and Pleasants, M. E., 1980, Effect of diethyldithiocarbamate rescue on tumor response to cis-platinum in a rat model. *Proc. Natl Acad. Sci. USA*, **77**, 5441–5444.

Calvert, A. H., Harland, S. J., Newell, D. R., Siddik, Z. H., Jones, A. C., McElwain, T. J., Raju, S., Wiltshaw, E., Smith, I. E., Baker, J. M., Peckham, M. J. and Harrap, K. P., 1982, Early clinical studies with cis-diammine-1,1-cyclobutane-dicarboxylate platinum(II). *Cancer Chemother. Pharmacol.*, **9**, 140–147.

Campbell, A. B., Kalman, S. M. and Jacobs, C., 1983, Plasma platinum levels: relationship to cisplatin dose and nephrotoxicity. *Cancer Treat. Rep.*, **67**, 169–172.

Ciccarelli, R. B., Solomon, M. J., Varshavsky, A., and Lippard, S. J., 1985, In vivo effects of cis- and trans-diamminedichloroplatinum(II) on SV40 chromosomes: differential repair, DNA-protein cross-linking, and inhibition of replication. *Biochemistry*, **24**, 7533–7540.

Corden, B. J., Fine, R. L., Ozols, R. F. and Collins, J. M., 1985, Clinical pharmacology of high-dose cisplatin. *Cancer Chemother. Pharmacol.*, **14**, 38–41.

Creaven, P. J., Madajewicz, S., Pendyala, L., Mittelman, A., Pontes, E., Spaulding, M., Arbuck, S. and Solomon, J., 1983, Phase I clinical trial of *cis*-dichloro-*trans*-dihydroxy-bis-isopropylamine platinum(IV) (CHIP). *Cancer Treat. Rep.*, **67**, 795–800.

Curt, G. A., Grygiel, J. J., Corden, B. J., Ozols, R. F., Weiss, R. B., Tell, D. T., Myers, C. E. and Collins, J. M., 1983, A phase I and pharmacokinetic study of diamminecyclobutanedicarboxylatoplatinum (NSC 241240). *Cancer Res.*, **43**, 4470–4473.

Daley-Yates, P. T. and McBrien, D. C. H., 1982 a, The mechanism of renal clearance of cisplatin (cis-dichlorodiammine platinum II) and its modification by furosemide and probenecid. *Biochem. Pharmacol.*, **31**, 2243–2246.

Daley-Yates, P. T. and McBrien, D. C. H., 1982 b, The inhibition of renal ATPase by cisplatin and some biotransformation products. *Chem. Biol. Interactions*, **40**, 325–334.

Daley-Yates, P. T. and McBrien, D. C. H., 1983, Cisplatin metabolites: a method for their separation and for measurement of their renal clearance in vivo. *Biochem. Pharmacol.*, **32**, 181–184.

Daley-Yates P. T. and McBrien, D. C. H., 1984, Cisplatin metabolites in plasma, a study of their pharmacokinetics and importance in the nephrotoxic and anti-tumour activity of cisplatin. *Biochem. Pharmacol.*, **33**, 3063–3070.

Daley-Yates, P. T. and McBrien, D. C. H., 1985 a, The renal fractional clearance of platinum antitumour compounds in relation to nephrotoxicity. *Biochem. Pharmacol.*, **34**, 1423–1428.

Daley-Yates, P. T. and McBrien, D. C. H., 1985 b, A study of the protective effect of chloride salts on cisplatin nephrotoxicity. *Biochem. Pharmacol.*, **34**, 2363–2369.

Dedon, P. C., Qazi, R. and Borch, R. F., 1986, Potential mechanisms of cisplatin toxicity and diethyldithiocarbamate rescue. In *Biochemical Mechanisms of Platinum Antitumour Drugs*, edited by D. C. H. McBrien (Oxford: IRL Press), pp. 199–225.

Dedon, P. C. and Borch, R. F., 1987, Characterization of the reactions of platinum antitumor agents with biologic and nonbiologic sulfur-containing nucleophiles. *Biochem. Pharmacol.* (in the press).

Douple, E. B., 1984, Cis-diamminedichloroplatinum(II): effects of a representative metal coordination complex on mammalian cells. *Pharmacol. Ther.*, **25**, 297–326.

Drasga, R. E., Einhorn, L. H. and Williams, S. D., 1982, The chemotherapy of testicular cancer. *CA-A Cancer Journal for Clinicians*, **32**, 65–77.

Eastman, A., 1983, Characterization of the adducts produced in DNA by cis-diamminedichloroplatinum(II) and cis-dichloro(ethylenediamine) platinum(II). *Biochemistry*, **22**, 3927–3933.

Eastman, A., 1985, Interstrand cross-links and sequence specificity in the reaction of *cis*-dichloro(ethylenediamine) platinum(II) with DNA. *Biochemistry*, **24**, 5027–5032.

Eastman, A., 1986, Reevaluation of cis-dichloro(ethylenediamine)platinum(II) with DNA. *Biochemistry*, **25**, 3912–3915.

Egorin, M. J., Van Echo, D. A., Tipping, S. J., Olman, E. A., Whitacre, M. Y., Thompson, B. W. and Aisner, J., 1984, Pharmacokinetics and dosage reduction of *cis*-diammine(1,1-cyclobutanedicarboxylato)platinum in patients with impaired renal function. *Cancer Res.*, **44**, 5432–5438.

Endreson, L., Schjerven, L, and Rugstad, H. E., 1984, Tumors from a cell strain with a high content of metallothionein show enhanced resistance against *cis*-dichlorodiammine platinum. *Acta Pharmacol Tox.*, **55**, 183–187.

Ervin, T. J., Clark, J. R. and Weichselbaum, R. R., 1985, Multidisciplinary treatment of advanced squamous carcinoma of the head and neck. *Seminars in Oncology*, **12**, (Suppl. 6), 71–78.

Evans, B. D., Raju, K. S., Calver, A. H., Harland, S. J. and Wiltshaw, E., 1983, Phase II study of JM8, a new platinum analog, in advanced ovarian carcinoma. *Cancer Treat. Rep.*, **67**, 997–1000.

Fichtinger-Schepman, A. M. J., vanderVeer, J. L., denHartog, J. H. J., Lohman, P. H. M., and Reedijk, J., 1985, Adducts of the antitumor drug *cis*-diammine-dichloroplatinum(II) with DNA: formation, identification, and quantitation. *Biochemistry*, **24**, 707–713.

Gastaut, J. L. and Pellissier, J. F., 1985, Cisplatinum-induced peripheral neuropathy: a clinical neurophysiological and pathological study. *Revue Neurologique* (Paris), **141**, 614–626.

Glover, D., Glick, J. H., Weiler, C., Yuhas, J. and Kligerman, M. M., 1984, Phase I trials of WR-2721 and cis-platinum. *Int. J. Radiat. Oncol. Biol. Biophys.*, **10**, 1781–1784.

Gonias, S. L. and Pizzo, S. V., 1983, Complexes of serum albumin and cis-dichlorodiammineplatinum(II). *J. Biol. Chem.*, **258**, 5764–5769.

Gonias, S. L., Oakley, A. C., Walther, P. J. and Pizzo, S. V., 1984, Effects of diethyldithiocarbamate and nine other nucleophiles on the intersubunit protein cross-linking and inactivation of purified human α_2-macroglobulin by *cis*-diamminedichloroplatinum(II). *Cancer Res.*, **44**, 5764–5770.

Greco, F. A., Johnson, D. H., Hainsworth, J. D. and Wolff, S. N., 1985, Chemotherapy of small-cell lung cancer. *Seminars in Oncology*, **12** (Suppl. 6), 31–37.

Green, J. A., Vistica, D. T., Young, R. C., Hamilton, T. C., Rogan, A. M. and Ozols, R. F., 1984, Potentiation of melphalan cytotoxicity in human ovarian cancer cell lines by glutathione depletion. *Cancer Res.*, **44**, 5427–5431.

Guthrie, D., 1985, Chemotherapy of cervical cancer. *Clin. Obst. Gynec.*, **12**, 229–246.

Hacker, M. P., Douple, E. B. and Krakoff, I. H. (editors), 1984, *Platinum Coordination Compounds in Cancer Chemotherapy* (Boston: Martinus Nijhoff).

Hamilton, T. C., Winker, M. A., Louie, K. G., Batist, G., Behrens, B. C., Tsuruo, T., Grotzinger, K. R., McKoy, W. M., Young, R. C. and Ozols, R. F., 1985, Augmentation of adriamycin, melphalan, and cisplatin cytotoxicity in drug-resistant and -sensitive human ovarian carcinoma cell lines by buthionine sulfoximine mediated glutathione depletion. *Biochem. Pharmacol.*, **34**, 2583–2586.

Hamilton, T. C., Young, R. C., Maasuda, H., Grotzinger, K. R., McKoy, W. and Ozols, R. F., 1986, Effect of buthionine sulfoximine on the activity of anticancer drugs in vitro and in vivo in human ovarian cancer. *Proc. Am. Ass. Cancer Res.*, **27**, 393.

Harland, S. J., Newell, D. R., Siddik, Z. H., Chadwick, R., Calver, A. H. and Harrap, K. R., 1984, Pharmacokinetics of *cis*-diammine-1,1-cyclobutane dicarboxylate platinum(II) in patients with normal and impaired renal function. *Cancer Res.*, **44**, 1693–1697.

Harrap, K. R., Jones, M., Wilkinson, C. R., Clink, H. M., Sparrow, S., Mitchley, B. C. V., Clarke, S. and Veasey, A., 1980, Antitumor, toxic, and biochemical properties of cisplatin and eight other platinum complexes. In *Cisplatin: Current Status and New Developments*, edited by A. W. Prestayko, S. T. Crooke, and S. K. Carter (New York: Academic Press), pp. 193–212.

Harrison, R., McAuliffe, C. A., Zaki, A., Baer, J., Sharma, H., Smith, A., Jackson,

H. and Fox, B. W., 1983, A comparative study of the distribution in the male rat of platinum-labelled *cis*-dichlorodiammine platinum(II), *cis-trans*-1-dichlorodihydroxy-bis-(Isopropylamine)platinum(IV), and *cis*-dichloro-bis-cyclopropylamine platinum(II). *Cancer Chemother. Pharmacol.*, **10**, 90–95.

Hayes, D. M., Cvitkovic, E., Golbey, R. B., Scheiner, E., Helson, L. and Krakoff, I. H., 1977, High dose *cis*-platinum diammine dichloride amelioration of renal toxicity by mannitol diuresis. *Cancer*, **39**, 1372–1381.

Heidemann, H.Th., Gerkens, J. F., Jackson, E. K. and Branch, R. A., 1985, Attenuation of cisplatinum-induced nephrotoxicity in the rat by high salt diet, furosemide and acetazolamide. *Arch. Pharmacol.*, **329**, 201–205.

Himmelstein, K. J., Patton, T. F., Belt, R. J., Taylor, S., Repta, A. J. and Sternson, L. A., 1981, Clinical kinetics of intact cisplatin and some related species. *Clin. Pharmacol. Exp. Ther.*, **29**, 658–664.

Howell, S. B., Pjeifle, C. E., Wung, W. E. and Olshen, R. A., 1983, Intraperitoneal *cis*-diamminedichloroplatinum with systemic thiosulfate protection. *Cancer Res.*, **43**, 1426–1431.

Howell, S. B. and Taetle, R., 1980, Effect of sodium thiosulfate on *cis*-dichlorodiammineplatinum II toxicity and antitumor activity in L1210 leukemia. *Cancer Treat. Rep.*, **64**, 611–616.

Jacobs, C., 1986, The handling of platinum by the human kidney. In *Biochemical Mechanisms of Platinum Antitumour Drugs*, edited by D. C. H. McBrien (Oxford: IRL Press), pp 147–170.

Jacobs, C., Kalman, S. M., Tretton, M. and Weiner, M. W., 1980, Renal handling of *cis*-diamminedichloroplatinum II. *Cancer Treat. Rep.*, **64**, 1223–1226.

Jacobs, C., Coleman, C. N., Rich, L., Hirst, K. and Weiner, M. W., 1984, Inhibition of *cis*-diamminedichloroplatinum secretion by the human kidney with probenecid. *Cancer Res.*, **44**, 3632–3635.

Jensen, K. H., 1939, Über die Sauerstarken der stereoisomeren Diaquo-diammineplatoionen. *Zeitsch. Anorg. Allg. Chemie*, **242**, 87–91.

Johnson, N. P., Hoeschele, J. D. and Rahn, R. O., 1980, Kinetic analysis of the in vitro binding of radioactive *cis*- and *trans*-dichloroammineplatinum(II) to DNA. *Chem. Biol. Interactions*, **30**, 151–169.

Johnson, N. P., Mazard, A. M., Escalier, J. and Macquest, J. P., 1985, Mechanism of the reaction between cis-$[PtCl_2(NH_3)_2]$ and DNA in vitro. *J. Am. Chem. Soc.*, **107**, 6376–6380.

Klastersky, J. and Sculier, J. P., 1985, Chemotherapy of non-small-cell lung cancer. *Seminars in Oncology*, **12** (Suppl. 6), 38–48.

Knox, R. J., Friedlos, F., Lydall, D. A. and Roberts, J. J, 1986, Mechanism of cytotoxicity of anticancer platinum drugs: evidence that *cis*-diamminedichloroplatinum(II) and *cis*-diammine-(1,1-cyclobutanedicarboxylato)platinum(II) differ only in the kinetics of their interaction with DNA. *Cancer Res.*, **46**, 1972–1979.

Kosower, N. S. and Kosower, E. M., 1978, The glutathione status of cells. *Int. Rev. Cytol.*, **54**, 109–160.

Kraker, A., Schmidt, J., Krezoski, S. and Petering, D. H., 1985, Binding of *cis*-dichlorodiammine platinum(II) to metallothionein in Ehrlich cells. *Biochem. Biophys. Res. Commun.*, **130**, 786–792.

Lagasse, L. D., Pretorius, R. G., Petrilli, E. S., Ford, L. C., Hoeschele, J. and Kean, C., 1981, The metabolism of *cis*-dichlorodiammineplatinum(II): distribution, clearance, and toxicity. *Am. J. Obst. Gynec.*, **139**, 791–798.

Lee, K. W. and Martin, D. S. Jr., 1976, Aquation equilibria and isotopic exchange of chloride ligands with free chloride ion and tetrachloroplatinate(II). *Inorg. Chim. Acta*, **17**, 105–110.

Levi, J., Jacobs, C., Kalman, S. M., McTigue, M. and Weiner, M. W., 1980,

Mechanism of cis-platinum nephrotoxicity: I. Effects of sulfhydryl groups in rat kidneys. *J. Pharmacol. Exp. Ther.*, **213**, 545–550.

Leyland-Jones, B., Morrow, C., Tate, S., Urmacher, C., Gorden, C. and Young, C., 1983, *cis*-Diamminedichloroplatinum II nephrotoxicity and its relationship to renal γ-glutamyl transpeptidase. *Cancer Res.*, **43**, 6072–6076.

Lippard, S. J., 1982, New chemistry of an old molecule: cis-[$Pt(NH_3)_2Cl_2$]. *Science*, **218**, 1075–1082.

Lippard, S. J. (editor), 1983, *Platinum, Gold, and Other Metal Chemotherapeutic Agents*, ACS Symposium Series No. 209 (Washington: American Chemical Society).

Litterst, C. L., 1981, Alterations in the toxicity of *cis*-dichlorodiammineplatinum II and in tissue localization of platinum as a function of NaCl concentration in the vehicle of administration. *Toxic. Appl. Pharmacol.*, **61**, 99–108.

Litterst, C. L., 1984, Cisplatinum: a review, with special reference to cellular and molecular interactions. *Agents and Actions*, **15**, 520–524.

Litterst, C. and Uozumi, J., 1986, Correlation between cisplatin toxicity and chemically-induced alterations in tissue glutathione levels. *Proc. Am. Ass. Cancer Res.*, **27**, 287.

Litterst, C. L., Torres, I. J. and Guarino, A. M., 1977, Plasma levels and organ distribution of platinum in the rat, dog, and dogfish following intravenous administration of cis-DDP(II). *J. Clin. Hematol. Oncol.*, **7**, 169–178.

Litterst, C. L., Tong, S., Hirokata, Y. and Siddik, Z. H., 1982, Alterations in hepatic and renal levels of glutathione and activities of glutathione S-transferases from rats treated with *cis*-dichlorodiammineplatinum-II. *Cancer Chemother. Pharmacol.*, **8**, 67–71.

Loehrer, P. J. and Einhorn, L. H., 1984, Cisplatin. *Ann. Int. Med.*, **100**, 704–713.

Mansy, S., Chu, G. Y. H., Duncan, R. E., and Tobias, R. S., 1978, Heavy metal nucleotide interactions. 12. Competitive reactions in systems of four nucleotides with *cis*- or *trans*-diammineplatinum(II). Raman difference spectrophotometric determination of the relative nucleophilicity of guanosine, cytidine, adenosine, and uridine monophosphates as well as the analogous bases in DNA. *J. Am. Chem. Soc.*, **100**, 607–616.

Mason, R., Edwards, I. R. and McLaren, S. J., 1984, Interaction of platinum with metallothionein-like ligands in the rat kidney after administration of cis-dichlorodiammineplatinum II. *Chem. Biol. Interactions*, **49**, 165–176.

Micetich, K. C., Barnes, D. and Erickson, L. C., 1985, A comparative study of the cytotoxicity and DNA-damaging effects of *cis*-(diammino)(1,1-cyclobutanedicarboxylato)platinum(II) and *cis*-diamminedichloroplatinum(II) on L1210 cells. *Cancer Res.*, **45**, 4043–4047.

Murphy, M. P., Andrews, P. A. and Howell, S. B., 1985, Metallothionein mediated cisplatin and melphalan resistance in human ovarian carcinoma. *Proc. Am. Ass. Cancer Res.*, **26**, 344.

Murray, D., Jenkins, W. T. and Meyn, R. E., 1985, Kinetics of DNA cross-linking in normal and neoplastic mouse tissues following treatment with *cis*-diamminedichloroplatinum(II) in vivo. *Cancer Res.*, **45**, 6446–6452.

Naganuma, A., Satoh, M., Koyama, Y. and Imura, N., 1985, Protective effect of metallothionein inducing metals on lethal toxicity of *cis*-diamminedichloroplatinum in mice. *Toxic. Lett.*, **24**, 203–207.

Nagy, B., Dale, P. J. and Grdina, D. J., 1986, Protection against cisdichlorodiammineplatinum cytotoxicity and mutagenicity in V79 cells by 2[(aminopropyl)amino]ethanethiol. *Cancer Res.*, **46**, 1132–1135.

Nechay, B. R. and Neldon, S. L., 1984, Characteristics of inhibition of human renal adenosine triphosphatases by cisplatin and chloroplatinic acid. *Cancer Treat. Rep.*, **68**, 1135–1141.

Nelson, J. A., Santos, G. and Herbert, B. H., 1984, Mechanisms for the renal secretion of cisplatin. *Cancer Treat. Rep.*, **68**, 849–853.

Osman, N. M., Copley, M. P. and Litterst, C. L., 1984 b, Amelioration of cisplatin-induced nephrotoxicity by the diuretic acetazolamide in F344 rats. *Cancer Treat. Rep.*, **68**, 999–1004.

Osman, N. M., Copley, M. P. and Litterst, C. L., 1984 a, Effects of the diuretics mannitol or acetazolamide on nephrotoxicity and physiological disposition of cisplatin in rats. *Cancer Chemother. Pharmacol.*, **13**, 58–62.

Osman, N. M., Copley, M. P. and Litterst, C. L., 1984 b, Amelioration of cisplatin-induced nephrotoxicity by the diuretic acetazolamide in F344 rats. *Cancer Treat. Rep.*, **68**, 999–1004.

Ozols, R. F., Deisseroth, A. B., Javadpour, N., Barlock, A., Messerschmidt, J. and Young, R. C., 1983, Treatment of poor prognosis nonseminomatous testicular cancer with a "high-dose" platinum combination chemotherapy regimen. *Cancer*, **51**, 1803–1807.

Ozols, R. F., Corden, B. J., Jacob, J., Wesley, M. N., Ostchega, Y. and Young, R. C., 1984, High-dose cisplatin in hypertonic saline. *Ann. Int. Med.*, **100**, 19–24.

Ozols, R. F. and Young, R. C., 1984, Chemotherapy of ovarian cancer. *Seminars in Oncology*, **11**, 251–263.

Ozols, R. F. and Young, R. C., 1985, High-dose cisplatin therapy in ovarian cancer. *Seminars in Oncology*, **112**, Suppl. 6, 21–30.

Patton, T. F., Himmelstein, K. J., Belt, R., Bannister, S. J. Sternson, L. A. and Repta, A. J., 1978, Plasma levels and urinary excretion of filterable platinum species following bolus injection and iv infusion of *cis*-dichlorodiammineplatinum(II) in man. *Cancer Treat. Rep.*, **62**, 1359–1362.

Pendyala, L., Cowens, J. W. and Creaven, P. J., 1982, Studies on the pharmacokinetics and metabolism of *cis*-dichloro-*trans*-dihydroxy bis-isopropylamine platinum(IV) in the dog. *Cancer Treat. Rep.*, **66**, 509–516.

Pendyala, L., Greco, W., Cowens, J. W., Madajewicz, S. and Creaven, P. J., 1983, Pharmacokinetics of *cis*-dichloro-*trans*-dihydroxy-bis-isopropylamine platinum(IV) (CHIP) in patients with advanced cancer. *Cancer Chemother. Pharmacol.*, **11**, 23–28.

Pendyala, L., Madajewicz, S. and Creaven, P. J., 1985, Effect of renal function impairment on iproplatin pharmacokinetics and relation to toxicity. *Cancer Res.*, **45**, 5936–5938.

Pfeifle, C. E., Howell, S. B., Felthouse, R. D., Woliver, T. B. S., Andrews, P. A., Markman, M. and Murphy, M. P., 1985, High-dose cisplatin with sodium thiosulfate protection. *J. Clin. Oncol.*, **3**, 237–244.

Pinto, A. L. and Lippard, S. J., 1985 a, Binding of the antitumour drug *cis*-diamminedichloroplatinum(II) (cisplatin) to DNA. *Biochim. Biophys. Acta*, **780**, 167–180.

Pinto, A. L. and Lippard, S. J., 1985 b, Sequence-dependent termination of in vitro DNA synthesis by *cis*- and *trans*-diamminedichloroplatinum(II). *Proc. Natl Acad. Sci. USA*, **82**, 4616–4619.

Prestayko, A. W., Crooke, S. T. and Carter, S. K. (editors), 1980, *Cisplatin: Current Status and New Developments* (New York: Academic Press).

Rahn, R. O., 1984, Chromatographic analysis of the adducts formed in DNA complexed with *cis*-diamminedichloroplatinum(II). *J. Inorg. Biochem.*, **21**, 311–321.

Reece, P. A., Stafford, I., Russell, J. and Hill, P. G., 1985, Nonlinear renal clearance of ultrafilterable platinum in patients treated with *cis*-diamminedichloroplatinum (II). *Cancer Chemother. Pharmac.*, **15**, 295–299.

Reishus, J. W. and Martin, D. S., 1961, *Cis*-dichlorodiammineplatinum(II). Acid hydrolysis and isotopic exchange of the chloride ligands. *J. Am. Chem. Soc.*, **83**, 2457–2462.

Repta, A. J. and Long, D. F., 1980, Reactions of cisplatin with human plasma and plasma fractions. In *Cisplatin: Current Status and New Developments*, edited by A. W. Prestayko, S. T. Crooke, and S. K. Carter (New York: Academic Press), pp. 285–304.

Roberts, J. J. and Friedlos, F., 1982, The frequency of interstrand cross-links in DNA following reaction of *cis*-diamminedichloroplatinum(II) with cells in culture or DNA in vitro: stability of DNA cross-links and their repair. *Chem. Biol. Interactions*, **39**, 181–189.

Robins, A. B., 1982, The binding of platinum ethylenediamine dichloride to proteins in vitro and in vivo. *Chem. Biol. Interactions*, **38**, 349–356.

Rooney, M., Kish, J., Jacobs, J., Kinzie, J., Weaver, A., Crissman, J. and Al-Sarraf, M., 1985, Improved complete response rate and survival in advanced head and neck cancer after three-course induction therapy with 120-hour 5-FU infusion and cisplatin. *Cancer*, **55**, 1123–1128.

Rose, W. C., Schurig, J. E., Huftalen, J. B. and Bradner, W. T., 1982, Antitumor activity and toxicity of cisplatin analogs. *Cancer Treat. Rep.*, **66**, 125–146.

Rosenberg, B., VanCamp, L. and Krigas, T., 1965, Inhibition of cell division in *Escherichia coli* by electrolysis products frrom a platinum electrode. *Nature*, **205**, 698–699.

Rosenberg, B., VanCamp, L., Trosko, J. E. and Mansour, V. H., 1969, Platinum compounds: a new class of potent antitumor agents. *Nature*, **222**, 385–386.

Rosenberg, B., 1985, Fundamental studies with cisplatin. *Cancer*, **55**, 2303–2316.

Ross, D. A. and Gale, G. R., 1979, Reduction of the renal toxicity of *cis*-dichlorodiammineplatinum II by Probenecid. *Cancer Treat. Rep.*, **63**, 781–787.

Safirstein, R., Daye, M. and Guttenplan, J. B., 1983, Mutagenic activity and identification of excreted platinum in human and rat urine and rat plasma after administration of cisplatin. *Cancer Lett.*, **18**, 329–338.

Safirstein, R., Miller, P. and Guttenplan, J. B., 1984, Uptake and metabolism of cisplatin by rat kidney. *Kidney International*, **25**, 753–758.

Salles, B., Butour, J. L., Lesca, C. and Macquet, J. P., 1983, *Cis* $Pt(NH_3)_2Cl_2$ and *trans* $Pt(NH_3)_2Cl_2$ inhibit DNA synthesis in cultured L1210 leukemia cells. *Biochem. Biophys. Res. Commun.*, **112**, 555–563.

Segal, E. and LePecq, J.-B., 1985, Role of ligand exchange processes in the reaction kinetics of the antitumor drug *cis*-diamminedichloroplatinum(II) with its targets. *Cancer Res.*, **45**, 492–498.

Sharma, R. P. and Edwards, I. R., 1983, cis-Platinum: subcellular distribution and binding to cytosolic ligands. *Biochem. Pharmacol.*, **32**, 2665–2669.

Sherman, S. E., Gibson, D., Wang, A. H.-J. and Lippard, S. J., 1985, X-ray structure of the major adduct of the anticancer drug cisplatin with DNA: *cis*$[Pt(NH_3)_2\{d(pGpG)\}]$. *Science*, **230**, 412–417.

Siddik, Z. H., Dible, S. E., Boxall, F. E. and Harrap, K. R., 1986, Renal pharmacokinetics of cisplatin and carboplatin. In *Biochemical Mechanisms of Platinum Antitumor Drugs*, edited by D. C. H. McBrien (Oxford, IRL Press), pp. 171–198.

Smith, I. E., Harland, S. J., Robinson, B. A., Evans, B. D., Goodhart, L. C., Calvert, A. H., Yarnold, J., Glees, J. P., Baker, J. and Ford, H. T., 1985, Carboplatin: a very active new cisplatin analog in the treatment of small cell lung cancer. *Cancer Treat. Rep.*, **69**, 43–46.

Strandberg, M. C., Bresnick, E. and Eastman, A., 1982, The significance of DNA cross-linking to *cis*-diamminedichloroplatinum(II)-induced cytotoxicity in sensitive and resistant lines of murine leukemia L1210 cells. *Chem. Biol. Interactions*, **39**, 169–180.

Thatcher, N., Sharma, H., Harrison, R., Smith, A., Zaki, A., McAuliffe, C. A., Crowther, D. and Fox, B. W., 1982, Blood clearance of three radioactively labelled platinum complexes in patients with malignant disease. *Cancer Chemother. Pharmacol.*, **9**, 13–16.

Uozumi, J., Ishizawa, M., Iwanmoto, Y. and Baba, T., 1984, Sodium thiosulfate inhibits *cis*-diamminedichloroplatinum II activity. *Cancer Chemother. Pharmacol.*, **13**, 82–85.

Uozumi, J. and Litterst, C. L., 1985, The effect of cisplatin on renal ATPase activity in vivo and in vitro. *Cancer Chemother. Pharmacol.*, **15**, 93–96.

Uozumi, J. and Litterst, C. L., 1986, Antagonizing action of sodium thiosulfate against cisplatin in vitro and in vivo. *Proc. Am. Ass. Cancer Res.*, **27**, 287.

Ushay, H. M., Tullius, T. D. and Lippard, S. J., 1981, Inhibition of the BamHI cleavage and unwinding of pBR322 deoxyribonucleic acid by the antitumor drug *cis*-dichlorodiammineplatinum(II). *Biochemistry*, **20**, 3744–3748.

Williams, P. D. and Hottendorf, G. H., 1985, Effect of cisplatin on organic ion transport in membrane vesicles from rat kidney cortex. *Cancer Treat. Rep.*, **69**, 875–880.

Von Hoff, D. D., Schilsky, R., Reichert, C. M., Reddick, R. L., Rozencweig, M., Young, R. C. and Muggia, F. M., 1979, Toxic side effects of *cis*-dichlorodiammineplatinum(II) in man. *Cancer Treat. Rep.*, **63**, 1527–1531.

Winston, J. A. and Safirstein, R., 1985, Reduced renal blood flow in early cisplatin-induced acute renal failure in the rat. *Am. J. Physiol.*, **249**, F490–F496.

Wolf, W. and Manaka, R. C., 1976, Synthesis and distribution of ^{195m}Pt *cis*-dichlorodiammine platinum (II). *J. Clin. Hematol. Oncol.*, **7**, 79–95.

Yagoda, A., 1983, Chemotherapy for advanced urothelial cancer. *Seminars in Urology*, **1**, 60–74.

Yuhas, J. M. and Culo, F., 1980, Selective inhibition of nephrotoxicity of *cis*-dichlorodiammineplatinum(II) by WR-2721 without altering its anti-tumor properties, *Cancer Treat. Rep.*, **64**, 57–64.

Zelazowski, A. J., Garvey, J. S. and Hoeschele, J. D., 1984, In vivo and in vitro binding of platinum to metallothionein. *Arch. Biochem. Biophys.*, **229**, 246–252.

Zunino, F., Tofanetti, O., Besati, A., Cavalletti, E. and Savi, G., 1983, Protective effect of reduced glutathione against *cis*-dichlorodiammine platinum (II)-induced nephrotoxicity and lethal toxicity. *Tumori*, **69**, 105–111.

7. Metabolism of bleomycin and bleomycin-like compounds

John S. Lazo, Said M. Sebti and Andrew E. Filderman

Brief historical introduction

The identification of bleomycin as an effective antineoplastic agent arose from the extensive screening program of Umezawa and colleagues (Umezawa, 1979). In 1956, a group of water-soluble natural products called phleomycins were identified as effective antibacterial agents (Maeda *et al.*, 1956). Within several years, sufficient quantities of the phleomycins became available to allow a clear demonstration of antineoplastic activity with transplantable tumours (Umezawa *et al.*, 1962; Bradner and Pindell, 1962). Unfortunately, preclinical studies in dogs indicated extensive renal toxicity that precluded the clinical use of the phleomycins. A search for "second-generation" phleomycins led to identification of structurally similar compounds that lacked renal toxicity. Called bleomycins, these compounds were extracted from cultures of *Streptomyces verticillus* as a copper-containing mixture that could be separated by ion exchange chromatography into at least 11 compounds (Umezawa *et al.*, 1966; Umezawa, 1979). In initial studies with Ehrlich carcinoma, the therapeutic effectiveness of the individual copper-containing compounds was inferior to results obtained with the mixture of bleomycins (Umezawa, 1979). The reasons for this apparent synergistic interaction among bleomycins remain unclear. Nonetheless, further preclinical and clinical development of this class of compounds focused upon a mixture comprising 55–70% bleomycin A_2, 25–30% bleomycin B_2, and small quantities of a variety of other bleomycins. The current clinically used bleomycin sulphate is formulated in this manner and is copper-free, due to early observations that inclusion of copper produced significant phlebitis (Umezawa, 1979).

Numerous analogues of bleomycin have been developed since the introduction of bleomycin into the clinic. The two most promising compounds now undergoing clinical trials are peplomycin and talisomycin S_{10b}. The chemical structures of these compounds and some of the bleomycins are shown in Figure 1.

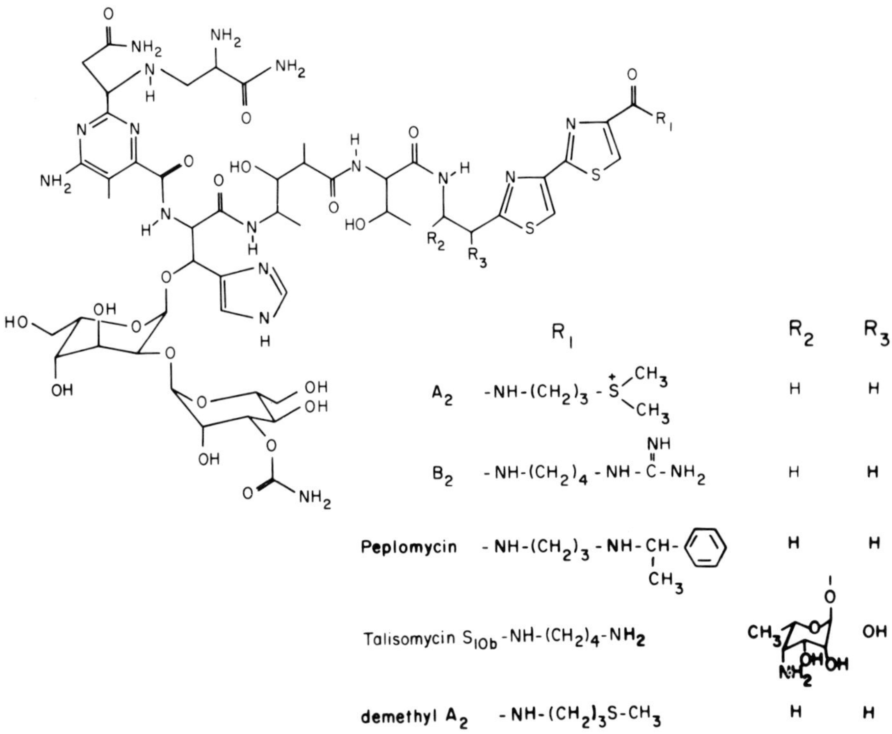

Figure 1. Structure of bleomycin and bleomycin-like compounds.

Clinical usage

Bleomycin has been used in the treatment of a variety of malignancies including Hodgkin's and non-Hodgkin's lymphomas, testicular carcinomas and squamous cell carcinomas of the head and neck, oesophagus, penis, and cervix (Blum *et al.*, 1973). While the drug has limited efficacy as a single agent, it comprises an important part of several combination chemotherapeutic regimens. One of the more unusual and valuable features of this class of compounds is a lack of significant bone marrow, hepatic or renal toxicity (Bennett and Reich, 1979). Thus, overlapping toxicity between bleomycin and other antineoplastic drugs is uncommon. In addition, tumour cells resistant to a variety of other antineoplastic agents may be more responsive to bleomycin (Gupta, 1985).

Bleomycin is an essential component of regimens that are curative against germ-cell and testicular carcinomas and lymphomas. Bleomycin combined with vinblastine and *cis*-diamminedichloroplatinum has been reported to produce a greater than 70% complete response rate and disease-free survival in testicular carcinoma (Einhorn and Donohue, 1977). In Hodgkin's disease, the addition of doxorubicin, bleomycin, vinblastine, dacarbazine (ABVD) alternating with the more traditional mechlorethamine, vincristine, procarbazine, prednisone (MOPP) regimen has improved complete response rates to 92% and five-year disease-free survival to 84% (Bonadonna and Santoro, 1982). Bleomycin, when added to cyclophosphamide, doxorubicin, vincristine, prednisone (CHOP) chemotherapy for diffuse histocytic lymphoma results in over 85% complete response rate and four-year disease-free survival (Newcomer *et al.*, 1982).

Certain types of squamous cell carcinomas have responded to a moderate degree to bleomycin-containing regimens. For example, overall response rates in head and neck carcinomas have been as high as 30–40% (Bennett and Reich, 1979). Less success has been observed with tumours of the oesophagus, lung and penis. Other tumours in which bleomycin has some activity include ovarian, cervical (Krebs *et al.*, 1980), choriocarcinoma (Schlaerth *et al.*, 1980), thyroid carcinoma (Poster *et al.*, 1981), and mycosis fungoides (Grozea *et al.*, 1979).

Structural features

Although first reported in 1966, the exact chemical structure of bleomycin required more than a decade to be established. Bleomycin A_2 has now been chemically synthesized (Takita *et al.*, 1982; Aoyagi *et al.*, 1982 b), which has greatly extended our understanding of the complex chemistry associated with this class of compounds.

Bleomycinic acid, the common structure of all bleomycins, is a glycopeptide comprising two sugars and five amino acids, one of which contains a bithiazole moiety that confers intrinsic fluorescence (Figure 1). In contrast, the phleomycins have a double bond in one of the thiazoles reduced. The bleomycins are different from each other in their C-terminal amine. In general, the terminal amine is highly cationic. Bleomycin A_2, for example, contains a dimethyl sulphonium propylamine linked to bleomycinic acid, peplomycin has a phenethylamine propylamine as the C-terminal group, while bleomycin B_2 contains an agmatine moiety (Figure 1). The search for newer bleomycins has led to the isolation of hundreds of bleomycin analogues with various C-terminal substitutions, although few have been well characterized (Umezawa, 1979). The talisomycins contain the bithiazole and both a hydroxyl and a talose sugar in close proximity to the bithiazole moiety. In addition, bleomycins lacking the sugar moieties also have been synthesized (Aoyagi *et al.*, 1982 a) and a few analogues with modifications proximal to the bithiazole region have been reported (Henichart *et al.*, 1985).

Mechanism of biological activity

Bleomycin has two structural domains: (*a*) the DNA-binding portion comprising the terminal amine and the bithiazole moiety and (*b*) a distinct metal-binding region located between the bithiazole moiety and the end terminal β-aminoalanine. A variety of metals, such as Zn(II,III), Cu(I,II), Co(II,III), Ni(II,III) and Fe(II,III), can bind to bleomycin (Dabrowiak, 1980). Potentiometric studies suggest that the divalent metal complexes of bleomycin have a similar coordination core, although their stabilities differ with the following order: Fe(II) < Co(II) < Ni(II) < Cu(II) (Sugiura, 1980). Spectroscopic and X-ray crystallographic studies are consistent with a square-pyramidal structure in which the basal plane comprises the secondary amine nitrogen, the N-4 pyrimidine ring nitrogen, the deprotonated peptide bond nitrogen of the histidine residue and the histidine imidazole nitrogen. The fifth axial donor is the α-amino nitrogen of the β-aminoalanine (Sugiura, 1980; Antholine *et al.*, 1984; Umezawa, 1979) (Figure 2). ESR spectroscopy of the iron–bleomycin complex indicates that the sixth axial coordination site is occupied by oxygen (Sugiura, 1980).

The *in vivo* metal association of the clinically used bleomycin, which is metal-free upon injection, has been only poorly examined. The limited studies that have addressed this question suggest that bleomycin is complexed with Cu(II) in the circulating blood (Kanao *et al.*, 1973). The mode of bleomycin entry into cells is unknown, although Co(II)-bound peplomycin may enter cells more readily than metal-free or Cu(II)–peplomycin (Uehara *et al.*, 1982). It has been hypothesized that when the Cu(II)–bleomycin complex enters cells, the cupric ion is reduced and the resulting cuprous ion is abstracted by a sulphydryl-containing macromolecule (Takahashi *et al.*, 1977; Umezawa, 1979). Some of this metal-free drug could be inactivated and some may interact with cellular macromolecules, such as DNA. Definitive experimental

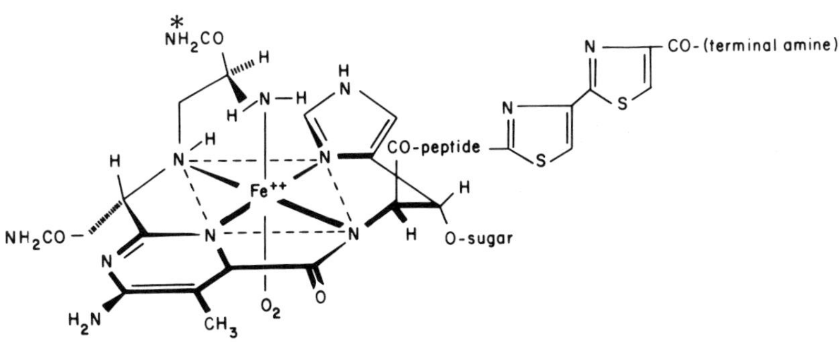

Bleomycin-ferrous-ion complex

Figure 2. Proposed metal coordination structure of bleomycin.

data determining the biologically active form of bleomycin within cells are not available. Cell-free *in vitro* data, however, strongly suggest that a bleomycin–ferrous ion complex is the biologically active species (Figure 2). In this rigid square-pyramidal coordination environment, oxygen binding is efficient and oxygen reduction is permitted. Both hydroxyl and superoxide radicals can be formed based upon spin-trapping data (Lown and Sim, 1977). In the presence of appropriate reductants, catalytic formation of radicals occurs. Caspary *et al.* (1979), for example, have reported that the reductive activation of bleomycin in cell-free *in vitro* conditions follows classic Michaelis–Menten kinetics ($V_{max} = 0{\cdot}27$ μmol/min/ml and $K_m = 1{\cdot}8$ mM) and that one mole of bleomycin turns over approximately 5000 moles of Fe(II) per min. In the absence of DNA, bleomycin may self-inactivate (Umezawa, 1979).

Considerable attention has focused upon the fate of these radicals; both cellular membranes and DNA have been identified as possible participants in the radical chemistry associated with bleomycin–ferrous ion–oxygen reactions (Sausville *et al.*, 1978; Umezawa, 1979). It is generally believed, however, that the antineoplastic activity (and antibacterial activity) of bleomycin is derived from its ability to induce single- and double-strand breaks in double-stranded DNA. The DNA binding portion of the molecule directs bleomycin to specific nucleotide sequences (e.g. 5′-GC-3′ and 5′-GT-3′). In addition to the nucleotide sequence specificity, the DNA breakage also appears to depend upon the overall DNA topology (Mirabelli *et al.*, 1983) and possibly the degree of DNA methylation (Hertzberg *et al.*, 1985). The association of bleomycin with DNA allows the metal chelated portion of the molecule to generate radicals in close proximity to DNA, which results in DNA strand scissions and base release. This is enhanced by sulphydryl compounds, ascorbate, peroxides and phosphate-containing compounds, such as ATP (Burger *et al.*, 1985). The chemistry of molecular oxygen bleomycin-mediated DNA strand scissions has been thoroughly studied using well defined DNA sequences and plasmid DNA (D'Andrea and Haseltine, 1978; Mirabelli *et al.*, 1983; Hertzberg *et al.*, 1985). Of particular interest is the production of base propenals from DNA, which appear to have toxic properties of their own (Grollman *et al.*, 1985).

Recent data suggest that sites other than DNA may also be important for the anti-tumour properties of bleomycin (Berry *et al.*, 1985). Bleomycin can both bind to the plasma membrane (Fujimoto, 1974) and affect the plasma membrane cellular functions (Sun and Crane, 1985), but the significance of these actions is not known. The biological targets responsible for pulmonary toxicity and the dose-limiting toxicity associated with bleomycin are also unclear. Both DNA and membrane damage may be important.

Metabolism in vivo

Umezawa and co-workers (1968, 1972) first studied the organ distribution of bleomycin in mice subcutaneously injected with ^{3}H-bleomycin. Radioactivity was found in all organs with the highest amounts of radioactivity being found in the homogenates from kidneys, urinary bladder and skin, and with lower amounts in heart and brain homogenates. The biological activity of the radiolabel-containing homogenates was evaluated using a growth inhibition assay of *Bacillus subtilis*. Comparisons between the radiolabel content and the biological activity indicated that a considerable fraction of the radiolabelled drug was inactive in all organs except skin and lungs, where high levels of the active form of bleomycin were found. These data suggested the possible metabolism of bleomycin. Furthermore, among all organs examined, only skin and lungs showed age-related differences in their bleomycin-inactivating activity. The youngest mice had the greatest ability to inactivate bleomycin one hour after subcutaneous injection of ^{3}H-bleomycin. Results from these bioassays must be reviewed with some caution due to the possible interference of components in the homogenates (Lazo and Humphreys, 1983; Thomas *et*

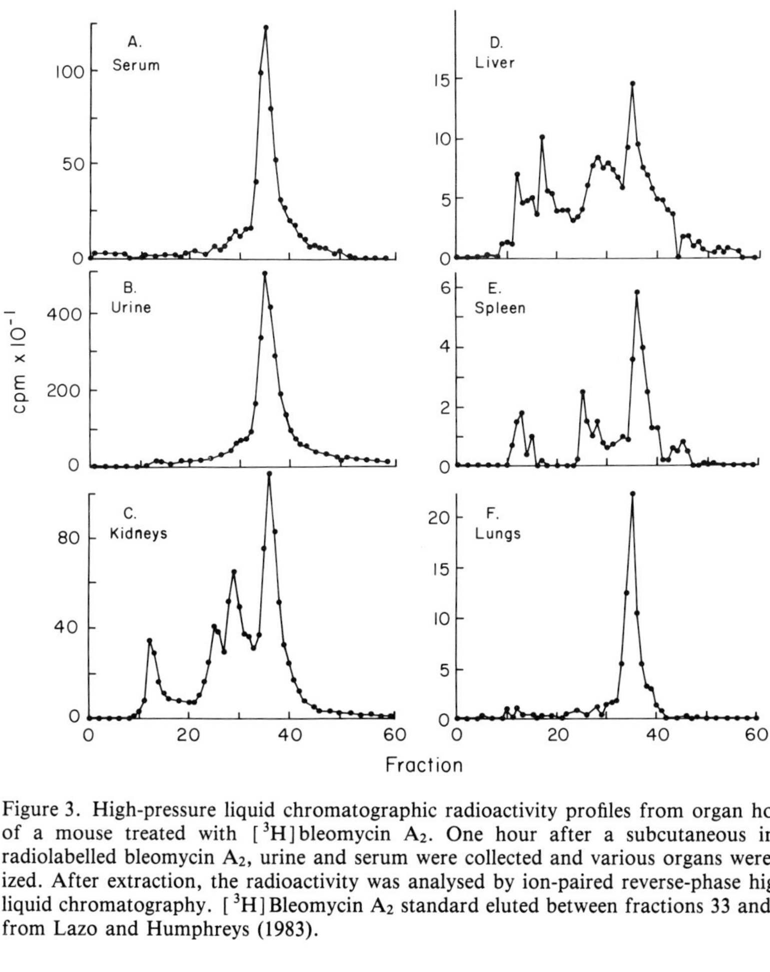

Figure 3. High-pressure liquid chromatographic radioactivity profiles from organ homogenates of a mouse treated with [^{3}H]bleomycin A_2. One hour after a subcutaneous injection of radiolabelled bleomycin A_2, urine and serum were collected and various organs were homogenized. After extraction, the radioactivity was analysed by ion-paired reverse-phase high-pressure liquid chromatography. [^{3}H]Bleomycin A_2 standard eluted between fractions 33 and 40. Taken from Lazo and Humphreys (1983).

al., 1984). Lazo and Humphreys (1983), however, used a high-pressure liquid chromatography system to separate bleomycin A_2 from its metabolites and demonstrated that ^{3}H-bleomycin was metabolized *in vivo*. Furthermore, they confirmed the conclusions derived from the bioassay methods. More than 40% of the radioactive material found in liver, kidneys, and spleen of C57BL/6 mice was metabolized one hour after subcutaneous drug injection (Figure 3). After two hours, less than 50% of the radiolabel co-migrated with bleomycin A_2. The *in vivo* metabolism of bleomycin in lung tissue was significantly less than that seen in other organs examined (Figure 3). No metabolites were seen in urine or serum. Twenty-four hours after an intratracheal injection of ^{3}H-bleomycin, however, metabolites could be detected in pulmonary tissue from C57BL/6 mice (Lazo and Pham, 1984).

The HPLC profile of radioactivity observed from tissues of mice treated with ^{3}H-bleomycin contained several peaks suggesting multiple metabolites (Figure 3). The relative peak areas changed with time after injection, although a clear precursor–product relationship could not be deciphered. The difficulty in assigning such a relationship among peaks could be related to possible differences in the efflux rates of the putative metabolites from the various organs. Both the HPLC and bioassay data do indicate, however, that bleomycin is extensively metabolized by a variety of organs. The chemical nature of most of the peaks is unknown, although one, deamidobleomycin (see below), has been clearly assigned.

Metabolism in vitro

Initial studies by Umezawa and co-workers (1972) demonstrated that incubation of bleomycin with organ homogenates greatly reduced the antibacterial activity of bleomycin. This loss of growth inhibitory activity appears to result from an enzymatic inactivation. Tissue homogenates from many murine and human organs possess this inactivating activity (Umezawa *et al.*, 1972; Ohnuma *et al.*, 1974; Umezawa, 1979). Although the relative levels of inactivating activity varied among organ homogenates, lung and skin homogenates frequently were the lowest. The inactivating activity was found in the high molecular weight ($>$25 000 dalton) postmicrosomal supernatant fraction suggesting a cytoplasmic location. A second low molecular weight ($<$25 000 dalton) substance that could inactivate the antibacterial activity of bleomycin was suggested by Yoshioka *et al.* (1978) but was not found in subsequent studies (Akiyama *et al.*, 1981).

Analysis of the chemical integrity of bleomycin after incubation with the postmicrosomal supernatant fraction from organ homogenates with inactivating activity, such as rat liver, suggested the formation of a single metabolite (Yoshioka *et al.*, 1978; Lazo *et al.*, 1982). Although the identification of the metabolite has been difficult due to the complexity of the bleomycin

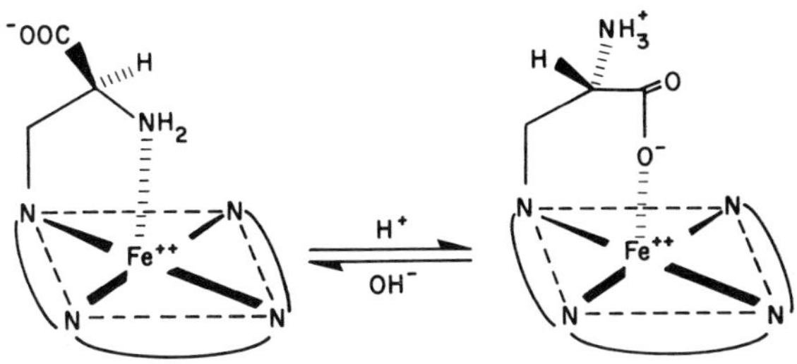

Figure 4. Coordination structure of deamidobleomycin as a function of pH 9 (left side) and pH 7 (right side).

structure, it is now believed that inactivation occurs primarily via the hydrolysis of the carboxyamide bond in the β-aminoalanine moiety (see Figure 2,*). The resulting metabolite contained a carboxylic acid rather than a carboxyamide and was named deamidobleomycin. This assignment is based upon the following observation using bleomycin B_2: (*a*) one mole of ammonia is released per mole of bleomycin hydrolysed, (*b*) hydrolysis of the isolated metabolite in 6 N HCl gives the same degradation products as those obtained from the parent compound, (*c*) the carbamoyl group on the mannose is found in the inactivated metabolite, and (*d*) the pK_a of the α-amino group of the β-aminoalanine is shifted to 9·4 from 7·4 (Umezawa *et al.*, 1972; Umezawa, 1979). Finally recent fast atom bombardment mass spectral analyses of the inactivated bleomycin A_2 are consistent with the proposed site of metabolism (S. M. Sebti and J. S. Lazo, unpublished observation).

The conversion of the carboxyamide of the β-aminoalanine to a carboxylic acid by the bleomycin-inactivating activity results in a more basic β-amino group of the β-aminoalanine, as shown by the shift in its pK_a from 7·4 to 9·4. Thus, at physiological pH the α-amino group is protonated in deamidobleomycin and the β-aminoalanine carboxylic acid rather than the α-amine occupies the fifth coordination site of the bleomycin–Fe(II) complex (Figure 4). This results in a decreased efficiency of binding of molecular oxygen to the sixth axial coordination site and a decreased ability to generate radicals. The ability of deamidobleomycin B_2 to generate radicals as well as to cleave DNA is 1/100th that of bleomycin B_2 (Sugiura, 1980). Deamidobleomycin B_2 is also 100-fold less active than bleomycin B_2 in inhibiting bacterial and tumour growth (Umezawa, 1979). Furthermore, deamidobleomycin A_2 is 1/100th as potent as bleomycin A_2 in killing murine L1210 cells in culture (Figure 5). Finally, in contrast to bleomycin A_2, deamidobleomycin A_2 does not produce pulmonary fibrosis or weight loss when repeatedly administered to mice (Lazo and Humphreys, 1983). Thus, the fifth axial coordination site is essential for effective O_2 binding and radical formation and, therefore, is very important for the biological activity of bleomycin.

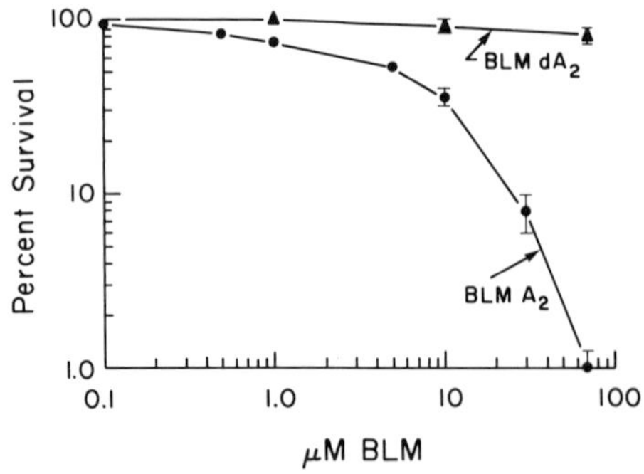

Figure 5. Cytotoxicity of deamidobleomycin A_2 and bleomycin A_2 to cultured L1210 cells. Cells were exposed to the drugs for 1 h, then washed free of drug and plated in soft agar as described by Lazo *et al.* (1985).

The inactivating activity that hydrolyses bleomycin and generates deamidobleomycin was termed bleomycin hydrolase by Umezawa *et al.* (1974). They suggested that bleomycin hydrolase was an aminopeptidase B-like enzyme, based upon its ability to cleave artificial substrates having lysine or arginine but not leucine on their N-termini and the ability of bleomycin B_2 to act as a competitive inhibitor of the aminopeptidase B reaction. This study, however, was carried out on a partially purified (27-fold) bleomycin hydrolase preparation. Further attempts to purify bleomycin hydrolase were hindered by the highly unstable character of the enzyme and the lack of a sensitive and rapid bleomycin hydrolase assay.

The recent development of high speed and fast protein liquid chromatography methods in our laboratory have allowed us to purify bleomycin hydrolase over 450-fold from rabbit lungs. Based upon these studies, it appears that the enzyme has an apparent molecular mass of 250 000 daltons, has no disulphide bonds, and has a pH optimum of 7·5 (Sebti and Lazo, 1986). Our results also indicate that although the major pulmonary aminopeptidase B and bleomycin hydrolase have affinity for mutual substrates, as demonstrated by affinity chromatography and inhibition studies, they are two distinct enzymes (Sebti and Lazo, 1986). This can be clearly demonstrated by anion exchange chromatography of the 105 000 *g* supernatant from rabbit lung homogenates (Figure 6). The substrate preference of bleomycin hydrolase remains to be established. Talisomycin S_{10b} and deglycobleomycin also appear to be metabolized by bleomycin hydrolase (S. M. Sebti and J. S. Lazo, unpublished results) and it has been stated that the enzyme recognizes the metal-free but not metal-bound form of bleomycin (Umezawa, 1979).

The physiological role of bleomycin hydrolase is unknown but it is tempting to speculate that it could function as an amidohydrolase, cleaving amide bonds of peptides capped with a carboxyamide at their C-termini. A large number of biologically active peptides have such a capped C-terminus and the hydrolysis of the amide results in their inactivation (Bauer, 1983).

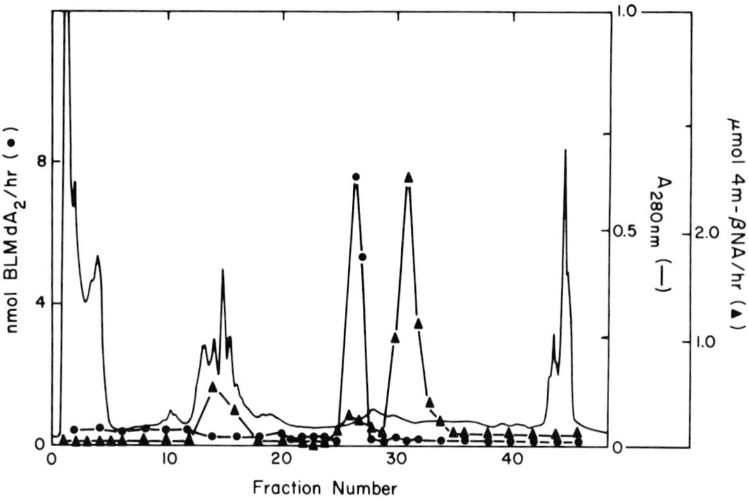

Figure 6. Anion exchange Mono *Q* column chromatography of 105 000 *g* supernatant fraction from rabbit lung homogenates. The column was washed with 10 ml of starting buffer (20 mM Tris, 0·2 nM DTT, pH 7·4). The sample (15 mg of 105 000 *g* supernatant fraction in 1·5 ml of starting buffer) was loaded and the column was eluted at 1 ml/min with 10 ml of starting buffer, 8 ml of starting buffer containing 0·2 M NaCl, followed by a linear gradient of 0·2 M to 0·4 M NaCl in 20 min. One ml fractions were collected and the absorbance at 280 nm was monitored. Bleomycin hydrolase activity was determinined by incubating 100 μl of each fraction with bleomycin A_2 (50 μM) for one hour at 37°C and the reaction mixture analysed for deamido-bleomycin A_2 (BLM dA_2) as described in Figure 3. Aminopeptidase B activity was assayed by incubating 100 μl of each fraction with L-arginyl-4-methoxy-β-naphthylamide (0·5 mM) for 30 min at 37°C. The reaction mixture was further incubated at room temperature with 0·25 volume of 1 mg/ml Fast Garnet. Based upon the absorbance at 520 nm, the amount of 4-methoxy-β-naphthylamine (4m-β NA) was then calculated.

Relationship between metabolism and organ toxicity

The level of bleomycin hydrolase activity in different tissues appears to play an important role in protecting organs from bleomycin-induced toxicity and may define the spectrum of organs sensitive to bleomycin. The potential importance of drug metabolism was suggested by Umezawa's studies of bleomycin inactivation in various murine tissues (Umezawa *et al.*, 1972). Drug inactivation was significantly lower in lung and skin, the two major sites of bleomycin-induced toxicity. This was in contrast to greater rates of inactivation in organs such as liver, kidney, spleen and bone marrow, which are resistant to bleomycin-induced toxicity. A similarly designed study by Ohnuma *et al.* (1974) also found inactivation of bleomycin to be low in the lungs and skin of mice, and elevated in liver, intestine, kidney and spleen. In a limited screen of human tissue (Ohnuma *et al.*, 1974), skin was shown to have a lower metabolic capacity than liver, erythrocytes and spleen.

Lazo and Humphreys (1983) studied the activity of bleomycin hydrolase in lung homogenates from rabbits, a species known to be less sensitive to the

Table 1. *In vitro* pulmonary bleomycin hydrolase activity in murine strains

Strain	Sensitivity to bleomycin fibrosis	Bleomycin metabolism†
C57BL/6	High	0·27 ± 0·01‡
DBA/2	Intermediate	0·60 ± 0·05
BALB/c	Low	0·99 ± 0·03

Values taken from Filderman and Lazo (1985). Bleomycin metabolism was determined as described by Lazo and Humphreys (1983).
† μg deamidobleomycin A_2 formed h^{-1} mg protein^{-1}
‡ Mean values ± S.E.

pulmonary toxic effects of bleomycin. Consistent with the theory that bleomycin hydrolase is protective against organ toxicity, rabbit lungs were noted to have a significantly greater conversion of bleomycin to deamidobleomycin than a sensitive murine strain (C57BL/6). The finding of inversely related species differences in pulmonary bleomycin hydrolase activity and in sensitivity to bleomycin-induced pulmonary toxicity suggests that both of these characteristics may have a genetic basis. Results from Schrier *et al.* (1983) and our laboratory (J. H. Harrison and J. S. Lazo, unpublished observations) demonstrated an inbred murine strain variation in sensitivity to bleomycin-induced lung fibrosis. Mice of the C57BL/6 strain were reported to be sensitive to bleomycin-induced lung fibrosis, with BALB/c mice being resistant, and DBA/2 being intermediate. Filderman and Lazo (1985) have examined the level of bleomycin hydrolase activity in lung homogenates from these murine strains and found a significant variation in enzyme activity, correlating inversely with pulmonary sensitivity to bleomycin (Table 1). Therefore, the current data show bleomycin hydrolase activity to be low in those organs clinically sensitive to bleomycin, and elevated in tissues unaffected by bleomycin. Furthermore, there appears to be a pharmacogenetic variation in pulmonary bleomycin metabolism that may be the ultimate determinant of clinical toxicity in human lungs.

The cellular site of pulmonary bleomycin metabolism remains to be established. Data from freshly isolated and cultured cells has shown bleomycin hydrolase activity to be heterogeneously distributed among pulmonary cell types (Lazo *et al.*, 1984). Rabbit pulmonary artery endothelial cells, fibroblasts, and alveolar macrophages were found to have significant amounts of enzyme activity, while type II pneumocytes had nearly undetectable activity. This finding may explain the observed sensitivity to bleomycin of type I epithelial cells (Adamson and Bowden, 1979), which are thought to be derived from the type II cell. In contrast to the results with rabbit lungs, bovine lungs appear to have endothelial cells with low bleomycin hydrolase activity. Thus, the pulmonary toxicity of bleomycin may be related to an initial adverse effect on either epithelial or endothelial cells lacking bleomycin hydrolase activity.

Secondary changes such as neutrophil accumulation and inflammatory product secretion may then amplify the lung injury. Based on these data, we have proposed a model in which the pulmonary endothelium acts as a physical and metabolic barrier to the entry of unmetabolized bleomycin into the pulmonary interstitium (Lazo *et al.*, 1983, 1984; Lazo and Pham, 1984). If the barrier were to be circumvented as with an intratracheal injection, it may be possible to produce pulmonary fibrosis with a single low dose of bleomycin. This is seen experimentally (Catravas *et al.*, 1983). Such factors as hyperoxia or radiation may injure the pulmonary endothelium and allow increased entry of unmetabolized bleomycin into the interstitium and thus result in enhanced bleomycin-related lung damage (Tryka *et al.*, 1982; Collis *et al.*, 1983). Advanced age in mice may diminish bleomycin hydrolase activity (Umezawa *et al.*, 1972) and this finding may partially explain the greater sensitivity of elderly patients to bleomycin-induced lung toxicity. Whether other variables, such as concomitant or prior chemotherapy, poor nutritional status, or diminished renal function, adversely affect bleomycin hydrolase activity is not known.

Relationships between metabolism and anti-tumour activity

Several studies have attempted to evaluate the relationship between metabolism and sensitivity to anti-tumour activity. Umezawa *et al.* (1972) have suggested that bleomycin hydrolase activity may be a major determinant of tumour cell responsiveness. For example, murine tumours sensitive to bleomycin have significantly lower levels of bleomycin-inactivating activity than tumours that are resistant to the drug (Umezawa *et al.*, 1972). These studies have relied on bioassays as a measure of inactivation of bleomycin and the limitations of this approach have been addressed above. Muller *et al.* (1977), using an *in vitro* DNA polymerase assay, found that human carcinomas from head and neck region could inactivate bleomycin. Results from our laboratory (Lazo *et al.*, 1982) indicate that a variety of human tumours can metabolize bleomycin and that the enzyme activity varies at least 100-fold in freshly obtained gynaecological tumour samples from previously untreated patients. No relationship was seen between the differentiation stage and bleomycin hydrolase activity, in contrast to results previously reported by Muller *et al.* (1977), who found that the level of bleomycin inactivation varied according to the state of tumour differentiation. Tanaka (1984) and Akiyama *et al.* (1981) found that resistant Chinese hamster cells had higher levels of bleomycin hydrolase than sensitive Chinese hamster cells. A similar relationship was reported by Ueda *et al.* (1984) with peplomycin and cultured human gynaecological tumours. In contrast, no correlation was observed between bleomycin hydrolase activity and the sensitivity of either murine B16 melanoma cells (Zuckerman *et al.*, 1986) or human gynaecological tumour cells (Lazo *et al.*, 1982) to bleomycin as measured by colony formation in soft agar. These data suggest that other factors in addition to bleomycin metabolism might be important in determining the response of certain tumour cells to bleomycin. These factors might include endogenous inhibitors of enzyme activity, increased DNA repair, different DNA methylation states, poor bleomycin uptake or varying intracellular concentrations of thiols, Fe(II), or ATP. Further work is required to determine the importance of bleomycin metabolism in modulating the anti-tumour activity of bleomycin.

Future directions

Data from several laboratories suggest that metabolism may be important in determining the toxicity of bleomycin to normal tissue. In contrast, the role of metabolism in controlling the anti-tumour activity of bleomycin has not yet been established. If pulmonary toxicity is related to decreased bleomycin hydrolase activity, induction of the enzyme activity in lungs may provide protection for pulmonary tissue and permit the use of higher doses of bleomycin. Alternatively, efforts could be made to develop means to identify those patients with low pulmonary hydrolase activity and to synthesize compounds which are better substrates for bleomycin hydrolase.

The relationship between bleomycin metabolism in intact cells and tissues and bleomycin hydrolase activity as measured *in vitro* remains to be firmly established. Differences between *in vitro* data and that obtained from intact cells or tissues may reflect endogenous inhibitors removed during enzyme purification or may reflect differential subcellular localizations. The development of antibodies to bleomycin hydrolase should be useful in evaluating this. The recently described (Seki *et al.*, 1985) antibody to bleomycin that lacks cross-reactivity with the deamidobleomycin metabolite should also be a powerful reagent. Further work is required to determine whether metabolites other than deamidobleomycin exist. Other metabolites appear to be generated *in vivo* and efforts should be directed toward chemically evaluating these and determining their biological activity. Finally, bleomycin is commonly used in conjuction with other anti-tumour agents, which can potentially affect a variety of enzyme activities. Consequently, it would be interesting to determine whether some currently used anti-cancer agents influence the activity of bleomycin hydrolase.

The recent observation (Genilloud *et al.*, 1984; Mazodier *et al.*, 1985) that a gene coding for bleomycin resistance is harboured on the bacterial transposon 5 suggests that other, as yet undefined, factors could control cellular responsiveness to bleomycin. It is possible that the small (approximately 14 000 dalton) protein coded for by this gene participates in the metabolic inactivation of bleomycin.

References

Adamson, I. Y. R. and Bowden, D. H., 1979, Bleomycin-induced injury and metaplasia of alveolar type 2 cells. *Am. J. Path*, **96**, 531–538.

Akiyama, S.-I., Ikezaki, K., Kuramochi, H., Takahashi, K. and Kuwano, M., 1981, Bleomycin-resistant cells contain increased bleomycin-hydrolase activities. *Biochem. Biophys. Res. Commun.*, **101**, 55–60.

Antholine, W. E., Riedy, G., Hyde, J. S., Basosi, R. and Petering, D., 1984, ESR parameters for cupric bleomycin in the mobilized state. *J. Biomol. Struct. Dynamics*, **2**, 469–480.

Aoyagi, Y., Suguna, H., Murugesan, N., Ehrenfeld, G. M., Chang, L.-H., Shekhani, M. S., Kirkup, M. P. and Hecht, S. M., 1982a, Deglycobleomycin: Total synthesis and oxygen transfer properties of an bleomycin analogue. *J. Am. Chem. Soc.*, **104**, 5237–5239.

Aoyagi, Y., Katano, K., Suguna, H., Primeau, J., Chang, L.-H. and Hecht, S. M., 1982 b, Total synthesis of bleomycin. *J. Am. Chem. Soc.*, **104**, 5537–5538.

Bauer, K., 1983, Biochemical properties of TRH-inactivating enzymes. In *Thyrotropin-Releasing Hormone*, edited by E. C. Griffiths and G. W. Bennett (New York: Raven Press), pp. 103–108.

Bennett, J. M. and Reich, S. D., 1979, Bleomycin. *Ann. Int. Med.*, **90**, 945–948.

Berry, D. E., Kilkuskie, R. E. and Hecht, S. M., 1985, DNA damage induced by bleomycin in the presence of dibucaine is not predictive of cell growth inhibition. *Biochemistry*, **24**, 3214–3219.

Blum, R. H., Carter, S. K. and Agre, K., 1973, A clinical review of bleomycin: A new antineoplastic agent. *Cancer*, **31**, 903–914.

Bonadonna, G. and Santoro, A., 1982, ABVD chemotherapy in the treatment of Hodgkins disease. *Cancer Treat. Rev.*, **9**, 21–35.

Bradner, W. T. and Pindell, M. H., 1962, Antitumour properties of phleomycin. *Nature*, **196**, 682–683.

Burger, R. M., Horwitz, S. B. and Peisach, J., 1985, Stimulation of iron(II) bleomycin activity by phosphate-containing compounds. *Biochemistry*, **24**, 3623–3629.

Caspary, W. S., Niziak, C., Lanzo, D. A., Friedman, R. and Bachur, N. B., 1979, Bleomycin A_2: A ferrous oxidase. *Mol. Pharmacol.*, **16**, 256–260.

Catravas, J. D., Lazo, J. S., Dobuler, K. J., Mills, L. R. and Gillis, C. N., 1983, Pulmonary endothelial dysfunction in the presence or absence of interstitial injury induced by intratracheal injection of bleomycin to rabbits. *Am. Rev. Resp. Dis.*, **128**, 740–746.

Collis, C. H., Down, J. D., Pearson, A. E. and Steel, G. G., 1983, Bleomycin and radiation-induced lung damage in mice. *Br. J. Radiol.*, **56**, 21–26.

Dawbrowiak, J. C. 1980, The coordination chemistry of bleomycin: A review. *J. Inorg. Biochem.*, **13**, 317–337.

D'Andrea, A. D. and Haseltine, W. A., 1978, Sequence specific cleavage of DNA by the antitumor antibiotics neocarcinostatin and bleomycin. *Proc. Natl. Acad. Sci. USA*, **75**, 3608–3612.

Einhorn, L. H. and Donohue, J., 1977, *Cis*-diamminedichloroplatinum, vinblastine, and bleomycin combination chemotherapy in disseminated testicular cancer. *Ann. Int. Med.*, **87**, 293–298.

Filderman, A. E. and Lazo, J. S., 1985, Murine strain variation in bleomycin (BLM) metabolism *in vitro*. *Am. Rev. Resp. Dis.*, **131**, A381.

Fujimoto, J., 1974, Radioautographic studies on the intracellular distribution of bleomycin ^{14}C in mouse tumor cells. *Cancer Res.*, **34**, 2969–2974.

Genilloud, O., Garrido, M. C. and Moreno, F., 1984, The transposon Tn5 carries a bleomycin-resistance determinant. *Gene*, **32**, 225–233.

Grollman, A. P., Takeshita, M., Pillai, K. M. R. and Johnson, F., 1985, Origin and cytotoxic properties of base propenals derived from DNA. *Cancer Res.*, **45**, 1127–1131.

Grozea, P. N., Jones, S. E., McKelvey, E. M., Coltman, C. A., Fisher, R. and Haskins, C. L., 1979, Combination chemotherapy for mycosis fungoides: A Southwest Oncology Group Study. *Cancer Treat. Rep.*, **63**, 647–653.

Gupta, R. S., 1985, Cross-resistance of vinblastine- and taxol-resistant mutants of Chinese hamster ovary cells to other anticancer drugs. *Cancer Treat. Rep.*, **69**, 515–521.

Henichart, J. P., Bernier, J. L., Houssin, R., Lohez, M., Kenani, A. and Catteau, J.-P., 1985, Copper(II)- and iron(II)-complexes of methyl 2-(2-aminoethyl)-aminomethyl-pyridine-6-carboxyl-histidinate (AMPHIS), a peptide mimicking the metal-chelating moiety of bleomycin. An ESR investigation. *Biochem. Biophys. Res. Commun.*, **126**, 1036–1041.

Hertzberg, R. P., Caranfa, M. J. and Hecht, S. M., 1985, DNA methylation diminishes bleomycin-mediated strand scission. *Biochemistry*, **24**, 5285–5289.

Kanao, M., Tomita, S., Ishida, S., Murakami, A. and Okada, H., 1973, Chelation of bleomycin with copper *in vivo. Chemotherapy* (*Tokyo*), **21**, 1305–1310.

Krebs, H.-B., Girtanner, R. E., Nordqvist, S. R. B., Mineau, I., Helmkamp, B. F. and Averette, H. E., 1980, Treatment of advanced cervical cancer by combination of bleomycin and mitomycin-C. *Cancer*, **46**, 2159–2161.

Lazo, J. S. and Humphreys, C. J., 1983, Lack of metabolism as the biochemical basis of bleomycin-induced pulmonary toxicity. *Proc. Natl. Acad. Sci. USA*, **80**, 3064–3068.

Lazo, J. S. and Pham, E. T., 1984, Pulmonary fate of [^{3}H]bleomycin A_2 in mice. *J. Pharmacol. Exp. Ther.*, **228**, 13–18.

Lazo, J. S., Boland, C. J. and Schwartz, P. E., 1982, Bleomycin hydrolase activity and cytoxicity in human tumors *Cancer Res.*, **42**, 4026–4031.

Lazo, J. S., Merrill, W. W., Pham, E. T., Lynch, T. J., McCallister, J. and Ingbar, D. H., 1984, Bleomycin hydrolase activity in pulmonary cells. *J. Pharmacol. Exp. Ther.*, **231**, 583–588.

Lazo, J. S., Braun, I. D., Meandzija, B., Kennedy, K. A., Pham, E. T. and Smaldone, L. F., 1985, Lidocaine potentiation of bleomycin A_2 cytotoxicity and DNA strand breakage. *Cancer Res.*, **45**, 2103–2109.

Lown, J. W. and Sim, S.-K., 1977, The mechanism of the bleomycin-induced cleavage of DNA. *Biochem. Biophys. Res. Commun.*, **77**, 1150–1157.

Maeda, K., Kosaka, H., Yagishita, K. and Umezawa, H., 1956, A new antibiotic, phleomycin. *J. Antibiotic* (*Tokyo*) *Ser. A.*, **9**, 82–85.

Mazodier, P., Cossart, P., Girand, E. and Gasser, F., 1985, Completion of the nucleotide sequence of the central region of Tn5 confirms the presence of three resistance genes. *Nucleic Acid Res.*, **13**, 195–205.

Mirabelli, C. K., Huang, C.-H. and Crooke, S. T., 1983, Role of deoxyribonucleic acid topology in altering the site/sequence specificity of cleavage of deoxyribonucleic acid by bleomycin and talisomycin. *Biochemistry*, **22**, 300–306.

Muller, W. E. G., Schmidseder, R., Rohde, H. J., Zahn, R. K. and Scheunemann, H., 1977, Bleomycin sensitivity test: Application for human squamous cell carcinoma. *Cancer*, **40**, 2787–2791.

Newcomer, L. N., Cadman, E. C., Nerenberg, M. I., Chen, M., Bertino, J. R., Farber, L. R. and Prosnitz, L. R., 1982, Randomized study comparing doxorubicin, cyclophosphamide, vincristine, methotrexate with leucovorin rescue, and cytarabine (ACOMLA) with cyclophosphamide, doxorubicin, vincristine, prednisone and bleomycin (CHOP-B) in the treatment of diffuse histiocytic lymphoma. *Cancer Treat. Rep.*, **66**, 1279–1284.

Ohnuma, T., Holland, J. F., Masuda, H., Waligunda, J. A. and Goldberg, G. A., 1974, Microbiological assay of bleomycin: Inactivation, tissue distribution and clearance. *Cancer*, **33**, 1230–1238.

Poster, D. S., Bruno, S., Penta, J., Pina, K. and Catane, R., 1981, Current status of chemotherapy in the treatment of advanced carcinoma of the thyroid gland. *Cancer Clin. Trials*, **4**, 301–307.

Sausville, E. A., Stein, R. W., Peisach, J. and Horwitz, S. B., 1978, Properties and products of the degradation of DNA by bleomycin and iron(II). *Biochemistry*, **17**, 2746–2754.

Schlaerth, J. B., Morrow, C. P. and DePetrillo, A. D., 1980, Sustained remission of choriocarcinoma with cis-platinum, vinblastine, and bleomycin after failure of conventional combination drug therapy. *Am. J. Obst. Gynecol.*, **136**, 983–985.

Schrier, D. J., Kunkel, R. G. and Pham, S. H., 1983, The role of strain variation in murine bleomycin-induced pulmonary fibrosis. *Am. Rev. Resp. Dis.*, **127**, 63–66.

Sebti, S. M. and Lazo, J. S., 1986, Separation of pulmonary bleomycin hydrolase from pulmonary aminopeptidases. *Fed. Proc.*, **44**, 30213.

Seki, T., Muraoka, Y., Takahashi, K., Horinishi, H. and Umezawa, H., 1985, Radioimmunoassay of bleomycins. *J. Antibiotics (Tokyo) Ser. A.*, **38**, 1251–1256.

Sugiura, Y., 1980, Bleomycin-iron complexes. Electron spin resonance study, ligand effect, and implication for action mechanism. *J. Am. Chem. Soc.*, **102**, 5208–5215.

Sun, I. L. and Crane, F. L., 1985, Bleomycin control of transplasma membrane redox activity and proton movement in Hela cells. *Biochem. Pharmacol.*, **34**, 617–622.

Tanaka, N., 1984, Studies on the mechanism of drug resistance in tumor cells and a new antitumor antibiotic. *Gan To Kagaku Ryoho*, **11**, 2666–2676.

Takahashi, K., Yoskioka, O., Matsuda, A. and Umezawa, H., 1977, Intracellular reduction of the cupric ion of bleomycin copper complex and transfer of the cuprous ion to a cellular protein. *J. Antibiotics (Tokyo) Ser. A*, **30**, 861–869.

Takita, T., Umezawa, Y., Saito, S., Morishima, H., Naganawa, H., Umezawa, H., Tsuchiya, T., Miyake, T., Kageyama, S., Umezawa, S., Muraoka, Y., Suzuki, M., Otsuka, M., Narita, M., Kobayashi, S. and Ohno, M., 1982, Total synthesis of bleomycin A_2. *Tetrahedron Lett.*, **23**, 521–524.

Thomas, A. H., Newland, P. and Sharma, N. R., 1984, Chromatographic methods for the analysis of bleomycin complex. *J. Chromatog.*, **291**, 219–230.

Tryka, A. F., Skornik, W. A., Godleski, J. J. and Braine, J. D., 1982, Potentiation of bleomycin-induced lung injury by exposure to 70% oxygen. *Am. Rev. Respir. Dis.*, **26**, 1074–1079.

Ueda, M., Nozawa, S., Ueki, M., Sano, T., Nagai, S., Sugimoto, O. and Kurihara, S., 1984, Peplomycin sensitivity of various types of human gynecological cultured tumor cells. *Nippon Sanka Fujinka Gakkai Zasshi*, **36**, 1867–1876.

Uehara, Y., Hori, M. and Umezawa, H., 1982, Specificity of transport of bleomycin and cobalt-bleomycin in L5178Y cells. *Biochem. Biophys. Res. Commun.*, **104**, 416–421.

Umezawa, H., 1979, In *Bleomycin: Chemical, Biochemical, and Biological Aspects*, edited by S. M. Hecht (New York: Springer-Verlag), pp. 24–36.

Umezawa, H., Hori, M., Ishizuka, M. and Takeuchi, T., 1962, Studies on the antitumor effect of phleomycin. *J. Antibiotics (Tokyo) Ser. A.*, **15**, 274–275.

Umezawa, H., Maeda, K., Takeuchi, T. and Okami, Y., 1966, New antibiotics, bleomycin A and B. *J. Antibiotics (Tokyo) Ser. A*, **19**, 200–209.

Umezawa, H., Ishizuka, M., Hori, S., Chimura, H. and Takeuchi, T., 1968, The distribution of [^{3}H]-bleomycin in mouse tissue. *J. Antibiotics* (*Tokyo*) *Ser. A.*, **21**, 638–642.

Umezawa, H., Takeuchi, T., Hori, S., Sawa, T. and Ishizuka, M., 1972, Studies on the mechanism of antitumor effect of bleomycin on squamous cell carcinoma. *J. Antibiotics* (*Tokyo*) *Ser. A.*, **25**, 409–420.

Umezawa, H., Hori, S., Tsutomu, S., Yoshioka, T. and Takeuchi, T., 1974, A bleomycin-inactivating enzyme in mouse liver. *J. Antibiotics* (*Tokyo*) *Ser. A*, **27**, 419–424.

Yoshioka, O., Amano, N., Takahashi, K., Matsuda, A. and Umezawa, H., 1978, Intracellular fate and activity of bleomycin, In *Bleomycin: Current Status and New Developments*, edited by S. K. Carter, S. T. Crooke, and H. Umezawa (New York: Academic Press) pp 35–56.

Zuckerman, J. E., Raffin, T. A., Brown, J. M., Etiz, B., and Sikic, B. I., 1986, *In vitro* selection and characterization of a bleomycin-resistant subline of B16 melanoma. *Cancer Res.*, **46**, 1748.

8. Anthracycline metabolism and free radical formation

Garth Powis

Historical perspective

The anthracycline glycosides were first studied in the late 1950s as pigmented antibiotics produced by different strains of *Streptomyces* (Brockmann, 1963). The era of anti-tumour anthracyclines began with the almost simultaneous isolation in 1963 by workers in France, Italy and the USSR of the anthracycline now known as daunorubicin from *S. coeroleorubidus* (Aubel-Sadron and Londos-Gagliardi, 1984) and *S. peucetius* (DiMarco *et al.*, 1963; Gause, 1964). The potent antileukaemic activity of daunorubicin led to the search for other anthracylines with anti-tumour activity and in 1969 doxorubicin was isolated from a chemically mutated strain *S. peucetius* var. *caesius* (Arcamone *et al.*, 1969). This new antibiotic had an enlarged spectrum of activity and greater efficacy than daunorubicin against solid tumours. Since its introduction for clinical use in the early 1970s, more than two million patients have received doxorubicin (Arcamone, 1985). Several hundred analogues of daunorubicin and doxorubicin have been obtained by partial or total synthesis and tested in experimental tumour models in an attempt to improve on the biological activity of the parent compounds (Arcamone, 1977, 1984; Henry, 1979; Naff *et al.*, 1982). In 1975 Japanese investigators isolated a substantially different type of anthracycline named aclacinomycin A from *S. galilaeus* (Oki *et al.*, 1975). Instead of a single sugar attached to the aglycone portion of the molecule, as with daunorubicin and doxorubicin, aclacinomycin A had three sugars linked in a carbohydrate chain. Since the discovery of aclacinomycin A, other anthracyclines with two or three saccharide carbohydrate chains, such as musettamycin and marcellomycin, have been isolated (Nettleton *et al.*, 1977; Oki, 1977).

Structural features

Active anthracyclines are composed of a tetracyclic aglycone chromophore, usually red, orange or yellow in colour, linked to a mono-, di- or tri-saccharide carbohydrate chain. The structures of some anthracyclines of clinical and

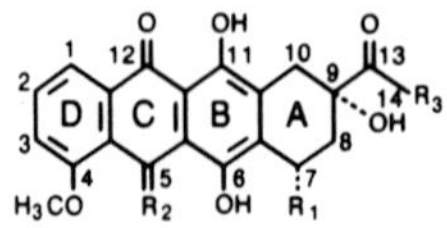

Compound	R_1	R_2	R_3
Doxorubicin	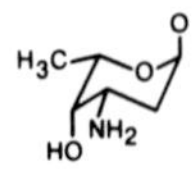	O	CH_2OH
4'-Epidoxorubicin	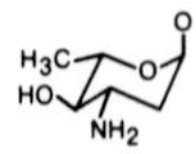	O	CH_2OH
Daunorubicin	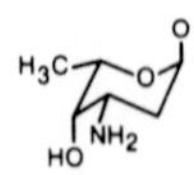	O	CH_3
5-Iminodaunorubicin	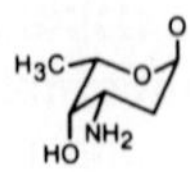	NH	CH_3
AD32	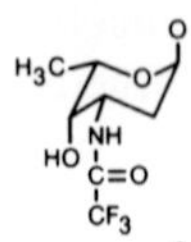	O	$CH_2OC(O)(CH_2)_3CH_3$
MRA-CN	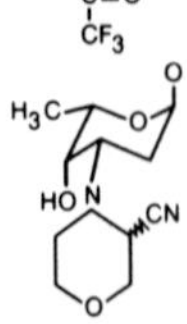	O	CH_2OH

Figure 1. Structures of some important anthracyclines.

experimental importance are shown in Figure 1. Changes in the structure of the aglycone moiety of anthracyclines, with the exception of alterations in the 9-acyl group, frequently result in inactive compounds (Brown, 1978; Arcamone, 1977). However, the C-4 methoxy group of daunorubicin and doxorubicin is not essential for anti-tumour activity and many active semisynthetic compounds have a C-4 hydroxyl group. The saccharide most frequently found attached to the anthracycline aglycone moiety is daunosamine, as in daunorubicin and doxorubicin, while a carbohydrate chain may contain L-rhodosamine, L-rhodinose, 2-deoxy-L-fucose, L-cinerulose A, L-cinerulose B, D-cinerulose A, L-amicetose and L-aculose as constituents (Oki *et al.*, 1977). Structural changes in the carbohydrate moiety of anthracyclines are

Figure 1 (*cont.*)

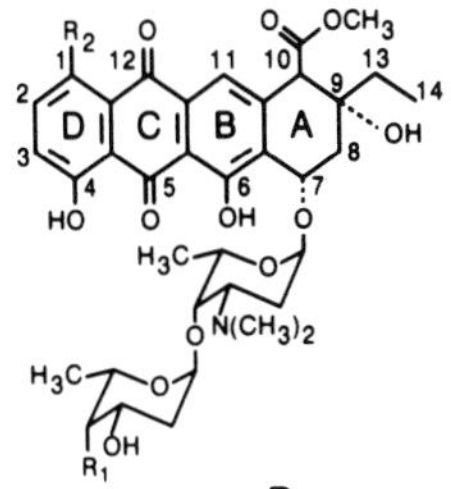

Compound	R_1	R_2
Aclacinomycin A	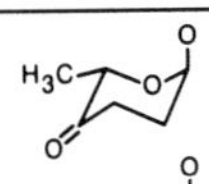	H
Marcellomycin	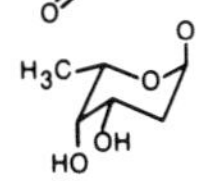	OH
Musettamycin	OH	OH
Menogaril	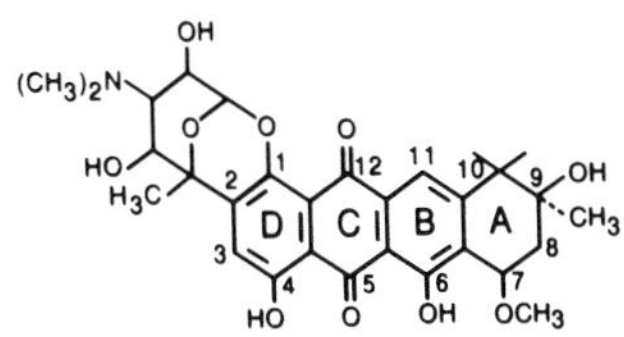	

compatible with retention of anti-tumour activity. 4′-Epidoxorubicin is an epimer of doxorubicin with a different configuration of the C-4′ hydroxyl group of daunosamine. *N*-Trifluoroacetyl doxorubicin 14-valerate (AD32) has a trifluoroacetyl group attached to the amino nitrogen of daunosamine. Incorporation of the amino nitrogen of daunosamine into a morpholino ring yields compounds that are more potent anti-tumour agents than the parent anthracycline. One such compound, 3′-deamino-3′-(3″-cyano-4″-morpholinyl) doxorubicin (MRA-CN), has a potency up to 1000 times greater than doxorubicin *in vitro* and *in vivo* (Acton *et al.*, 1984; Johnston *et al.*, 1983). Complete removal of the carbohydrate moiety from anthracyclines usually gives compounds that are devoid of anti-tumour activity (Henry, 1979). Menogaril is an active semisynthetic derivative of the naturally occurring nogalomycin and is unusual in having no C-7 carbohydrate moiety, but it does have a dimethylamine saccharide (glucopyranose) attached to the anthracycline D ring through both carbon–oxygen and carbon–carbon bonds (McGovren *et al.*, 1984).

A functional classification of anthracyclines based on their relative abilities to inhibit DNA and nuclear RNA synthesis has been proposed by Crooke *et al.* (1978). Class I anthracyclines, which includes daunorubicin, doxorubicin and carminomycin, inhibit DNA and RNA synthesis at similar concentrations, while Class II anthracyclines preferentially inhibit nucleolar RNA synthesis at concentrations several hundred-fold lower than required to inhibit DNA synthesis. Class II anthracyclines have a C-10 carbomethoxy group and a di- or tri-saccharide carbohydrate chain (DuVernay *et al.*, 1979; DuVernay and Crooke, 1980). Removal of the C-10 carbomethoxy group decreases the inhibition of nucleolar RNA synthesis as well as the *in vitro* and *in vivo* toxicity of Class II anthracyclines (Oki *et al.*, 1977). Because this classification of anthracyclines is based on a functional property and since only a limited number of anthracyclines have been studied, the classification cannot be considered comprehensive and there may be compounds whose structures do not fit within the above guidelines.

Clinical uses

Since the first clinical trials of daunorubicin and doxorubicin little more than a decade ago, they have gained rapid acceptance as major therapeutic agents in the treatment of cancer. Both drugs are widely used as part of combination chemotherapy regimens for the effective treatment of acute non-lymphocytic leukaemia, Hodgkin's and non-Hodgkin's lymphomas, breast cancer and sarcomas (Young *et al.*, 1981). Doxorubicin has shown a wide range of activity in human solid tumours including those of the breast, lung, ovary, head and neck, bladder, endometrium and prostate and it is the most effective single agent against soft-tissue sarcomas in adults, although it is rarely curative in the advanced disease. The use of doxorubicin for adjuvant chemotherapy of soft-tissue sarcomas is being actively studied.

Toxic effects of anthracyclines include myelosuppression, cardiomyopathy, nausea and vomiting, hair loss and, if the drug accidentally extravasates during administration, tissue necrosis (Young *et al.*, 1981). Myelosuppression, mainly in the form of neutropenia, is the acute dose-limiting toxicity of daunorubicin and doxorubicin while cardiomyopathy is the cumulative dose-limiting toxicity. The incidence of congestive heart failure is proportional to the dose. With doses of doxorubicin of 400 mg/m^2 or less, the incidence of cardiomyopathy is under 2%; for cumulative doses in excess of 700 mg/m^2 the incidence is greater than 20% (Olson *et al.*, 1974). The cardiac damage produced by doxorubicin does not undergo significant repair and once clinically overt cardiomyopathy is present the prognosis is grave, with mortality rates as high as 48% (Pratt *et al.*, 1978). Weekly, as opposed to every three weeks, administration of doxorubicin may result in less cardiotoxicity (Weiss and Manthel, 1977), as may continuous infusion of doxorubicin (Legha *et al.*, 1982). Attempts to lessen the cardiotoxicity of daunorubicin and doxorubicin have provided the main rationale for the extensive isolation and synthetic programmes of anthracycline analogues. Analogues that have been reported to have less cardiotoxicity and other toxicities in experimenal animals are 4′-epidoxorubicin, 4′-deoxydoxorubicin, aclacinomycin A, menogaril, 5-iminodaunorubicin, AD-32 and MRA-CN. It remains to be seen whether these agents will be better tolerated clinically and whether they will be as effective anti-tumour agents as daunorubicin and doxorubicin.

Metabolism

There are three types of anthracycline metabolic reactions: keto reduction, cleavage reactions and conjugation. In addition, during anthracycline cleavage to aglycone, an anthracycline free radical is formed which in the presence of molecular oxygen can undergo redox cycling to form reactive oxygen species. The metabolism of anthracyclines by each pathway will be reviewed from the viewpoint of, first, *in vitro*, and, second, *in vivo* studies. Free radical formation and alkylation will be dealt with separately.

Metabolism *in vitro*

Keto-reduction

All rat tissues studied except plasma contain a soluble enzyme that in the presence of NADPH is capable of reducing anthracyclines and anthracycline aglycones with a C-13 keto group to the corresponding C-13 alcohol (Bachur and Cradock, 1970; Bachur and Gee, 1971). A C-13 anthracycline alcohol is designated by the suffix -ol, for example, the C-13 alcohol of daunorubicin is daunorubicinol and the C-13 alcohol of doxorubicin is doxorubicinol. Liver, lung and kidney show the highest daunorubicin C-13 keto reductase activity. The enzyme has a molecular weight of 39 000 daltons (Felsted *et al.*, 1974) and belongs to a group of widely distributed enzymes classified as $NADP^+$ oxidoreductase (E.C. 1.1.1.2) (Felsted *et al.*, 1977; Turner and Hick, 1976). Activity of the enzyme is non-competitively inhibited by barbiturates, warfarin and diphenylhydantoin. The enzyme exhibits extensive activity with a variety of natural and foreign aldehydes, but has only limited activity with ketones as substrates. In fact, daunorubicin is the only ketone so far found to undergo reduction at a significant rate. Daunorubicin is a much better substrate than doxorubicin. The K_m of daunorubicin for the purified enzyme is 0.06 mM and the K_m of doxorubicin 0.19 mM (Felsted *et al.*, 1974). Except for daunorubicin and doxorubicin, which have a pH optimum of 8·5, other substrates have a pH optimum of 6·0 (Felsted *et al.*, 1977). 4-Demethoxydaunorubicin is a better substrate than doxorubicin for C-13 keto reduction by rat liver homogenate (Riggs and Schrader, 1985). 4′-Epidoxorubicin and 4′-deoxydoxorubicin have been reported to be both better (Weenen *et al.*, 1984) and poorer (Riggs and Schrader, 1985) substrates than doxorubicin for C-13 keto reduction by rat liver preparations.

Human and rabbit liver cytosol contain in addition to the pH 8·5 aldehyde daunorubicin reductase found in rodent liver, a pH 6·0 ketone daunorubicin reductase (Ahmed *et al.*, 1978 a, 1981). The enzyme has different properties to the pH 8·5 aldehyde daunorubicin reductase on isoelectric focusing, ion exchange and gel filtration chromatography and is not inhibited by barbiturates, although it is inhibited by the alkaloid quercitrin. Work by Schwartz and Parker (1981) suggests there may also be an anthracycline C-13 keto reductase in the rat hepatic microsomal fraction that is not removed by extensive washing. The properties of this enzyme have not been characterized.

The C-4‴ keto group of the terminal L-cinerulose of aclacinomycin A undergoes stereoselective reduction by cytosolic and microsomal reductases in rat liver (Komiyama *et al.*, 1978, 1979 b). Cytosolic cinerulose reductase requires NADPH and converts L-cinerulose to L-amicetose and L-rhodinose. Microsomal cinerulose reductase requires NADH and converts L-cinerulose to L-rhodinose only. Neither enzyme is capable of reducing the C-13 keto group of daunorubicin (Oki *et al.*, 1981).

The C-13 keto reduced metabolites of daunorubicin and doxorubicin, and the C-14‴ keto reduced metabolites of alacinomycin A retain anti-tumour activity comparable to that of the parent compounds (Henry, 1979; Oki *et al.*, 1981).

C-7 cleavage (aglycone formation)

DiMarco *et al.* (1967) first reported that daunorubicin incubated with homogenates of rat liver and kidney formed a much less polar metabolite and suggested it might be a modified aglycone of daunorubicin. In 1971 Bachur identified the metabolite as 7-hydroxydaunorubicinol aglycone and suggested it was formed by hydrolytic cleavage of daunorubicinol (Bachur and Cradock, 1970). Bachur and Gee (1971) reported that the enzyme responsible for the hydrolytic cleavage was found in the liver microsomal fraction, required NADPH but not NADH and, significantly, was equally active under aerobic or anaerobic conditions. In 1972 Asbell *et al.* reported that different aglycone metabolites were formed from daunorubicin under anaerobic conditions by NADPH fortified rat liver and kidney homogenate. The aglycones were the products of reductive cleavage, 7-deoxydaunorubicin aglycone and 7-deoxydaunorubicinol aglycone. Doxorubicin formed corresponding 7-deoxyaglycone metabolites. The enzyme responsible for reductive cleavage was found in the liver microsomal fraction, required NADPH but not NADH, was induced by phenobarbital and was reversibly inhibited by oxygen (Bachur and Gee, 1972, 1976). This explained why previous studies conducted under aerobic conditions had not seen 7-deoxyaglycone formation. In fact, formation of 7-hydroxyaglycones is now recognized as a minor pathway of anthracycline metabolism and may result from hydroxy radical generated during redox cycling of anthracyclines reacting with radical precursors of 7-deoxyaglycone (Schwartz and Paul, 1984).

A clue to the identity of the microsomal enzyme catalysing 7-deoxyaglycone formation came in 1976 when Handa and Sato (1976) found that catalytic amounts of daunorubicin and doxorubicin stimulated the oxidation of NADPH by a partly purified preparation of the microsomal flavoenzyme NADPH–cytochrome P-450 reductase (E.C. 1.6.2.4.). Confirmation that the microsomal enzyme responsible for reductive cleavage of anthracyclines was NADPH–cytochrome P-450 reductase was provided by Oki *et al.*, (1977), who showed that the purified enzyme catalysed the conversion of a number of anthracyclines to the 7-deoxyaglycones (Table 1). The enzyme had a broad substrate specificity and also reduced 7-hydroxyaglycones to 7-deoxyaglycones, although Bachur and Gee (1976) had previously reported that 7-hydroxyaglycones were not substrates for reduction by rat liver microsomes. 6-Deoxy-4-demethoxydaunorubicin is not a substrate for reductive cleavage by rat liver preparations (Arcamone, 1985). This confirms expectations from electrochemical reduction studies where compounds such as 10-β-methoxydaunorubicin and 11-deoxydaunorubicin, with the same α conformation of the A ring as daunorubicin, are readily reduced in a two-step process to the corresponding 7-deoxyaglycone, while 10-α-methoxydaunorubicin and 6-deoxydaunorubicin, with a β conformation of the A ring, do not undergo reductive deglycosidation and in polar solvents form only the hydroquinone glycoside (Malatesta *et al.*, 1984). The reason for the different behaviour of β-anthracyclines is thought to be the lack of conjugative electron delocalization due to the large dihedral angle with respect to the pi-type orbital(s) of the anthraquinone system compared to α-anthracyclines. Anthracyclines are only one group of a large number of quinones that undergo single-electron reduction by NADPH–cytochrome P-450 reductase. An important factor in determining the rate of quinone reduction by the enzyme is the one-electron reduction potential (E^1) of the quinone (Powis and Appel, 1980). E^1 values for several anthracyclines are around -300 mV (Powis and Svingen, 1981) and

Table 1. Reductive cleavage of anthracycline antibiotics by NADPH–cytochrome P-450 reductase.

Substrate	Products	Rate (relative to daunorubicin)
Daunorubicin	7-Deoxydaunorubicin aglycone	1·00
Doxorubicin	7-Deoxydoxorubicin aglycone	0·46
Aclacinomycin A	7-Deoxyaklavinone aglycone	0·04
	7-Deoxyaklavinone aglycone dimer	0·04
Daunorubicinol	7-Deoxydaunorubicin aglycone	0·30
Aklavinone	7-Deoxyaklavinone aglycone	0·12
	7-Deoxyaklavinone aglycone dimer	0·17
Daunorubicinone	7-Deoxydaunorubicin aglycone	0·40
Doxorubicinone	7-Deoxydoxorubicin aglycone	0·71

Data from Oki *et al.* (1977)

E^1 is probably not a major factor in determining relative rates of reduction of different anthracyclines by NADPH–cytochrome P-450 reductase.

Other flavoenzymes that catalyse single-electron reduction will support reductive cleavage of anthracyclines under anaerobic conditions. The enzymes include xanthine oxidase (xanthine : oxidase oxygen oxidoreductase, E.C. 1.2.3.2.), mitochondrial NADH-dehydrogenase (E.C. 1.6.99.3) and nitrate reductase from *Neurospora* (E.C. 1.6.6.3) (Komiyama *et al.*, 1979 a; Pan and Bachur, 1980; Pan *et al.*, 1981 a; Schwartz, 1983). Flavoenzymes catalysing two-electron reduction have been reported not to support reductive cleavage of anthracyclines (Pan *et al.*, 1981 a), although Komiyama *et al.* (1979 a) found that quinone reductase (NAD(P)H : quinone oxidoreductase, E.C. 1.6.99.2, also known as DT-diaphorase), which catalyses only two-electron reduction of quinones (Iyanagi and Yamazaki, 1970), cleaved doxorubicin to 7-deoxydoxorubicin aglycone.

Reductive cleavage of anthracyclines is associated with formation of a free radical intermediate. Free radical formation is discussed in detail in the section on Free Radical Formation. Although a free radical intermediate appears to be obligatory, the exact mechanism of reductive cleavage is not known. Mason (1979) and Sinha (1980) have suggested a mechanism involving a carbon-centred C-7 anthracycline free radical. Houée-Levin *et al.* (1984) have proposed that the anthracycline semiquinone radical disproportionates to an unstable hydroquinone which loses its sugar moiety by heterolytic bond cleavage.

C-4 cleavage

Schwartz and his colleagues (Schwartz and Parker, 1981; Schwartz and Paul, 1984) have shown C-4 cleavage as an additional pathway of anthracycline metabolism by rat liver microsomes under anaerobic conditions. Daunorubicin aglycone undergoes C-4 reductive cleavage to 4-deoxydaunorubicin aglycone, as well as C-4-*O*-demethylation to 4-hydroxydaunorubicin aglycone. Both reactions require NADPH and because they were inhibited by SKF 525A (β-diethylaminoethyl diphenylpropylacetate), it was suggested that C-4 reductive cleavage and C-4-*O*-demethylation were catalysed by microsomal cytochrome P-450. SKF 525A is not, however, a specific inhibitor of cytochrome P-450-catalysed reactions and it is possible that other microsomal enzyme(s) are involved in C-4 cleavage.

A complete reaction sequence for formation of aglycone metabolites from daunorubicin by rat liver microsomes as proposed by Schwartz and Paul (1984) is shown in Figure 2. The first step, based on kinetic evidence, is C-7 reductive cleavage of daunorubicin to 7-deoxydaunorubicin aglycone with smaller amounts of C-7 hydrolytic cleavage to 7-hydroxydaunorubicin aglycone. This is followed by C-13 keto reduction and C-4 cleavage.

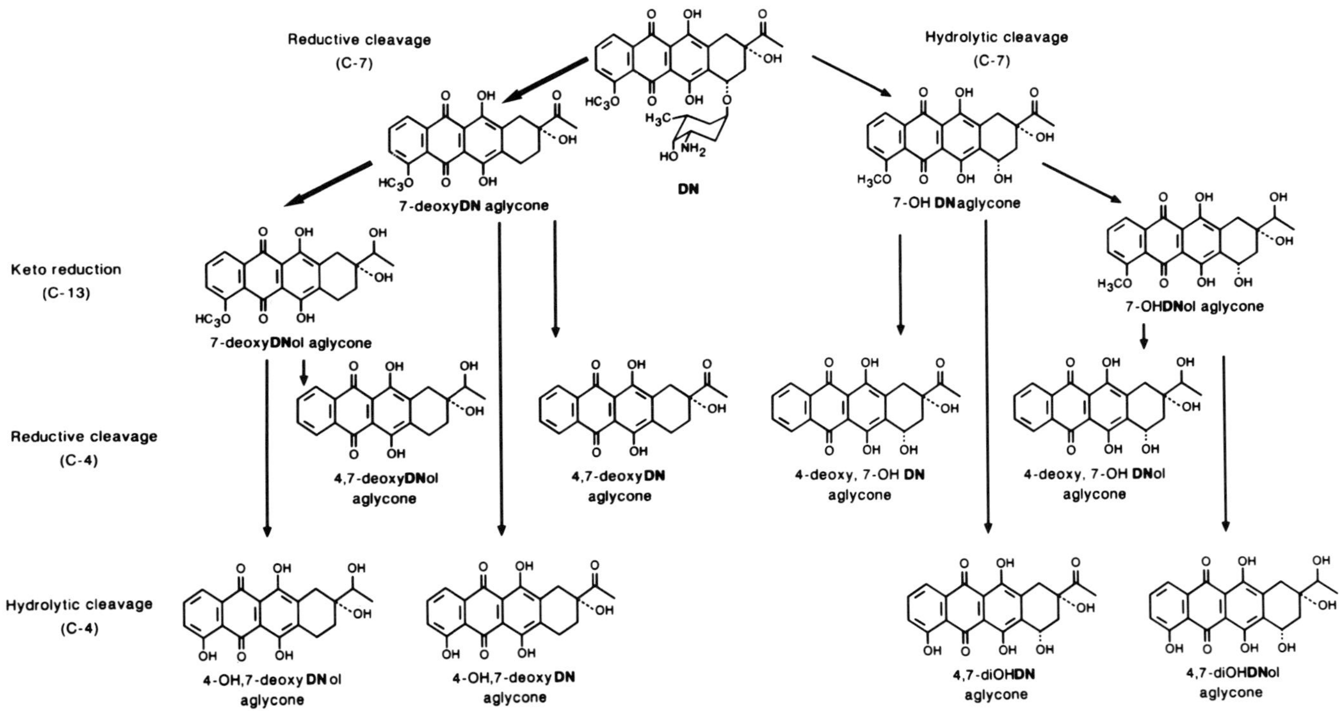

Figure 2. Formation of aglycone metabolites of daunorubicin (DN) by rat liver microsomes and NADPH under anaerobic conditions. Dark arrows indicate major pathways. Adapted from Schwartz and Paul (1984).

Miscellaneous metabolic reactions

Glutathione–anthracycline adducts are formed when reduced glutathione is included in incubations of daunorubicin or doxorubicin with NADPH and rat liver microsomes (Oki, 1977). A 7, 7′-dimer of 7-deoxyaklavinone has been identified as one of the products of the reductive cleavage of aclacinomycin A by purified NADPH–cytochrome P-450 reductase (Oki *et al.*, 1977). Both of

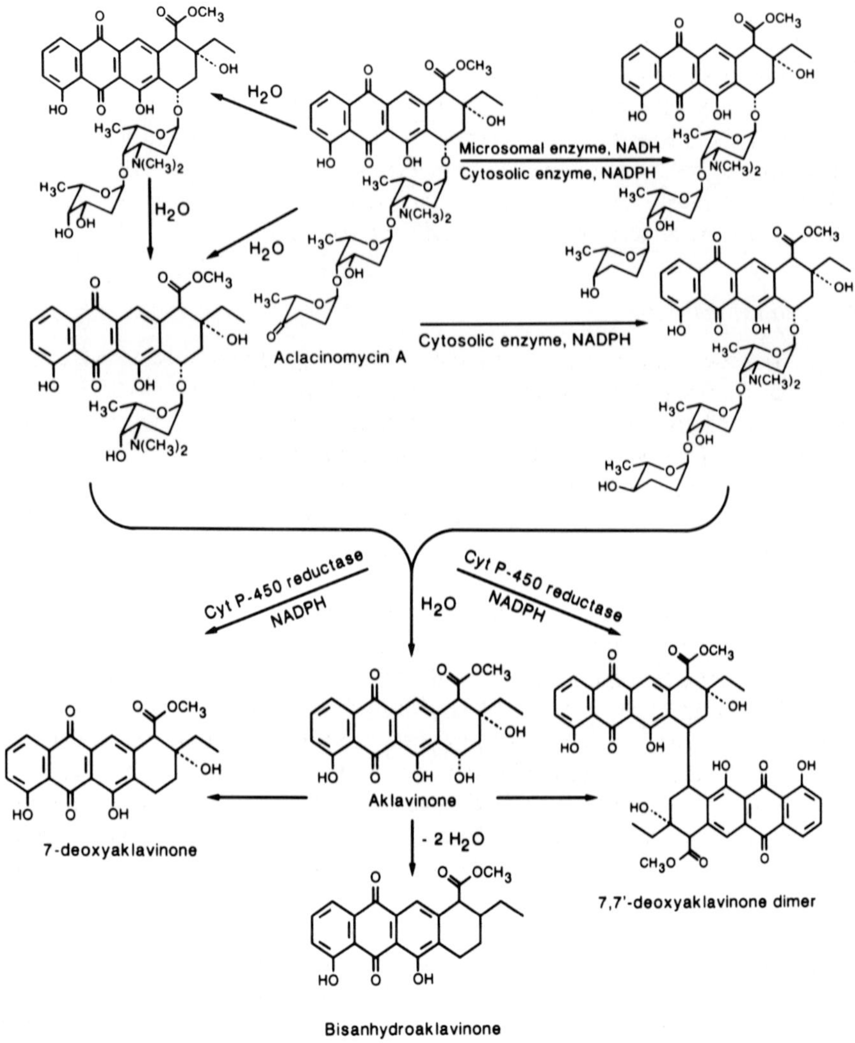

Figure 3. Metabolism of aclacinomycin A by liver, kidney and heart homogenate under aerobic (upper panel) and anaerobic (lower panel) conditions. Adapted from Oki (1977) and Komiyama *et al.*, (1979 a, b).

these reactions are thought to proceed through an anthracycline free radical intermediate. Aclacinomycin A undergoes a number of modifications of the carbohydrate chain (Oki, 1977). A suggested reaction sequence for *in vitro* metabolism of aclacinomycin A is shown in Figure 3. Xanthine oxidase using xanthine as an electron donor converts 7-deoxydaunorubicin aglycone to a non-fluorescent metabolite (Dodion *et al.*, 1984). Analogy to metabolism of dihydroxyanthraquinone, which is converted by xanthine oxidase to tetrahydroxyanthracene, suggests that the non-fluorescent metabolite of 7-deoxydaunorubicin aglycone might be a dihydroquinone derivative. Marcellomycin is converted to a non-fluorescent metabolite upon prolonged incubation with NADPH fortified rat liver microsomes or cytosol under anaerobic conditions, probably through 7-deoxypyrromycin aglycone (Chang *et al.*, 1983). The same non-fluorescent metabolite is formed from 7-deoxypyrromycin aglycone by xanthine oxidase and xanthine, and by rat liver cytosol and NADPH or NADH, under anaerobic conditions. The metabolite may be 7-deoxypyrromycin dihydroquinone aglycone (Dodion *et al.*, 1984).

Free radical formation

Simple quinones are known to undergo flavoenzyme-catalysed one-electron reduction to semiquinone free radicals (Iyanagi and Yamazaki, 1969; Powis and Appel, 1980). It is not surprising to find, therefore, that anthracyclines also undergo flavoenzyme-catalysed one-electron reduction to free radicals. Handa and Sato (1975) first reported that daunorubicin and doxorubicin incubated with rat liver microsomes and NADPH under aerobic conditions formed a free radical that was capable of initiating sulphite oxidation. Inhibition of the reaction by superoxide dismutase suggested that the radical species being formed was the superoxide anion radical ($O_2^{\cdot-}$). Two years later simultaneous reports appeared that conclusively demonstrated the formation of anthracycline semiquinone free radicals during anthracycline metabolism using electron spin resonance (ESR) spectroscopy. Sato *et al.* (1977) reported ESR spectra due to the anthracycline semiquinone free radical when daunorubicin and doxorubicin were incubated with NADPH-fortified rat liver microsomes or with Ehrlich ascites tumour cells. The anthracycline semiquinone free radical was rapidly auto-oxidized and the ESR signal appeared only when dissolved oxygen in the reaction mixture had been exhausted. Bachur *et al.* (1977) also reported an ESR signal when daunorubicin was incubated with NADPH fortified rat liver microsomes under conditions where dissolved oxygen in the incubation medium was probably depleted. Subsequently, a number of other anthracyclines have been shown to undergo enzymatic one-electron reduction to form ESR-detectable semiquinone free radicals (Table 2).

The ESR spectra obtained by reduction of anthracyclines can be observed for up to several hours. The long duration of the signal is probably due to the

Table 2. Free radical formation by anthracyclines

Compound	Drug radical	Oxygen radical
Doxorubicin	ESR (Bachur *et al.*, 1978; Berlin and Haseltine, 1981; Pietronigro *et al.*, 1979, 1983; Pollakis *et al.*, 1984; Sato *et al.*, 1977; Sinha and Chignell, 1979)	ESR/spin trap (Davies *et al.*, 1983; Gutierrez *et al.*, 1983; Goormaghtigh and Ruysschaert, 1983; Kalyanaraman *et al.*, 1980, 1984; Komiyama *et al.*, 1982; Nohl and Jordan, 1983; Sinha *et al.*, 1984). Chemical (Adachi *et al.*, 1983; Doroshow, 1983 a, c; Komiyama *et al.*, 1982; Powis *et al.*, 1981; Tobia *et al.*, 1985).
N-Acetyldoxorubicin	ESR (Pollakis *et al.*, 1984)	
Daunorubicin	ESR (Bachur *et al.*, 1977; Kalyanaraman *et al.*, 1984; Sinha and Chignell, 1979)	ESR/spin trap (Kalyanaraman *et al.*, 1980, 1984) Chemical (Doroshow, 1983 a,)
Aclacinomycin A	ESR (Bachur *et al.*, 1978; Kodama *et al.*, 1983)	ESR/spin trap (Komiyama *et al.*, 1982) Chemical(Doroshow, 1983 a, b)
Rubidazone		Chemical (Doroshow, 1983 a, b)

Techniques used to demonstrate free radical formation are electron spin resonance (ESR), with or without spin-trapping, and chemical assay.

well known disproportionation–comproportionation equilibrium between quinone (Q) and hydroquinone (QH_2) which continually destroys and reforms the semiquinone free radical ($Q^{\bar{\cdot}}$) (reaction 1) (Michaelis, 1946).

$$2Q^{\bar{\cdot}} + 2H^+ \rightleftharpoons Q + QH_2 \qquad (1)$$

Aqueous solutions of doxorubicin spontaneously form doxorubicin semiquinone free radical at physiological pH, although the rate is much slower than the enzyme-catalysed rate (Pietronigro *et al.*, 1979). This is probably due to intramolecular electron transfer between the hydroquinone B ring and the quinone C ring of the anthracycline.

An unusual feature of ESR spectra of doxorubicin and daunorubicin is that they change with time (Figure 4) (Kalyanaraman *et al.*, 1980; Pan *et al.*, 1980,

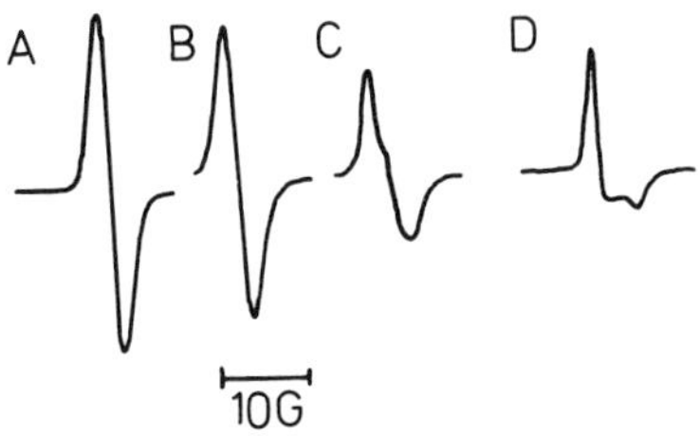

Figure 4. Electron spin resonance signals obtained when daunorubicin (1 mg/ml) is incubated with rat liver microsomes (1·5 mg protein/ml) and an NADPH-generating system. GSH was also present at a 10-fold molar excess over drug but had no effect on signal formation. A to D show progressive immobilization of the signal. A, 2 min (receiver gain 4×10^3); B, 10 min (receiver gain 8×10^3); C, 30 min (receiver gain 8×10^3); and D, 2·0 h (receiver gain $1{\cdot}6 \times 10^4$). From Sinha and Gregory (1981) with permission.

1981 b; Pollakis *et al.*, 1984; Sinha *et al.*, 1984). The first signal that appears is symmetrical with a spectroscopic splitting constant (g) of 2·0036 (Kalyanaraman *et al.*, 1980; Pan *et al.*, 1980, 1981 b). With time the spectrum evolves into one with asymmetry and g anisotropy, $g_1 = 2{\cdot}0046$ to 2·0052, $g_{11} = 2{\cdot}0023$ (Gutierrez *et al.*, 1983; Kalyanaraman *et al.*, 1980; Pan *et al.*, 1981 b), characteristic of a highly immobilized free radical. The immobilized signal has been suggested to be produced by either the 7-deoxyaglycone semiquinone free radical or an anthracycline polymerization product (Kalyanaraman *et al.*, 1980). The best evidence is that the anisotropic signal is that of the 7-deoxyaglycone semiquinone free radical. Appearance of anthracycline 7-deoxyaglycone in the incubation mixture precedes the appearance of the anisotropic signal (Gutierrez *et al.*, 1983), and the fully developed anisotropic signal has the same parameters as the signal obtained with 7-deoxyaglycone as substrate (Pan *et al.*, 1980). Other anthracyclines, such as *N*-acetyldoxorubicin, also give an ESR signal that shows anisotropy with time (Pollakis *et al.*, 1984). Daunosamine, the sugar cleaved from the anthracycline, does not give rise to an ESR signal (Pan *et al.*, 1980).

The properties of anthracycline semiquinone free radicals have been studied by pulse radiolysis. In this technique an aqueous solution of anthracycline is irradiated with a short burst of high energy electrons in the presence of a trapping agent to remove oxidizing species formed by the radiolysis of water. The anthracycline is reduced by aqueous electrons to a semiquinone free radical whose decay can be followed spectrophotometrically (Svingen and Powis, 1981). E^1 for the anthracycline can be calculated from the rates of electron transfer between the anthracycline and a redox indicator of known E^1. Measurements made by an approach to equilibrium method have given E^1 (at pH 7.0) for daunorubicin as -305 mV and doxorubicin as -292 mV (Svingen and Powis, 1981). Measurements made at equilibrium have given E^1 for doxorubicin as -328 mV (Land *et al.*, 1983). An E^1 of -430 mV has been calculated from the rate of disproportionation of doxorubicin semiquinone

(Houée-Levin *et al.*, 1985). Values in this range indicate that anthracyclines such as doxorubicin and daunorubicin have a low E^1 compared to simple quinones, which may explain the relatively slow rate of reduction of anthracyclines by NADPH–cytochrome P-450 reductase and other flavoenzymes compared to simple quinones (Svingen and Powis, 1981). Pulse radiolysis studies have shown that the doxorubicin semiquinone free radical reacts rapidly with oxygen with a bimolecular rate constant of $3 \times 10^8 \text{M}^{-1} \text{s}^{-1}$ (Butler *et al.*, 1985; Land *et al.*, 1985).

The ability of catalytic amounts of anthracycline to stimulate NADPH oxidation and oxygen utilization by microsomes from liver (Goodman and Hochstein, 1977; Bachur *et al.*, 1977) and a variety of tissues including tumour cells (Bachur *et al.*, 1978), as well as by purified NADPH–cytochrome P-450 reductase (Handa and Sato, 1975; Bachur *et al.*, 1979) is well known. Levels of anthracycline remain constant until all the dissolved oxygen has been depleted, when there is a rapid conversion of anthracycline to the 7-deoxyaglycone (Figure 5). These, and other observations discussed previously, are consistent with the concept of redox cycling of the anthracycline to the semiquinone free radical and back, with molecular oxygen as the final electron acceptor. The initial species formed by reduction of molecular oxygen by the anthracycline semiquinone free radical is the superoxide anion radical. This has been shown by chemical assays and by ESR studies using dimethyl-1-pyrroline-1-oxide (DMPO) to spin trap the superoxide anion radical as a stable adduct (Table 2). Small amounts of a DMPO hydroxyl radical adduct are also occasionaly seen (Kalyanaraman *et al.*, 1980). Using another spin trapping agent, α-phenyl-*N*-butylnitrone (PBN), only hydroxyl radical trapped adduct is seen (Komiyama *et al.*, 1982; Sugioka *et al.*, 1984). Aqueous air-saturated solutions of daunorubicin and doxorubicin at physiological pH spontaneously form oxygen radicals at a slow rate. A solution of doxorubicin incubated with PBN gives an ESR signal that can be attributed to either the superoxide anion radical or hydroxyl radical adduct (Dickinson *et al.*, 1984). Photoirradiation of an aqueous solution of daunorubicin or doxorubicin at 438 nm stimulates the formation of superoxide anion radical, detected as the spin-trapped adduct with 4-(*N*-methylpyridinium)-t-butylnitrone, and of hydroxyl radical, detected as the spin-trapped adduct with DMPO (Carmichael *et al.*, 1983). In these studies the DMPO hydroxyl radical adduct was not formed by direct addition of hydroxyl radical to DMPO, and may have arisen from decomposition of a DMPO superoxide anion radical adduct.

Superoxide anion radical is a common respiratory intermediate of aerobic cells (Fridovich, 1976), as well as being formed by redox cycling of anthracyclines. It has been pointed out that the superoxide anion radical might react with anthracycline to give rise to reactive intermediates (Sawyer *et al.*, 1983). Studies of the interaction of superoxide anion radical with daunorubicin and its aglycones in aprotic media have shown that superoxide anion radical can

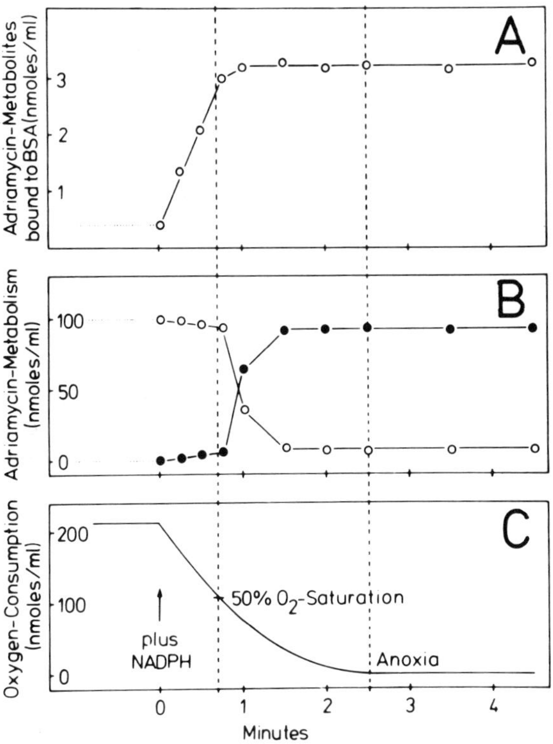

Figure 5. Simultaneous determination of (A) covalent binding of [^{3}H]doxorubicin metabolites to bovine serum albumin, (B) formation of 7-deoxydoxorubicin aglycone (●) from doxorubicin (○) and (C) oxygen consumption when [^{3}H]doxorubicin (0·1 mM) was incubated with rat liver microsomes (2 mg/ml) bovine serum albumin (0·2 mM) and an NADPH-generating system. From Scheulen *et al.* (1982) with permission.

extract a proton from one of the weakly acidic anthracycline C-6 or C-11 phenolic groups to generate a phenolate anion (Nakazawa *et al.*, 1985). The phenolate anion is then oxidized by molecular oxygen to give a B ring semiquinone free radical, or breaks down to unidentified products. This interpretation of the interaction is in contrast to earlier studies, where the interaction was attributed to direct electron transfer from superoxide anion radical to the anthracycline to give a D ring semiquinone free radical (Afanas'ev *et al.*, 1980). The findings raise the possibility that interaction of superoxide anion radical, generated spontaneously or drug-induced, with anthracycline in a hydrophobic region of the cell, for example, a lipid bilayer, might give rise to species important for the biological activity of the anthracycline (Nakazawa *et al.*, 1985).

The superoxide anion radical formed by redox cycling of anthracycline (reactions 2 and 3) is not a particularly reactive species but can give rise to hydroxyl radical, a powerful oxidizing species that can lead to oxidation of polyunsaturated fatty acids (Goodman and Hochstein, 1977; Mimnaugh *et al.*, 1983 a), degradation of deoxyribose (Bates and Winterbourn, 1982; Gutteridge and Quinlan, 1985) and DNA strand breaks (Rowley and Halliwell, 1983; Sinha *et al.*, 1984; Sugioka *et al.*, 1984). Hydroxyl radical is formed from superoxide anion radical only in the presence of catalytic amounts of a transition metal ion, in biological systems usually provided by iron salts. The first step is spontaneous dismutation of two molecules of superoxide anion radical to give hydrogen peroxide (reaction 4). Hydrogen peroxide then reacts with superoxide anion radical in the presence of trace amounts of iron salts to form hydroxyl radical (reaction 5). Reaction 5 is sometimes referred to as an iron-catalysed Haber–Weiss reaction (Halliwell and Gutteridge, 1984). Haemoproteins may be able to replace iron in catalysing anthracycline-induced hydroxyl radical formation from superoxide anion radical (Komiyama *et al.*, 1985). Inhibition of hydroxyl radical formation by superoxide dismutase is believed to be due to a lowered steady-state concentration of superoxide anion radical which also pulls reaction 3 to the right, consuming semiquinone free radical (Winterbourn *et al.*, 1978). Superoxide dismutase does not always inhibit anthracycline-induced hydroxyl radical formation (Gutteridge and Quinlan, 1985). In this case superoxide anion radical may be serving as a precursor for hydrogen peroxide which reacts with Fe(II) ion to generate hydroxyl radical by a Fenton reaction (reaction 6). Fe(III) ion is reduced to Fe(II) ion, probably by anthracycline semiquinone free radical (reaction 7).

$$Q \xrightarrow{e} Q^{\overline{\cdot}} \tag{2}$$

$$Q^{\overline{\cdot}} + O_2 \rightarrow O_2^{\overline{\cdot}} + Q \tag{3}$$

$$2O_2^{\overline{\cdot}} + 2H^+ \rightarrow H_2O_2 + O_2 \tag{4}$$

$$O_2^{\overline{\cdot}} + H_2O \xrightarrow[\text{catalysis}]{\text{Fe salt}} O_2 + HO^- + HO\cdot \tag{5}$$

$$H_2O_2 + Fe(II) \rightarrow HO^- + HO\cdot + Fe(III) \tag{6}$$

$$Q^{\overline{\cdot}} + Fe(III) \rightarrow Fe(II) + Q \tag{7}$$

Hydroxyl radical can also be formed by direct reaction of anthracycline semiquinone free radical with hydrogen peroxide without the need for iron catalysis. Several organic free radicals react with hydrogen peroxide in this way to give a hydroxyl radical-like species (Elstner *et al.*, 1980; Youngman and Elstner, 1981; Youngman *et al.*, 1982 b). Winterbourn and her colleagues (Bates, 1982; Winterbourn, 1981) first demonstrated the reaction of doxorubicin semiquinone free radical with hydrogen peroxide under aerobic conditions to give a species with reactivity similar to that of hydroxyl radical. Formation of this species was not inhibited by chelating agents, ruling out a

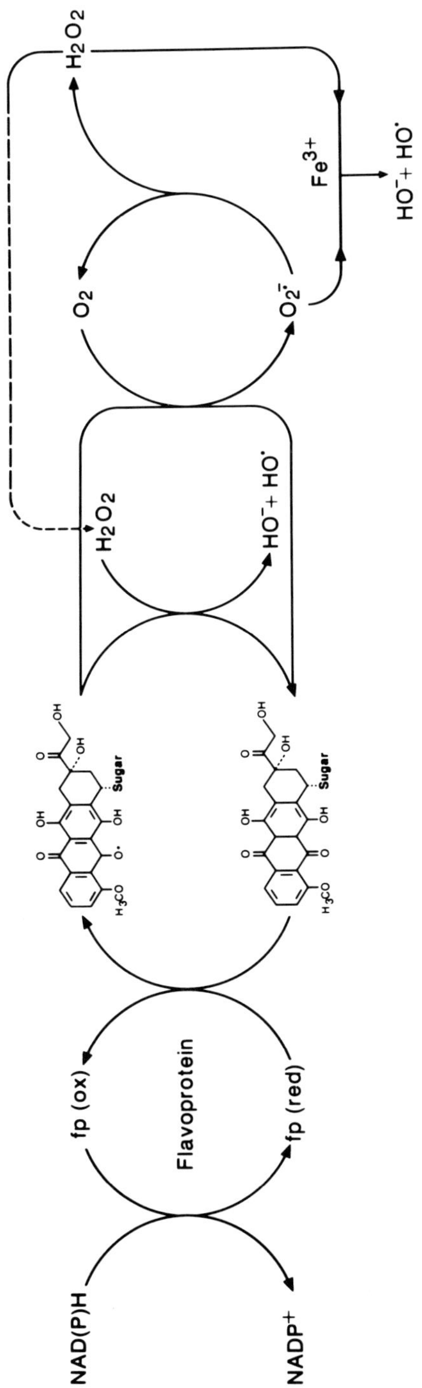

Figure 6. Pathways for formation of oxygen radicals during redox cycling of doxorubicin. For explanation see the text.

Haber–Weiss or Fenton type reaction, but was inhibited by oxygen. This is apparently because the rate of reaction of doxorubicin semiquinone free radical with hydrogen peroxide, 10^4 to $10^5\ \text{M}^{-1}\ \text{s}^{-1}$ (Kalyanaraman *et al.*, 1984), cannot effectively compete with the reaction of oxygen with doxorubicin semiquinone free radical, $3 \times 10^8\ \text{M}^{-1}\ \text{s}^{-1}$ (Land *et al.*, 1985). Evidence that the species formed by reaction of doxorubicin semiquinone free radical with hydrogen peroxide might be hydroxyl radical was provided by ESR and spin-trapping with DMPO (Bannister and Thornalley, 1983; Kalyanaraman *et al.*, 1984). However, unlike the breakdown of deoxyribose produced by systems known to generate hydroxyl radical, breakdown of deoxyribose by doxorubicin semiquinone free radical and hydrogen peroxide was not inhibited by hydroxyl radical scavenging agents (Winterbourn and Sutton, 1984). This suggests that an intermediate species with a more limited reactivity than hydroxyl radical may be formed. The formation of a species which mimics the hydroxyl radical but is more discriminating in its reactivity has been described for the reaction of paraquat anion free radical (Youngman and Elstner, 1981) and nitrofurantoin free radical (Youngman *et al.*, 1982 a) with hydrogen peroxide under limiting oxygen concentrations. The species has been termed a crypto-hydroxyl radical. A similar species may be formed by reaction of doxorubicin semiquinone free radical with hydrogen peroxide. A summary of the pathways for the formation of oxygen radicals during metabolism of anthracyclines is shown in Figure 6.

Anthracycline iron complexes

Several studies have indicated that anthracycline-mediated lipid peroxidation occurs only in the presence of trace amounts of iron (Doroshow, 1983 a; Mimnaugh *et al.*, 1983 a; Sterrenberg *et al.*, 1984; Sugioka *et al.*, 1981; Sugioka and Nakano, 1982). The iron in such systems might be catalysing a Haber–Weiss type or Fenton reaction to form hydroxyl radical as already discussed. Alternatively, a mechanism involving direct reaction of iron with the anthracycline could be involved, as suggested by the fact that a mixture of doxorubicin and Fe(III) chloride stimulates lipid peroxidation without the need for redox cycling of doxorubicin (Gutteridge, 1983, 1984; Sterrenberg *et al.*, 1984; Sugioka *et al.*, 1981). Anthracyclines, such as doxorubicin, daunorubicin and carminomycin, form very strong complexes with Fe(III) in which three molecules of anthracycline are bound to one Fe(III), each anthracycline molecule probably being chelated through one carbonyl and one phenolate oxygen to form a six-membered ring (Beraldo *et al.*, 1985; Fiallo and Garnier-Suillerot, 1985). The stability constant of such a complex is around 10^{28} to 10^{33} (Beraldo *et al.*, 1985; Fiallo and Garnier-Suillerot, 1985), which is among the highest reported for any Fe(III) complex. Doxorubicin can even extract iron from ferritin, the major storage form of iron in cells (Demant, 1984). Unlike the parent anthracyclines, anthracycline–iron complexes are poor stimulants of superoxide anion radical formation by redox cycling (Beraldo *et al.*, 1985).

Sugioka *et al.*, (1981) first proposed that a doxorubicin–Fe(III) complex might undergo self-reduction to a Fe(II) complex by a process involving intramolecular electron transfer. ESR evidence for such a mechanism has recently been provided by Zweier and his colleagues (1983, 1985). Doxorubicin slowly reduces bound Fe(III) to Fe(II), giving a complex with a one-electron oxidized doxorubicin semiquinone free radical (Gianni *et al.*, 1983 a; Zweier, 1983, 1985). In the presence of air, bound Fe(II) is rapidly oxidized back to Fe(III). Oxygen is presumed to bind to Fe(II) and an electron transferred from Fe(II) to oxygen (Zweier, 1983). The rate-limiting step in the redox cycle is reduction of Fe(III) to Fe(II) by doxorubicin, which may explain why preparations of Fe(II) or Fe(III) added to doxorubicin in air give only the Fe(III)–doxorubicin complex.

In the presence of thiols such as cysteine or glutathione (Gianni *et al.*, 1983 a; Myers *et al.*, 1982), or membrane protein thiol groups (Muindi *et al.*, 1985 a), the doxorubicin–Fe(III) complex is rapidly reduced and catalyses oxygen consumption and the formation of superoxide anion radical and hydrogen peroxide. Catalysis is inhibited by the specific Fe(II) chelator 4,7-diphenyl-1,10-phenanthroline sulphonate, indicating that Fe(II) is formed during the catalytic cycle (Gianni *et al.*, 1983 a). When doxorubicin–Fe(III) complex is reduced by thiol, no oxidized doxorubicin semiquinone free radical ESR signal is seen, suggesting that glutathione reduces Fe(III) directly, bypassing the doxorubicin-mediated reduction step (Zweier, 1985). Unlike the enzymatic reduction of doxorubicin to 7-deoxydoxorubicin aglycone, reduction of doxorubicin–Fe(III) complex by glutathione is not associated with loss of doxorubicin or with aglycone formation (Myers *et al.*, 1982). Reactive oxygen species generated by doxorubicin–Fe(III) complex in the presence of thiol lead to cell membrane lipid peroxidation (Myers *et al.*, 1982). Superoxide dismutase and catalase are weak inhibitors of the membrane lipid peroxidation, while the hydroxyl radical scavengers dimethylsulphoxide and mannitol are more effective inhibitors, suggesting involvement of a hydroxyl radical-like species (Myers *et al.*, 1982; Muindi *et al.*, 1985 a).

The doxorubicin–Fe(III) complex also cleaves DNA (Muindi *et al.*, 1985 b) by a process that is stimulated by thiol (Eliot *et al.*, 1983). DNA cleavage is inhibited by catalase, suggesting the involvement of hydrogen peroxide (Eliot *et al.*, 1983; Muindi *et al.*, 1985 b) probably generated by reduction of iron by doxorubicin (Zweier, 1983). ESR spectroscopy and spin-trapping with DMPO have demonstrated the formation of small amounts of free hydroxyl radical when hydrogen peroxide is mixed with doxorubicin–Fe(III) complex (Muindi *et al.*, 1984). The hydroxyl radical scavengers ethanol and dimethylsulphoxide inhibit DMPO–hydroxyl radical adduct formation. 5-Iminodaunorubicin–Fe(III) complex and hydrogen peroxide also give a DMPO–hydroxyl radical adduct, but ethanol and dimethylsulphoxide do not inhibit adduct formation and there is no cleavage of DNA (Lown *et al.*, 1982). This suggests that in this case free hydroxyl radical is not formed. Addition of DNA stimulates hydroxyl radical formation by doxorubicin–Fe(III) complex and hydrogen peroxide over 250% (Muindi *et al.*, 1984, 1985 b; Lown *et al.*, 1982). Stimulation of hydroxyl radical formation by DNA is also seen with iron complexes of 4-demethoxydaunorubicin and carminomycin, but not with daunorubicin (Muindi *et al.*, 1985 b) or 5-iminodaunorubicin (Lown *et al.*, 1982). Since all of these anthracyclines form a ternary complex with DNA and iron (Muindi *et al.*, 1985 b), this ability alone cannot explain why DNA enhances hydroxyl radical formation. Recently it has been shown that doxorubicin may be released from its strong coordination with Fe(III) and intercalate between the base pairs of DNA (Beraldo *et al.*, 1985). The importance of a ternary complex of drug, Fe(III) and DNA in DNA cleavage remains an unanswered question.

Unlike doxorubicin–Fe(III) complex-dependent cleavage of DNA, doxorubicin–Fe(III)-dependent degradation of deoxyribose is not inhibited by catalase or superoxide dismutase (Gutteridge, 1984). Furthermore, the process is inhibited by hydroxyl radical scavengers, such as mannitol and thiourea, but not by others, including benzoate and formate. The reactive oxygen species responsible for cleavage of deoxyribose by doxorubicin–Fe(III) complex may be a crypto-hydroxyl radical rather than free hydroxyl radical.

A summary of possible pathways for formation of reactive oxygen species by anthracycline iron complexes is given in Figure 7. The exact nature of the oxygen radical species, whether a free hydroxyl or a hydroxyl radical-like-species, remains to be established. The relationship of the reactions shown in Figure 7 to anthracycline anti-tumour activity is not known. Gianni *et al.*

$$\text{Dox H}_2 + \text{Fe(III)} \longrightarrow \text{Dox}^{-}\text{-Fe(III)} + 2\text{H}^{+}$$

$$\text{Dox}^{-}\text{-Fe(III)} \longleftrightarrow \text{Dox}^{\bullet}\text{-Fe(II)} \longleftrightarrow \text{Fe(II)} + \text{Dox}^{\bullet}$$

$$\text{Fe(II) (or Dox}^{\bullet}\text{-Fe(II))} + \text{O}_2 \longrightarrow \text{Fe(III)-O}_2^{\bullet -}$$

$$\text{Fe(III)-O}_2^{\bullet -} \longrightarrow \text{Fe(III)} + \text{O}_2^{\bullet -}$$

$$2\text{O}_2^{\bullet -} + 2\text{H}^{+} \longrightarrow \text{H}_2\text{O}_2 + \text{O}_2$$

$$\text{Fe(II) (or Dox}^{\bullet}\text{-Fe(II))} + \text{H}_2\text{O}_2 \longrightarrow \text{Fe(III)} + \text{HO}^{-} + [\text{HO}\cdot]$$

$$\text{Dox}^{\bullet} + \text{H}_2\text{O}_2 \xrightarrow[\text{catalysis}]{\text{Fe}} \text{Dox}^{+} + \text{HO}^{-} + [\text{HO}\cdot]$$

Figure 7. Reactions contributing to the reactivity of the doxorubicin-iron complex (Gutteridge, 1984). $DoxH_2$ is doxorubicin; Dox· the semiquinone free radical formed by oxidation of doxorubicin; [HO·] is hydroxyl radical or a species with similar reactivity to hydroxyl radical. The first two reactions are the self-reduction of doxorubicin–Fe(III) complex described by Sugioka and Nakano (1982).

(1983 b) have hypothesized that doxorubicin–Fe(III) complex might be the active form of the drug.

It is interesting that a combination of doxorubicin and iron has received clinical trial, under the name quelamycin, because of claims of reduced cardiotoxicity and other toxicities (Brugarolas *et al.*, 1978). Unfortunately, quelamycin was found to produce severe non-cardiac as well as cardiac toxicity (Brugarolas *et al.*, 1978; Cortes-Funes *et al.*, 1979). Quelamycin is a colloidal mixture of doxorubicin–Fe(III) complex and polymeric ferric hydroxide (Bachur *et al.*, 1984; Beraldo *et al.*, 1985) rather than a distinct triferric–doxorubicin complex as originally claimed (Gosalvez *et al.*, 1978). Quelamycin probably acts as an intravascular slow release form of doxorubicin (Bachur *et al.*, 1984), which might explain indications of less extensive metabolism of quelamycin than doxorubicin with less C-13 keto reduction and less aglycone formation (Reich and Gordon, 1977).

Alkylation by anthracyclines

In addition to giving free radicals when reduced, anthracyclines also form alkylating species that can bind covalently to protein, lipid and DNA. Reduction of daunorubicin and doxorubicin with a limiting amount of sodium borohydride under anaerobic conditions (Sinha and Chignell, 1979), or reduction by NADPH-fortified rat liver or heart microsomes under aerobic or anaerobic conditions (Scheulen *et al.*, 1982; Sinha, 1980; Sinha and Gregory, 1981) results in covalent binding of anthracycline residues to microsomal proteins and to added DNA. Incubation of doxorubicin with rat hepatic nuclei and NADPH under anaerobic conditions results in covalent binding of anthracycline residues to nuclear DNA (Sinha *et al.*, 1984). Covalent binding of doxorubicin residues to cardiolipin has been demonstrated in a reconstituted system of doxorubicin, cardiolipin, mitochondrial NADH–cytochrome c reductase and NADH (Goormaghtigh *et al.*, 1983; Pollakis *et al.*, 1983). 5-Iminodaunorubicin, which is not reduced by NADH–cytochrome c reductase, showed minimal binding to cardiolipin under the same conditions. A carbon-centred C-7 anthracycline free radical has been proposed to be a common intermediate in covalent binding and in reductive cleavage of anthracyclines to deoxyaglycones (Mason, 1979; Sinha, 1980). Reduced glutathione, which has no effect on the formation of anthracycline semiquinone free radicals (Sinha and Gregory, 1981), considerably decreased drug binding to protein (Scheulen *et al.*, 1982) and DNA (Sinha and Gregory, 1981). This was accompanied by the formation of a glutathione adduct, suggesting that reduced glutathione reacts with a species derived from the anthracycline semiquinone free radical, thereby reducing the concentration available for alkylation. Scheulen *et al.*, (1982) have shown that covalent binding of [^{3}H]doxorubicin to bovine serum albumin by NADPH-fortified rat liver microsomes occurs most readily under aerobic conditions before there is formation of 7-deoxydoxorubicin aglycone, suggesting that covalent binding can compete effectively with oxygen for the common intermediate (see Figure 5). The nature of the anthracycline residue in anthracycline–DNA adducts has not been elucidated (Sinha, 1980). Activated doxorubicin has a greater affinity for DNA than activated daunorubicin and gives rise to adducts with one drug molecule bound per 12 to 15 nucleotides, compared to one drug molecule per 135 nucleotides with daunorubicin (Sinha, 1980). Studies with synthetic polynucleotides suggest that activated anthracyclines have a high preference for guanine and cytosine regions of DNA.

Two-electron reduction of doxorubicin with an excess of sodium borohydride also results in covalent binding of anthracycline residues to DNA, although less than with single-electron reduction (Sinha and Chignell, 1979). Moore (1977) has proposed a mechanism for bioactivation of anthracyclines involving two-electron reduction of the anthracycline and elimination of the C-7 sugar group to give a quinone methide. In addition to binding covalently to nucleic acids and proteins, a C-7 quinone methide could form 7-deoxyaglycone and dimerization products through a H-transfer and Michael addition. Evidence for the enzymatic generation of a C-7 quinone methide has been sought in the ability of rat liver cytosol and NADH to covalently link daunorubicin and doxorubicin to DNA under anaerobic conditions (Sinha and Gregory, 1981). Binding was almost as great as with a microsomal system and the two-electron activation of anthracycline was ascribed to quinone reductase (Sinha and Gregory, 1981). Cytosol contains other enzymes that could metabolize anthracyclines and most important, dicoumarol, an inhibitor of quinone reductase, produced only slight inhibition of covalent binding. Covalent binding of anthracycline by cytosol could conceivably involve a free radical mechanism. The slow formation of an ESR-detectable anthracycline semiquinone free radical signal has been reported when daunorubicin is incubated with rat liver cytosol and NADPH under anaerobic conditions (Sinha and Gregory, 1981). This might be due to two-electron reduction of daunorubicin by an enzyme such as quinone reductase, and comproportionation of the resulting anthracycline hydroquinone with quinone to give an anthracycline semiquinone free radical. Whether two-electron reduction of anthracycline results in covalent binding independent of a mechanism involving an anthracycline free radical remains to be established.

In vivo metabolism

Daunorubicin

Daunorubicin is rapidly cleared from plasma by uptake into tissues in all species so far examined, including mouse, rat, hamster, dog and man (Alberts *et al.*, 1971; Huffman *et al.*, 1972; Yesair *et al.*, 1972). The drug is then slowly excreted, mostly as metabolites, in bile and in smaller amounts in urine. In rat

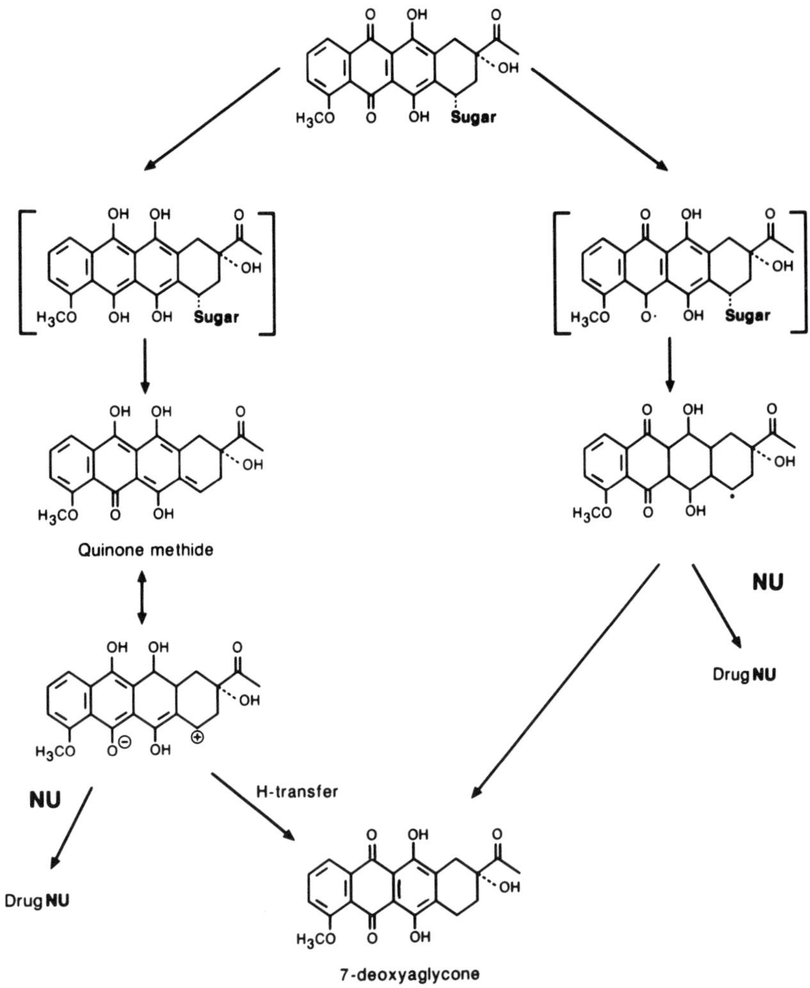

Figure 8. Proposed mechanisms for formation of reactive species from daunorubicin through either two-electron reduction to the quinone methide or through one-electron reduction to the semiquinone free radical. The nature of drug–nucleophile (Nu) adducts has not been elucidated.

8 h after administering drug 10–16% of daunorubicin fluorescence is excreted in the bile and 6–10% in the urine (Cradock *et al.*, 1973; Yesair *et al.*, 1972). In rabbit 17% of daunomycin fluorescence is excreted in the bile and 2% in the urine in 8 h (Bachur *et al.*, 1974). In human 7 to 17% of daunomycin fluorescence is excreted in the urine in 24 h (Alberts *et al.*, 1971; Huffman *et al.*, 1972). The primary metabolite of daunorubicin in all species is daunorubicinol. In rat daunorubicinol accounts for 53% of daunorubicin-derived fluorescent compounds excreted in the bile, unchanged drug for 32%

and polar metabolites for a further 13% (Cradock *et al.*, 1973). In urine the corresponding values are 57% for daunorubicinol, 40% for unchanged drug, 1% for aglycones and no measurable polar metabolites. Treatment of the polar metabolites from rat bile with β-glucuronidase yielded daunorubicin, daunorubicinol and the 7-hydroxy and 7-deoxyaglycones of daunorubicin, suggesting all were excreted as glucuronide conjugates. Such glucuronide conjugates are apparently degraded in the gastrointestinal tract, since only aglycones are found in faeces. Dog and rabbit excrete an even greater fraction of metabolites as daunorubicinol than does rat (Bachur *et al.*, 1974; Yesair *et al.*, 1972). In rabbit daunorubicinol accounts for 84% of daunorubicin-derived fluorescent compounds in bile, unchanged daunorubicin for 1·3%, polar metabolites for 12·4% and aglycones for 0·2% (Bachur *et al.*, 1973).

Takanashi and Bachur (1975) have reported a number of fluorescent metabolites of daunorubicin in 5 day urine of patients receiving doxorubicin for acute leukaemia. Comparison to reference compounds suggested the metabolites were daunorubicinol, 7-hydroxydaunorubicinol aglycone, 7-deoxydaunorubicin aglycone, 7-deoxydaunorubicinol aglycone; C-4-*O*-demethyl-7-deoxydaunorubicinol aglycone, and the conjugates 7-deoxydaunorubicinol aglycone-13-*O*-β-glucuronide, C-4-*O*-demethyl-7-deoxydaunorubicinol aglycone-4-*O*-β-glucuronide and C-4-O-demethyl-7-deoxydaunorubicinol aglycone-4-*O*-sulphate. Other metabolites were isolated but not identified. The pathways proposed by Takanashi and Bachur (1975) to explain formation of these metabolites are shown in Figure 9. As might be expected, the major metabolite of daunorubicin found in plasma of patients receiving daunorubicin is daunorubicinol, generally at concentrations higher than those of parent drug (Bolanowska *et al.*, 1983; Huffman *et al.*, 1972). Also found

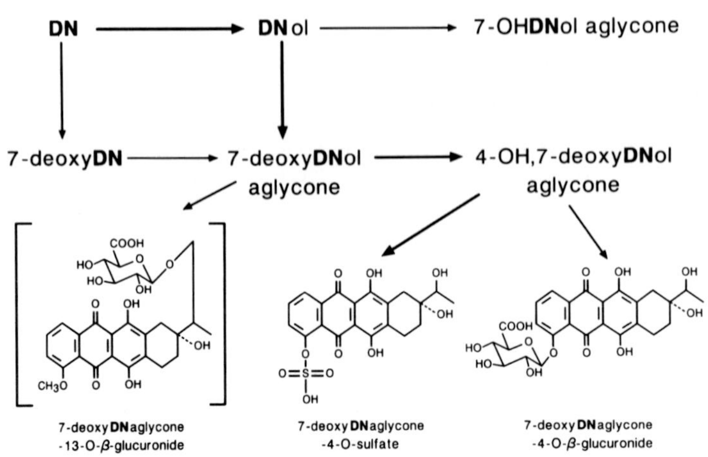

Figure 9. Proposed pathways for daunorubicin metabolism in man. Dark arrows indicate major pathways. Adapted from Takanashi and Bachur (1975).

in plasma in smaller amounts are 7-deoxydaunorubicinol and 7-deoxydaunorubicin aglycone. Tissues of animals administered daunorubicin have been found to contain substantial quantities of daunorubicinol but aglycone metabolites have been found only in liver, kidney and small intestine (Asbell *et al.*, 1972; Bachur *et al.*, 1973, 1974).

Doxorubicin

Clearance of doxorubicin from plasma and tissues is slower than for daunorubicin (Bachur *et al.*, 1973, 1974; DiFronzo *et al.*, 1971; Hartman *et al.*, 1982; Mhatre *et al.*, 1972; Oosterbaan *et al.*, 1984; Rosso *et al.*, 1972; Yesair *et al.*, 1972) and doxorubicin undergoes less metabolism than daunorubicin. Approximately 10% of an administered dose of doxorubicin fluorescence is excreted in rat bile in 24 h and 6% in urine, mostly as unchanged drug (Yesair *et al.*, 1972). In some early studies no evidence could be found for doxorubicin metabolism in rat and mouse (Bachur *et al.*, 1973; DiFronzo *et al.*, 1971; Yesair *et al.*, 1972). However, subsequent studies using improved analytical techniques have shown low levels of doxorubicin metabolism. Little or no doxorubicinol is excreted in rat bile or urine or is found in plasma (Broggini *et al.*, 1980; Hartman *et al.*, 1982; Israel *et al.*, 1978; Shinozawa and Oda, 1981), but small amounts of doxorubicin aglycone metabolites have been detected in rat bile (Hartman *et al.*, 1982; Shinozawa and Oda, 1981). Studies with [14-^{14}C]doxorubicin have shown unchanged drug to be the major form excreted in rat bile and urine, with small amounts of doxorubicinol (Arcamone *et al.*, 1984). Interestingly, expired air contained about 5% of total radioactivity indicating degradation of the C-14 side-chain. Hydrolysis of bile with β-glucuronidase showed there are small amounts of conjugated aglycone metabolites. Other animal species metabolize doxorubicin more extensively than rat and mouse, but still to a lesser extent than daunorubicin. Polar and aglycone doxorubicin metabolites have been found in tissue of hamsters administered doxorubicin (Bachur *et al.*, 1974). Rabbits excrete 17% of a dose of doxorubicin fluorescence in bile in 8 h, 60% as doxorubicinol, 30% as unchanged drug, 7% as polar metabolites and the remainder as aglycones (Bachur *et al.*, 1973). 2% of doxorubicin fluorescence is excreted in urine in 8 h, 60% as unchanged drug, 35% as doxorubicinol and 2% as polar metabolites. Doxorubicinol is the major metabolite of doxorubicin in rabbit plasma but concentrations never exceed more than one-third those of parent drug (Johansen *et al.*, 1984).

Doxorubicinol is the major metabolite of doxorubicin in human plasma but is present at concentrations well below those of parent drug (Andrews *et al.*, 1980; Pierce and Jatlow, 1979; Bolanowska *et al.*, 1983; Gill *et al.*, 1983). Recent studies have detected low levels of other doxorubicin metabolites in human plasma, including 7-hydroxydoxorubicin aglycone, 7-deoxydoxorubicin aglycone, 7-deoxydoxorubicinol aglycone (Brenner *et al.*, 1985;

Cummings, 1985), and other unidentified non-polar metabolites (Brenner *et al.*, 1985). Biliary excretion of doxorubicin in human is 50% of the administered dose over five days and urinary excretion 10% (Benjamin *et al.*, 1973, 1974). A pattern of doxorubicin metabolites qualitatively similar to that for daunorubicin has been reported in human urine by Takanashi and Bachur (1976). This was except for the absence of a 7-deoxydoxorubicin aglycone 13-*O*-β-glucuronide and the presence of 7-hydroxydoxorubicin aglycone. The formation of 7-hydroxyaglycones was thought to be artifactual due to the chemical breakdown of the parent glycosides. While with daunorubicin the amount of 4-*O*-sulphated conjugate of 4-*O*-demethyl-7-deoxydaunorubicinol aglycone exceeded 4-O-glucuronide conjugate nearly 2-fold, with 4-*O*-demethyl-7-deoxydoxorubicinol aglycone, almost equal amounts of 4-*O*-glucuronide and 4-*O*-sulphate conjugates were found (Takanashi and Bachur, 1976). In contrast to the report of Takanashi and Bachur (1976), where silicic acid chromatography and β-glucuronidase hydrolysis was used to identify glucuronide conjugates, more recent studies by Cassinelli *et al.* (1984) using improved extraction procedures for glucuronides could find no evidence for glucuronide conjugates of doxorubicin in urine of patients receiving the drug.

4′-Epidoxorubicin

Studies with 4′-epi[14-^{14}C]doxorubicin in rat have shown a similar pattern of metabolism to doxorubicin, except that bile contains less unchanged 4′-epidoxorubicin and more 4′-epidoxorubicin glucuronide (Arcamone *et al.*, 1984). Studies in human with 4′-epidoxorubicin have shown formation of 4-*O*-demethyl-4′-epidoxorubicinol, 7-deoxydoxorubicin aglycone, 7-hydroxydoxorubicin aglycone, 7-deoxydoxorubicinol aglycone, as well as 4′-epidoxorubicin glucuronide conjugates (Cassinelli *et al.*, 1984; Deesen and Leyland-Jones, 1984; Robert *et al.*, 1985; Speyer *et al.*, 1982; Weenen *et al.*, 1983, 1984). 4′-Epidoxorubicin glucuronide was the major metabolite of 4′-epidoxorubicin in plasma and exceeded the concentration of parent drug (Robert *et al.*, 1985). Attachment of the glucuronide group was shown by Cassinelli *et al.* (1984) to be at the C-4′-hydroxyl of daunosamine which in 4′-epidoxorubicin is in an equatorial orientation. Steric hindrance of the axial C-4′-hydroxyl of doxorubicin by the adjacent *cis*-equatorial 3′-amino group may explain the relative lack of glucuronide formation by doxorubicin compared to 4′-epidoxorubicinol (Cassinelli *et al.*, 1984). In human urine 4′-epidoxorubicin accounts for 57% of 4′-epidoxorubicin-derived fluorescent compounds, 4′-*O*-(β-D-glucuronyl)-4′-epidoxorubicin for 32%, 4′-epidoxorubicinol for 7% and 4′-*O*-(β-D-glucuronyl)-4′-epidoxorubicinol for 3% (Cassinelli *et al.*, 1984). No sulphate conjugates of 4′-epidoxorubicin have been detected (Deesen and Leyland-Jones, 1984). It has been suggested that glucuronidation may enhance the rate of elimination of 4′-epidoxorubicin compared to doxorubicin (Weenen *et al.*, 1984) and may be related to a lower incidence of toxic side-effects of 4′-epidoxorubicin (Arcamone, 1985).

AD-32

Metabolism of AD-32 has been studied in animals only. The drug is extensively excreted in bile, with 80% of the administered dose appearing in the bile in 24 h in rat and 2% in urine (Israel *et al.*, 1978). AD-32 undergoes rapid de-esterification of the C-14 side-chain to *N*-trifluoroacetyldoxorubicin by non-specific esterases in rat serum (Israel *et al.*, 1976). Approximately 18% to 22% of a dose is excreted in bile as *N*-trifluoroacetyldoxorubicin and 18 to 23% as *N*-trifluoroacetyldoxorubicinol (Israel *et al.*, 1976, 1981). Glucuronide conjugates form the major fraction of biliary metabolites, with about 20% unidentified polar metabolites. Only small amounts of aglycone metabolites have been detected (Israel *et al.*, 1976, 1981), although studies in rat with AD-32 labelled with ^{14}C at the carbonyl carbon on the *N*-trifluoroacetyl group have shown relatively large amounts of non-fluorescent radioactive metabolites in plasma and tissues, thought to be *N*-trifluoroacetyl daunosamine. This would suggest extensive C-7 reductive cleavage of AD-32. In rats given AD-32, only small amounts of doxorubicin (less than 0·2% of the total dose) have been detected in urine (Israel *et al.*, 1978) and tissue extracts (Zini *et al.*, 1984). AD-32 is not considered a pro-drug of doxorubicin.

Aclacinomycin A

The aglycone metabolites of aclacinomycin A, bisanhydroaklavinone, 7-deoxyaklavinone and the 7,7′-dimer of 7-deoxyaklavinone, have been found in liver and kidney of mouse administered the drug (Dodion *et al.*, 1985 a). In human aclacinomycin A is metabolized to the L-amicetose glycoside (Oki *et al.*, 1981), to bisanhydroaklavinone which persists in plasma for a long time, and to an unidentified metabolite (Arcamone *et al.*, 1984; Egorin *et al.*, 1982). Urinary excretion of unchanged aclacinomycin A in human is 0·6% in 24 h, with 4% as glycoside metabolites (Oki *et al.*, 1981). Egorin *et al.* (1983) analysed the urine of patients who had received aclacinomycin A and found 11 metabolites, including the metabolites identified *in vitro* by Oki *et al.* (1977) and Komiyama *et al.* (1979 a, b) shown in figure 3. An additional metabolite was identified as bisanhydroaklavinic acid, probably resulting from hydrolysis of the methyl ester of bisanhydroaklavinone, while another metabolite was converted to bisanhydroaklavinic acid by β-glucuronidase, suggesting it to be a glucuronide conjugate. The previously unidentified plasma metabolite was identical with the urinary metabolite identified as bisanhydroaklavinic acid.

Marcellomycin

Marcellomycin is metabolized by mouse to four fluorescent metabolites in plasma. Dodion *et al.* (1983) assigned structures to these metabolites as musettamycin, pyrromycin, 7-hydroxypyrromycin aglycone and 7-deoxypyrromycin aglycone. A contaminant present with the parent drug, possibly with a rhodinose sugar replacing the terminal deoxyfucose of marcellomycin, was also present in plasma. In liver an aglycone, tentatively identified as 7-deoxypyrromycin aglycone, was observed, initially at concentrations equal to those of marcellomycin but falling rapidly to be undetectable by 8 h. In other organs 7-deoxypyrromycin aglycone was observed in smaller quantities. In human, marcellomycin undergoes metabolism to an aglycone, probably bisanhydropyrromycinone, and a conjugate, both of which are found in plasma. The conjugate resisted hydrolysis by arylsulphatase and β-glucuronidase but was converted by acid hydrolysis to marcellomycin. 7–8% of a dose of marcellomycin is excreted in the urine over 72 h in man, with parent drug being the predominant component at a high dose, and bisanhydropyrromycinone the predominant component at a lower dose (Dodion *et al.*, 1985 b).

Metabolism by tumour cells

Anthracyclines are cytotoxic to cultured tumour cells *in vitro* at therapeutically achievable concentrations. It is, therefore, of interest to investigate anthracycline metabolism by tumour and other cells to see if cytotoxicity might be modified by metabolism. Some studies have found little or undetectable metabolism of anthracyclines by normal or tumour cells (DeGregorio *et al.*, 1984; Skovsgaard, 1977; Yesair *et al.*, 1980; Zenebergh *et al.*, 1984) while other studies have reported variable low levels of anthracycline metabolism. There are reports of between 5 and 30% conversion of daunorubicin to daunorubicinol after 4 to 24 h incubation by Ehrlich ascites cells (Londos-Gagliardi *et al.*, 1982), murine leukaemia L1210 cells (Baurain *et al.*, 1980; Yesair *et al.*, 1980), human promyelocytic HL-60 and leukaemic cells from patients with acute non-lymphocytic leukaemia (DeGregorio *et al.*, 1982). Aglycones, if formed, account for 1% or less of intracellular anthracyclines (Baurain *et al.*, 1980). No difference in daunorubicinol formation has been found between daunorubicin-resistant and sensitive cell lines (Baurain *et al.*, 1980) and no consistent pattern has emerged of levels of daunorubicin reductases in a number of murine and human tumour cell lines (Vasanthakumar and Ahmed, 1985). Claims have been made of a positive correlation between daunorubicin reductase in leukaemic myeloblasts and the response of the patients of chemotherapy (Gola, 1979; Huffman and Bachur, 1972), and that levels of daunorubicin and metabolites in leukaemic cells may be of more relevance in evaluating clinical outcome than monitoring plasma levels of drug

(DeGregorio *et al.*, 1982). Such suggestions are intriguing but need considerably more evaluation before their worth can be judged. The weight of available evidence suggests that cellular metabolism of anthracyclines to C-13 alcohols is not a major factor in determining cytotoxicity.

Free radical formation and biological activity

Anti-tumour activity

Three mechanisms have been proposed to account for the cytotoxicity of anthracyclines. The first and most studied mechanism is the high-affinity binding of anthracyclines to DNA through intercalation of the aglycone moiety between adjacent base pairs in the DNA double helix (Pigram *et al.*, 1972) leading to blockage of DNA, RNA and protein synthesis, DNA protein-associated strand breaks and inhibition of DNA repair (Painter, 1978). DNA intercalation may not, however, be a primary mechanism of anthracycline toxicity (Myers, 1982). No correlation has been found between inhibition of DNA or RNA synthesis by doxorubicin and the extent of cell survival, except at very toxic drug concentrations (Siegfried *et al.*, 1983). A second mechanism for anthracycline cytotoxicity has focused on cell membrane effects of anthracyclines leading to altered membrane fluidity (Tritton *et al.*, 1978; Hickman *et al.*, 1985) and altered ion permeability (Santone *et al.*, 1986; Solie and Yuncker, 1978). The third possible mechanism for anthracycline cytotoxicity involves generation of free radicals.

Bachur *et al.* (1978, 1979) first proposed that activation of anthracyclines to semiquinone free radicals by NADPH–cytochrome P-450 reductase or other flavoenzymes might lead to site-specific damage to nuclear DNA. Intercalation of the semiquinone free radical with DNA was seen as leading to increased likelihood of damage to DNA by direct reaction of the semiquinone free radical in close proximity to the double-stranded DNA, or by generation of reactive oxygen species within the DNA helix. A potential problem with this mechanism is that since most flavoenzymes are located outside the nucleus, the anthracycline semiquinone free radical would have to be stable enough to diffuse from its site of formation outside the nucleus to its presumed site of action within the nucleus (Bachur *et al.*, 1982; Svingen and Powis, 1981). Most semiquinone free radicals and oxygen free radicals have very short lifetimes under physiological conditions (Hutchinson, 1957). Pulse radiolysis studies suggest that the doxorubicin semiquinone free radical may decay rapidly under anaeroboc conditions with a lifetime as short as $<0\cdot1$ ms (Svingen and Powis, 1981). Transient equilibrium between the parent anthracycline quinone and the hydroquinone might stabilize the semiquinone free radical for up to a millisecond (Land *et al.*, 1985; Houée-Levin *et al.*, 1985) and in this case a semiquinone free radical could conceivably have time to diffuse from its site of formation to a critical site within a cell. However, the doxorubicin semiquinone radical reacts rapidly with oxygen to form superoxide anion radical with a bimolecular rate constant of 3×10^8 $\text{M}^{-1}\,\text{s}^{-1}$ (Butler *et al.*, 1985; Land *et al.*, 1985), which further reduces the distance a doxorubicin semiquinone free radical is likely to travel in the cell. Kalyanaraman *et al.* (1980) have calculated that the half-life of an anthracycline semiquinone free radical, even at an oxygen concentration as low as 1 μM which might be found in some poorly perfused tumours, is of the order of 6 ms. They concluded that with the exception of electron transfer reactions, most chemical reactions of semiquinones will be too slow to be of significance at *in vivo* oxygen concentrations. Oxygen radicals formed by redox cycling of anthracyclines are unlikely to diffuse any further than the drug radicals. The mean effective radius for the action of radicals produced by ionizing radiation, principally hydroxyl radical and superoxide anion radical, in cells is 3 nm (Hutchinson, 1957). It appears that if anthracycline free radicals or anthracycline-derived oxygen radicals are to produce an effect on DNA in the nucleus, they will have to be produced in close proximity to the nucleus. It has been shown that isolated nuclei in the presence of NADPH can activate doxorubicin and daunorubicin to ESR-detectable semiquinone free radicals (Sinha *et al.*, 1984; Bachur *et al.*, 1982; Mimnaugh *et al.*, 1985) and, in the presence of oxygen, form superoxide anion and hydroxyl radicals (Sinha *et al.*, 1984; Mimnaugh *et al.*, 1985). There is also nuclear membrane lipid peroxidation (Mimnaugh *et al.*, 1985), covalent binding of doxorubicin to DNA (Sinha *et al.*, 1984) and DNA strand breakage (Berlin and Haseltine, 1981).

There is some evidence that hydroxyl radicals are involved in the cytotoxic effects of anthracyclines. Scavengers of hydroxyl radicals, such as dimethylsulphoxide, thiourea and sodium benzoate, the iron chelator deferoxamine, and catalase and superoxide have all been reported to reduce the *in vitro* cytotoxicity of doxorubicin to Ehrlich tumour cells (Doroshow, 1985; Doroshow and deVries, 1984). The effect of these agents was linked to effects on the generation of hydroxyl radical by doxorubicin (Doroshow and deVries, 1984; Doroshow, 1985). In the same system radical scavengers did not affect the cytotoxicity of 5-iminodaunorubicin, which did not form hydroxyl radical. A dose–response relationship between doxorubicin-induced hydroxyl radical formation and doxorubicin cytotoxicity in a human breast cancer cell line has been reported (Sinha *et al.*, 1985). Mimnaugh *et al.* (1985) have emphasized a role for anthracycline-induced nuclear membrane lipid peroxidation in the cytotoxicity of anthracyclines and have suggested that it may contribute to biochemical and morphological alterations in the nucleus following anthracycline treatment. The authors pointed out that such a mechanism could explain why anthracyclines such as AD-32 that do not bind to DNA and apparently do not enter the nucleus (Egorin *et al.*, 1980) can cause protein-associated DNA strand breaks and DNA-protein cross-links in tumour cells (Levin *et al.*, 1981).

DNA strand breakage after exposure to anthracycline has been observed in DNA isolated from tumours in mice (Schwartz, 1975) and in DNA of cultured cells (Kanter and Schwartz, 1979). DNA is known to undergo degradation by superoxide anion radical-generating systems, almost entirely due to the formation of hydroxyl radical from superoxide anion radical in the presence of trace amounts of iron salts (Brawn and Fridovich, 1981; Rowley and Halliwell 1983). It has been suggested that oxygen radicals formed by redox cycling of anthracycline bound to DNA may produce selective damage to the DNA (Lown *et al.*, 1982). However, intercalation of doxorubicin into double-stranded DNA prevents its enzymatic reduction and greatly decreases the yield of superoxide anion and hydroxyl radicals (Sato *et al.*, 1977; Kalyanaraman *et al.*, 1980; Rowley and Halliwell, 1983; Berlin and Haseltine, 1981). Because of this, it has been argued that oxygen radicals are unlikely to be responsible for doxorubicin-induced DNA damage *in vivo* (Rowley and Halliwell, 1983). Potmesil *et al.* (1984) have reported that although doxorubicin produces DNA single-strand breaks in cultured cells, thought to be due to oxygen radicals, this occurs only at concentrations of doxorubicin above those achievable therapeutically. At lower concentrations of doxorubicin only protein-associated DNA breaks, thought to be due to activation of the enzyme DNA topoisomerase II, are seen (Potmesil *et al.*, 1983, 1984). It should also be noted that many anti-tumour agents produce protein-associated DNA breaks by a mechanism that probably does involve free radical formation or binding of the drug to DNA (Younes *et al.*, 1985). 5-Iminodaunorubicin does not undergo redox cycling to form oxygen radicals (Pollakis *et al.*, 1984) but will bind to DNA and causes protein-associated DNA breaks (Pommier *et al.*, 1985). There are also anthracyclines that do not bind to DNA that still produce protein-associated DNA breaks (Levin *et al.*, 1981). Recent studies with DNA topoisomerase II suggest that anthracycline may stabilize the enzyme–DNA complex in an open (cleaved) conformation of DNA (Pommier *et al.*, 1985; Tewey *et al.*, 1984). Zwelling *et al.* (1982) could find no simple correlation between the drug-induced cytotoxicity of doxorubicin and 5-iminodaunorubicin and either single-strand or protein-associated DNA breaks. Thus, the significance of anthracycline-induced DNA breaks to anthracycline cytotoxicity has yet to be established.

In summary, although intriguing, the hypothesis that anthracycline free radicals or anthracycline-induced oxygen radicals are important for the cytotoxicity of anthracyclines remains to be shown. The evidence for a relationship is incomplete and often contradictory. Studies showing a relationship between anthracycline free radical or anthracycline-induced oxygen radical formation by intact cells and the growth inhibitory effects of anthracyclines would be useful evidence to support such a hypothesis.

Cardiotoxicity

The cardiotoxicity of anthracyclines is frequently linked with their ability to undergo redox cycling to form reactive oxygen species (Goodman and Hochstein, 1977; Doroshow, 1983 b; Thayer, 1977; Adachi *et al.*, 1983; D'Alessandro *et al.*, 1980). There are several pieces of evidence favouring such an association.

Doxorubicin, daunorubicin and other cardiotoxic anthracyclines stimulate formation of superoxide anion radical, hydrogen peroxide and hydroxyl radical by heart subcellular fractions (Adachi *et al.*, 1983; Doroshow, 1983 a; Gutierrez *et al.*, 1983; Thayer, 1977). The mitochondrial NADH dehydrogenase complex is probably the major site of anthracycline-induced oxygen radical formation in the heart (Adachi *et al.*, 1983; Davies *et al.*, 1983; Doroshow, 1983 b). Unlike the liver, where superoxide anion radical is the primary oxygen species formed, ESR and spin-trap studies suggest that in the heart hydroxyl radical may be a major oxygen radical species produced by redox cycling of anthracyclines. Pollakis *et al.* (1984) using an ESR flow technique observed short-lived DMPO spin-trapped adducts of hydroxyl radical and superoxide anion radical formed by respiring heart mitochondria and heart submitochondrial particles in the presence of anthracycline. Superoxide anion radical was the predominant species formed by intact mitochondria, and hydroxyl radical the predominant species formed by sonicated mitochondria. Thornalley and Dodd (1985) could not detect superoxide anion radical formation by rat heart sarcosomas incubated with NADPH and doxorubicin using ESR and spin-trapping with DMPO, although they did detect formation of hydroxyl radical. Hydroxyl radical formation was strongly inhibited by catalase, although not by superoxide dismutase, suggesting a direct reduction of hydrogen peroxide to hydroxyl radical. The authors, however, assumed that hydrogen peroxide was being formed via superoxide, and that their failure to detect superoxide was due to the much greater efficiency of trapping of hydroxyl radical by DMPO compared to trapping of superoxide anion radical. Nohl and Jordan (1983) were also unable to find ESR evidence for formation of superoxide anion radical by respiring rat heart mitochondria and doxorubicin using DMPO as a spin-trapping agent. However, a doxorubicin semiquinone free radical signal was seen which was unaffected by the presence of oxygen. The signal disappeared on addition of hydrogen peroxide and, concomitantly, there appeared a DMPO spin-trapped hydroxyl radical signal. The authors interpreted the results to indicate that doxorubicin semiquinone free radical was being produced during mitochondrial respiration, probably at the liphophilic phase of the mitochondrial inner membrane, in a way which precludes electron transfer to oxygen. This allows reaction of the anthracycline semiquinone free radical with hydrogen peroxide, probably present at relatively high concentrations in heart because of low levels of catalase (Herzog and Fahimi, 1974), to form hydroxyl radical.

A second piece of evidence linking cardiotoxicity and oxygen radical formation is that newer anthracycline analogues with reportedly less cardiotoxicity form less reactive oxygen species. Studies by Lown *et al.* (1982) have shown a positive relation between the cardiotoxicity of a series of anthracyclines in rat and the ease of generation reactive oxygen species by electrochemical reduction, which appears to be related to the ease with which the reduced anthracycline species are reoxidized. 5-Iminodaunorubicin, which is less cardiotoxic in animals than either daunorubicin or doxorubicin (Zbinden *et al.*, 1978; Tong *et al.*, 1979), does not form an anthracycline semiquinone free radical (Pollakis *et al.*, 1984) and does not produce superoxide anion radical or hydroxyl radical (Doroshow, 1983 b; Pollakis *et al.*, 1984). The decreased tendency of 5-iminodaunorubicin to undergo redox cycling is because of hydrogen bonding between the imine nitrogen and adjacent hydroxyl groups, which makes the compound more difficult to reduce and much more difficult to reoxidize (Lown *et al.*, 1979). 4′-Deoxydoxorubicin and 4-demethoxydaunorubicin, which also have less tendency for producing cardiotoxicity than the parent anthracyclines, fail to generate oxygen free radicals spontaneously in aerated aqueous solution (Dickinson *et al.*, 1984, 1985).

The heart may have a decreased capacity to detoxify oxygen radicals compared to other tissues, making it susceptible to anthracycline-induced oxygen radical damage. Compared to other tissues the heart has low levels of superoxide dismutase (Adachi *et al.*, 1983; Doroshow *et al.*, 1980), catalase (Thayer, 1977; Doroshow *et al.*, 1980) and non-selenium-dependent glutathione peroxidase (Doroshow *et al.*, 1980; Revis and Marusic, 1978).

Generation of anthracycline semiquinone free radicals in the heart could lead to damage to mitochondrial membranes by a covalent interaction of the anthracycline semiquinone free radical with the mitochondrial membrane (Pollakis *et al.*, 1983). Alternatively, reactive oxygen species might damage heart mitochondria or other organelles. Activation of doxorubicin by heart NADH dehydrogenase with formation of hydroxyl radical has been shown to lead to inhibition of Ca^{2+} uptake by heart sarcoplasmic reticulum (Harris and Doroshow, 1985). Evidence was presented that this might be related to free radical oxidation of critical sulphydryl groups, since *N*-acetylcysteine and reduced glutathione protected against the damage. Lipid peroxidation is another mechanism by which oxygen radicals can damage critical macromolecules. Studies with rat heart microsomes and NADPH have shown that anthracyclines stimulate lipid peroxidation, but only if the microsomes are prepared from rats fed a diet deficient in α-tocopherol (Mimnaugh *et al.*, 1981, 1982). Mouse heart microsomes, on the other hand, have low endogenous levels of α-tocopherol and exhibit a marked increase in lipid peroxidation in the presence of anthracyclines (D'Alessandro *et al.*, 1980; Mimnaugh *et al.*, 1983 a). Some workers have found that it is necessary to add ferrous ions to obtain appreciable levels of doxorubicin-stimulated lipid peroxidation in mouse heart microsomes (Daugherty *et al.*, 1982). Even though anthracyclines may stimulate lipid peroxidation *in vitro*, lipid peroxidation may not be a primary effect of anthracyclines *in vivo*. Reports of increased lipid peroxidation *in vivo* following anthracycline administration using malondialdehyde as an indicator of lipid peroxidation (D'Alessandro *et al.*, 1980; Lenzhofer *et al.*,

1983; Myers *et al.*, 1977; Stuart *et al.*, 1978; Yamanaka *et al.*, 1979) are ambiguous because malondialdehyde is not a good indicator for lipid peroxidation (Bus and Gibson, 1979). Studies by Muliawan *et al.* (1980) using ethane expiration, which is generally regarded as a more reliable indicator of lipid peroxidation *in vivo*, failed to find an increase in lipid peroxidation in rats given lethal doses of doxorubicin. However, several compounds that are believed to exert their toxic effects through generation of active oxygen species and lipid peroxidation, for example nitrofurantoin, paraquat, diquat and menadione, also do not increase ethane production *in vivo* (Younes *et al.*, 1985). Only when animals are pretreated with a low dose of Fe(II) salts is there an increase in ethane production by these compounds. Thus, the failure to demonstrate increased ethane production by doxorubicin *in vivo* should not be taken as evidence for a lack of lipid peroxidation at a specific site in the body, such as the heart.

Free radical scavenging agents such as α-tocopherol (Myers *et al.*, 1976; Mimnaugh *et al.*, 1979), butylated hydroxytoluene (Daugherty *et al.*, 1982), ascorbate (Fujita *et al.*, 1982), ubiquinone (Bertazzoli *et al.*, 1975; Folkers *et al.*, 1978) and methylene blue, a redox agent (Hrushesky *et al.*, 1985), protect against the acute cardiotoxicity of doxorubicin in animals. The level of intracellular reduced glutathione, which is an endogenous free radical scavenger, also appears to be important in anthracycline cardiotoxicity. Pretreatment of mice with diethyl maleate, which lowers intracellular glutathione, increases lethality of doxorubicin (Olsen *et al.*, 1983), while concurrent administration of cysteamine (Freeman *et al.*, 1980; Olsen *et al.*, 1983) and *N*-acetylcysteine pretreatment (Doroshow *et al.*, 1982) protect against doxorubicin lethality in mice.

It is important to distinguish two kinds of doxorubicin cardiotoxicity. First, there is acute cardiotoxicity which occurs within minutes of drug administration and is characterized by the occurrence of cardiac arrhythmias and non-specific electrocardiographic changes (Cortes *et al.*, 1973). Second, there is irreversible congestive heart failure which occurs after the cumulative dose of anthracyclines has been reached (Cortes *et al.*, 1973; Jaenke, 1976). While the radical scavenger α-tocopherol can protect animals against acute doxorubicin cardiotoxicity, it does not protect against delayed (Mimnaugh *et al.*, 1979) and chronic doxorubicin cardiotoxicity (Breed *et al.*, 1980; Van Vleet *et al.*, 1980). Similarly, *N*-acetylcysteine does not protect dogs against chronic doxorubicin cardiotoxicity (Unverferth *et al.*, 1985). Protection against chronic doxorubicin cardiotoxicity has been reported for ubiquinone (Domae *et al.*, 1981) and ascorbate (Fujita *et al.*, 1982). The evidence suggests that while anthracycline-induced oxygen radicals and lipid peroxidation may be important factors in the acute cardiotoxicity of anthracyclines, they play a lesser role in chronic cardiotoxicity. It is possible that the anthracycline semiquinone free radical itself is more important in chronic cardiotoxicity.

Extravasation

Accidental infiltration of doxorubicin into the area around an intravenous infusion site in patients can cause severe ulceration. A free radical mechanism for the ulcerogenic activity of doxorubicin is suggested by the ability of topically applied free radical scavenging agents, such as dimethylsulphoxide (Desai and Teres, 1982; Svingen *et al.*, 1981), α-tocopherol (Svingen *et al.*, 1981; Nobbs and Barr, 1983) and butylated hydroxytoluene (Daugherty and Khurana, 1985) to prevent the ulceration in some, although not all (Dorr and Alberts, 1983) animal species. There are anecdotal reports of protection by such treatments in man (Olver and Schwarz, 1983).

Conclusions

The anthracyclines are arguably the most intriguing of all cytotoxic anti-tumour agents. More effort has probably gone into studying the anthracyclines, their physical properties, distribution, transport, metabolism, elimination and mechanisms of action, than any other class of cytotoxic agents. The search for new anthracycline analogues continues unabated. This research effort reflects not only the undoubted clinical usefulness of the anthracyclines but also intellectual fascination with their multi-faceted actions. From the early beginnings, when it appeared that some anthracyclines underwent little or no metabolism, improved analytical techniques have revealed a multiplicity of anthracycline metabolites formed by the interplay of pathways for anthracycline reduction, cleavage and conjugation. While early studies lacked definitive means for assigning structures to anthracycline metabolites, modern techniques make unequivocal structure assignment possible which may lead to a reassessment of the relative importance of different pathways of anthracycline metabolism. Studies of the metabolism of anthracyclines have been aided by their unique fluorescence properties but the very power of the approach has led to a neglect of non-fluorescent metabolites that may be formed. This is a fertile area for future research.

Although anthracyclines undergo extensive biotransformation, the metabolites discovered to date appear to play only a minor role in the biological activity of anthracyclines. This does not mean, however, that some as yet undetected, perhaps non-fluorescent metabolite, might not be important for biological activity. It is the formation of free radicals by anthracyclines that currently attracts most attention and is advocated by some as an explanation for the cytotoxic actions of anthracyclines. Although intriguing, the evidence for an association between cytotoxicity and anthracycline-induced free radical formation, either drug radical or oxygen radical formation, is largely indirect. More work is needed to establish whether such an association exists. It will be particularly important to demonstrate a correlation between free radical formation by intact cells and the cytotoxicity of anthracyclines. The relationship between free radical formation and the acute cardiotoxicity of anthracyclines is more convincing. It is possible that newer anthracycline analogues with less free radical forming ability will overcome the worrisome cardiotoxicity of currently used anthracyclines. The ability of anthracyclines to be metabolized and form alkylating species should not be forgotten and may play a role in the biological effects of anthracyclines. The role of iron or other metals in the actions of anthracyclines has recently become a fertile area of research and raises the possibility that such complexes may be formed within the cell and contribute to the activity of the anthracyclines.

The anti-tumour anthracyclines have beguiled and intrigued biochemists, pharmacologists and oncologists since their isolation almost 20 years ago. Recent discoveries will ensure that the anthracyclines receive just as much, if not more, attention in the years to come.

Acknowledgements

The author's work described in this chapter was supported in part by NIH Grant CA33712.

References

Acton, M., Tong, G. L., Mosher, C. W. and Wolgemuth, R. L., 1984, Intensely potent morpholinyl anthracyclines. *J. Med. Chem.*, **27**, 638–645.

Adachi, T., Nagae, T., Ho, Y., Hirano, K. and Sugiura, M., 1983, Relation between cardiotoxic effect of adriamycin and superoxide anion radical. *J. Pharmacobiodyn.*, **6**, 114–123.

Afanas'ev, I. B., Polozova, N. I. and Samokhvalov, G. I., 1980, Investigation of the interaction of superoxide ion with adriamycin and the possible origin of cardiotoxicity of the anthracycline anticancer antibiotics. *Bioorg. Chem.*, **9**, 434.

Ahmed, N. K., Felsted, R. L. and Bachur, N. R., 1978 b, Comparison and characterization of mammalian xenobiotic ketone reductases. *J. Pharmacol. Exp. Ther.*, **209**, 12–19.

Ahmed, N. K., Felsted, R. L. and Bachur, N. R., 1978 b, Comparison and characterization of mammalian xenobiotic ketone reductases. *J. Pharmacol Exp. Ther.*, **209**, 12–19.

Ahmed, N. K., Felsted, R. L. and Bachur, N. R., 1981, Daunorubicin reduction mediated by aldehyde and ketone reductases. *Xenobiotica*, **11**, 131–136.

Alberts, D. S., Bachur, N. R. and Holtzman, J. L., 1971, The pharmacokinetics of daunomycin in man. *Clin. Pharmacol. Ther.*, **12**, 96–104.

Andrews, P. A., Brenner, D. E., Chou, F. T. E., Kubo, H. and Bachur, N. R., 1980, Facile and definitive determination of human adriamycin and daunorubicin metabolites by high-pressure liquid chromatography. *Drug Metab. Disp.*, **8**, 152–156.

Arcamone, F., 1977, New antitumor anthracyclines. *Lloydia*, **40**, 45–66.

Arcamone, F., 1984, Antitumor anthracyclines: recent developments. *Med. Res. Rev.*, **4**, 153–158.

Arcamone, F., 1985, Properties of antitumor anthracyclines and new developments in their application; Cain Memorial Award Lecture. *Cancer Res.*, **45**, 5995–5999.

Arcamone, F., Franceschi, G., Penco, S. and Selva, A., 1969, Adriamycin (14-hydroxydaunomycin), a novel antitumor antibiotic. *Tetrahedron Lett.*, **13**, 1007–1016.

Arcamone, F., Lazzati, M., Vicario, G. P. and Zini, G., 1984, Disposition of ^{14}C-labelled 4′-epidoxorubicin and doxorubicin in the rat. A comparative study. *Cancer Chemother. Rep.*, **12**, 157–166.

Asbell, M. A., Schwartzbach, E., Bullock, F. J. and Yesair, D. W., 1972, Daunomycin and adriamycin metabolism via glycoside cleavage. *J. Pharmacol. Exp. Ther.*, **182**, 63–69.

Aubel-Sadron, G. and Londos-Gagliardi, D., 1984, Daunorubicin and doxorubicin, anthracycline antibiotics, a physicochemical and biological review. *Biochimie*, **66**, 333–352.

Bachur, N., 1971, Daunorubicinol, a major metabolite of daunorubicin; isolation from human urine and enzymatic reactions. *J. Pharmacol. Exp. Ther.*, **177**, 573–578.

Bachur, N. R. and Cradock, J. C., 1970, Daunomycin metabolism in rat tissue slices. *J. Pharmacol. Exp. Ther.*, **175**, 331–337.

Bachur, N. R. and Gee, M., 1971, Daunorubicin metabolism by rat tissue preparations. *J. Pharmacol. Exp. Ther.*, **177**, 567–572.

Bachur, N. R. and Gee, M., 1972, Oxygen sensitive reductive cleavage of daunorubicin and adriamycin. *Fed. Proc.*, **31**, 835.

Bachur, N. R. and Gee, M., 1976, Microsomal reductive glycosidase. *J. Pharmacol. Exp. Ther.*, **197**, 681–686.

Bachur, N. R., Egorin, M. J. and Hildebrand, R., 1973, Daunorubicin and adriamycin metabolism in the golden Syrian hamster. *Biochem. Med.*, **8**, 352–361.

Bachur, N. R., Hildebrand, R. C. and Jaenke, R. S., 1974, Adriamycin and daunorubicin disposition in the rabbit. *J. Pharmacol. Exp. Ther.*, **191**, 331–340.

Bachur, N. R., Gordon, S. L. and Gee, M. L., 1977, Anthracycline antibiotic augmentation of microsomal electron transport and free radical formation. *Mol. Pharmacol.*, **13**, 901–910.

Bachur, N. R., Gordon, S. L. and Gee, M. V., 1978, A general mechanism for microsomal activation of quinone anticancer agents to free radicals. *Cancer Res.*, **38**, 1745–1750.

Bachur, N. R., Gordon, S. L., Gee, M. V. and Kon, H., 1979, NADPH cytochrome P-450 reductase activation of quinone anticancer agents to free radicals. *Proc. Natl. Acad. Sci.*, **76**, 954–957.

Bachur, N. R., Gee, M. V. and Friedman, R. D., 1982, Nuclear catalyzed antibiotic free radical formation. *Cancer Res.*, **42**, 1078–1081.

Bachur, N. R., Friedman, R. D. and Hollenbeck, R. G., 1984, Physicochemical characteristics of ferric adriamycin complexes. *Cancer Chemother. Pharmacol.*, **12**, 5–9.

Bannister, J. V. and Thornalley, P. J., 1983, The production of hydroxyl radicals by adriamycin in red blood cells. *FEBS Lett.*, **157**, 170–172.

Bates, D. A., 1982, Evidence for the production of hydroxyl radicals from the adriamycin semiquinone and H_2O_2. *FEBS Lett.*, **136**, 89–94.

Bates, D. A. and Winterbourn, C. C., 1982, Deoxyribose breakdown by the adriamycin semiquinone and H_2O_2: evidence for hydroxyl radical participation. *FEBS Lett.*, **145**, 137–142.

Baurain, R., Masquelier, M., Deprez-DeCampaneere, D. and Trouet, A., 1980, Amino acid and dipeptide derivatives of daunorubicin. 2. Cellular pharmacology and antitumor activity on L1210 leukemic cells in vitro and in vivo. *J. Med. Chem.*, **23**, 1171–1174.

Benjamin, R. S., Riggs, C. E. and Bachur, N. R., 1973, Pharmacokinetics and metabolism of adriamycin in man. *Clin. Pharmacol. Ther.*, **14**, 592.

Benjamin, R. S., Riggs, C. E., Serpick, A. A. and Bachur, N. R., 1974, Biliary excretion of adriamycin (A) in man. *Clin. Res.*, **22**, 483A.

Beraldo, H., Garnier-Suillerot, A., Tosi, L. and Lavelle, F., 1985, Iron(III)–adriamycin and iron(III)–daunorubicin complexes: physicochemical characteristics, interaction with DNA, and antitumor activity. *Biochemistry*, **24**, 284–289.

Berlin, V. and Haseltine, W. A., 1981, Reduction of adriamycin to a semiquinone-free radical by NADPH cytochrome P-450 reductase produces DNA cleavage in a reaction mediated by molecular oxygen. *J. Biol. Chem.*, **256**, 4747–4756.

Bertazzoli, C., Sala, L., Solcia, E. and Ghione, M., 1975, Antagonistic action of ubiquinone on the experimental cardiotoxicity of adriamycin in isolated rabbit heart. *Int. Res. Commun. Sup. Med. Sci.*, **3**, 467–452.

Bolanowska, W., Gessner, T. and Preisler, H., 1983, A simplified method for determination of daunorubicin, adriamycin, and their chief fluorescent metabolites in human plasma by high-pressure liquid chromatography. *Cancer Chemother. Pharmacol.*, **10**, 187–191.

Brawn, K. and Fridovich, I., 1981, DNA strand scission by enzymatically generated oxygen radicals. *Arch Biochem. Biophys.*, **206**, 414–419.

Breed, J. G., Zimmerman, A. N. E., Dormans, J. A. M. and Pinedo, H. M., 1980, Failure of the antioxidant vitamin E to protect against adriamycin-induced cardiotoxicity in the rabbit. *Cancer Res.*, **40**, 2033–2038.

Brenner, D. E., Galloway, S., Cooper, J., Noone, R. and Hande, K. R., 1985, Improved high-performance liquid chromatography assay of doxorubicin: Detection of circulating aglycones in human plasma and comparison with thin-layer chromatography. *Cancer Chemother. Pharm.*, **14**, 139–145.

Brockman, H., 1963, Anthracyclinones and anthracyclines (Rhodomycinone and Pyrromycinone and their glycosides). *Fortschr. Chem. Org. Naturst.*, **21**, 121–182.

Broggini, M., Colombo, T., Martini, A. and Danelli, M. G., 1980, Studies on the comparative distribution and biliary excretion of doxorubicin and 4′-epi-doxorubicin in mice and rats. *Cancer Treat. Rep.*, **64**, 897–904.

Brown, J. R., 1978, Adriamycin and related anthracycline antibiotics. *Prog. Med. Chem.*, **15**, 125–164.

Brugarolas, A., Pachon, N., Gosalvez, M., Llanderal, A. P., Lacave, A. I., Buesa, J. M. and Marco, M. G., 1978, Phase I clinical study of quelamycin. *Cancer Treat. Rep.*, **62**, 1527—1534.

Bus, J. S. and Gibson, J. E., 1979, In *Reviews in Biochemical Toxicology*, edited by E. Hodgson, J. R. Bend and R. M. Philpot (New York: Elsevier/North-Holland), pp. 125–149.

Butler, J., Hoey, B. M. and Swallow, A. J., 1985, Reactions of the semiquinone free radicals of anti-tumour agents with oxygen and iron complexes. *FEBS Lett.*, **182**, 95–98.

Carmichael, A. J., Mossoba, M. M. and Riesz, P., 1983, Photogeneration of superoxide by adriamycin and daunomycin. An electron spin resonance and spin trapping study. *FEBS Lett.*, **164**, 401–405.

Cassinelli, G., Confligliacchi, E., Penco, S., Rivola, G., Arcamone, F., Pacciarini, A. and Ferrari, L., 1984, Separation, characterization, and analysis of epirubicin (4′-epidoxorubicin) and its metabolites from human urine. *Drug Metab. Disp.*, **12**, 506–510.

Chang, P., Tamburini, J. M., Dodion, P., Riggs, C. E. and Bachur, N. R., 1983, In vitro metabolism of marcellomycin (M). *Proc. Am. Ass. Cancer Res.*, **24**, 258.

Cortes, E. P., Lutman, G., Wanka, J., Pickron, J., Wallace, J. and Holland, J. F., 1973, Adriamycin cardiotoxicity in adults with cancer. *Clin. Res.*, **21**, 412.

Cortes-Funes, H., Gosalvez, M., Moyano, A., Manas, A. and Mendiola, C., 1979, Early clinical trial with quelamycin. *Cancer Treat. Rep.*, **63**, 903–907.

Cradock, J. C., Egorin, M. J. and Bachur, N. R., 1973, Daunorubicin biliary excretion and metabolism in the rat. *Arch. Int. Pharmacodyn. Ther.*, **202**, 48–61.

Crooke, S. T., DuVernay, V. H., Galvan, L. and Prestayko, A. W., 1978, Structure-activity relationships of anthracyclines relative to effects on macromolecular syntheses. *Mol. Pharmacol.*, **14**, 290–298.

Cummings, J., 1985, Method for the determination of 4′-deoxydoxorubicin, 4′-deoxydoxorubicin and their 7-deoxyaglycones in human serum by high-performance liquid chromatography. *J. Chromatogr.*, **341**, 401–409.

D'Alessandro, N. D., Dusonchet, L., Crosta, L., Crescimanno, M. and Rausa, L., 1980, Does catalase play a role in adriamycin induced cardiotoxicity? *Pharmacol. Res. Commun.*, **12**, 441–446.

Daugherty, J. P., Wheat, M., Conley, S., Cooley, E., Vanzant, C., Loggins, L. and Durant, J. R., 1982, Involvement of reactive oxygen spieces in adriamycin (ADR) cardiotoxicity. *Proc. Am. Ass. Cancer Res.*, **23**, 171.

Daugherty, J. P. and Khurana, A., 1985, Amelioration of doxorubicin-induced skin necrosis in mice by butylated hydroxytoluene. *Cancer Chemother. Pharmacol.*, **14**, 243–246.

Davies, K. J. A., Doroshow, J. H. and Hochstein, P., 1983, Mitochondrial NADH dehydrogenase-catalyzed oxygen radical production by adriamycin, and the relative inactivity of 5-iminodaunorubicin. *FEBS Lett.*, **153**, 227–230.

Deesen, P. E. and Leyland-Jones, B., 1984, Sensitive and specific determination of the new anthracycline analog 4′-epidoxorubicin and its metabolites by high pressure liquid chromatography. *Drug Metab. Disp.*, **12**, 9–13.

Demant, E. J. F., 1984, Transfer of ferritin-bound iron to adriamycin. *FEBS Lett.*, **176**, 97–100.

DeGregorio, M. W., Carrera, C. J., Klock, J. C. and Wilbur, J. R., 1982, Uptake and metabolism of daunorubicin by human leukemia cells. *Cancer Chemother. Pharmacol.*, **10**, 29–32.

DeGregorio, M. W., Liu, G. M., Macher, B. A. and Wilbur, J. R., 1984, Uptake, metabolism, and cytotoxicity of doxorubicin in human Ewing's sarcoma and rhabdomyosarcoma cells. *Cancer Chemother. Pharmacol.*, **12**, 59–63.

Desai, M. H. and Teres, D., 1982, Prevention of doxorubicin-induced skin ulcers in the rat and pig with dimethyl sulfoxide (DMSO). *Cancer Treat. Rep.*, **66**, 1371–1374.

Dickinson, A. C., DeJordy, J. D. and Teres, D., 1984, Absence of generation of oxygen-containing free radicals with 4′-deoxydoxorubicin, a non-cardiotoxic anthracycline drug. *Proc. Am. Asss. Cancer Res.*, **25**, 296.

Dickinson, A. C., Boutin, M. G., Matsunaga, N. and Teres, D., 1985, 4′-Deoxydoxorubicin and 4-demethoxydaunorubicin do not generate oxygen free radicals. *Proc. Am. Ass. Cancer Res.*, **26**, 225.

DiFronzo, G., Gambetta, R. A. and Lenaz, L., 1971, Distribution and metabolism of adriamycin in mice. Comparison with daunomycin. *Rev. Eur. Etud. Clin. Biol.*, **16**, 572–576.

DiMarco, A., Gaetini, M., Dorigotti, L., Soldatti, M. and Bellini, O., 1963, Studi sperimentali sull'attivitá antineoplastica del nuovo antibiotico daunomicina. *Tumori*, **49**, 203–217.

DiMarco, A., Boretti, G. and Rusconi, A., 1967, Transformazione metabolica della daunomicina da parte di estratti di tessuti. *Farmaco* [*Sci.*], **22**, 535–542.

Dodion, P., Bernstein, A. L., Fox, B. M., Davis, T. A., Engisch, K. L. and Bachur, N. R., 1984, Enzymic catalysis of anthracyclines to non-fluorescent metabolites. *Proc. Am. Ass. Cancer Res.*, **25**, 298.

Dodion, P., Egorin, M. J., Tamburini, J. M., Riggs, C. F. and Bachur, N. R., 1983, The murine metabolism and disposition of marcellomycin. *Drug Metab. Disp.*, **12**, 209–216.

Dodion, P., Rozencweig, M., Nicaise, C., Watthieu, M., Tamburini, J. M., Riggs, C. E. and Bachur, N. R., 1985 b, Human pharmacokinetics of marcellomycin. *Cancer Chemother. Pharmacol.*, **14**, 42–48.

Dodion, P., Rozencweig, M., Nicajse, C., Watthieu, M., Tamburini, J. M., Riggs, C. E. and Bachur, N. R., 1985 b, Human pharmacokinetics of marcellomycin. *Cancer Chemother. Pharmacol.*, **14**, 42–48.

Domae, N., Sawada, H., Matsuyama, E., Konishi, T. and Uchino, H., 1981, Cardiomyopathy and other chronic toxic effects induced in rabbits by doxorubicin and possible prevention of coenzyme Q10. *Cancer Treat. Rep.*, **65**, 79–91.

Doroshow, J. H., 1983 a, Anthracycline antibiotic-stimulated superoxide, hydrogen peroxide, and hydroxyl radical production by NADH dehydrogenase. *Cancer Res.*, **43**, 4543–4551.

Doroshow, J. H., 1983 b, Effect of anthracycline antibiotics on oxygen radical formation in rat heart. *Cancer Res.*, **43**, 460–472.

Doroshow, J., 1983 c, Anthracycline (A)-stimulated hydroxyl radical (OH·) production in the heart. *Proc. Am. Ass. Cancer Res.*, **23**, 255.

Doroshow, J. H., 1985, Oxygen radical-induced tumor cell killing by anticancer quinones: A common mechanism of cytotoxicity. *Proc. Am. Ass. Cancer. Res.*, **26**, 225.

Doroshow, J. H. and deVries, L., 1984, Hydroxyl radical (·OH)-induced tumor cell killing by doxorubicin (D). *Proc. Am. Ass. Cancer Res.*, **25**, 300.

Doroshow, J. H., Locker, G. Y. and Myers, C. E., 1980, Enzymatic defenses of the mouse heart against reactive oxygen metabolites: alterations produced by doxorubicin. *J. Clin. Inv.*, **65**, 128–135.

Doroshow, J. H., Locker, G. Y., Ifrim, I. and Myers, C. E., 1982, Prevention of doxorubicin cardiac toxicity in the mouse by N-acetylcysteine. *J. Clin. Inv.*, **68**, 1053–1064.

Dorr, R. T. and Alberts, D. S., 1983, Failure of DMSO and vitamin E to prevent doxorubicin skin ulceration in the mouse. *Cancer Treat. Rep.*, **67**, 499–501.

DuVernay, V. H. and Crooke, S. T., 1980, Effects of several anthracycline antitumor antibiotics on the transcriptional activity of isolated nucleoli. *J. Antibiot.*, **33**, 1048–1053.

DuVernay, V. H., Essery, J. M., Doyle, T. W., Bradner, W. T. and Crooke, S. T., 1979, The antitumor effects of anthracyclines. The importance of the carbomethoxy-group at position-10 of marcellomycin and rudolfomycin. *Mol. Pharmacol.*, **15**, 341–356.

Egorin, M. J., Clawson, R. E., Ross, L. A., Chou, F. T., Andrews, P. A. and Bachur, N. R., 1980, Disposition and metabolism of N,N-dimethyldaunorubicin and N,N-dimethyladriamycin in rabbits and mice. *Drug Metab. Disp.*, **8**, 353–362.

Egorin, M. J., Van Echo, D., Fox, B. M., Whitacre, M. and Bachur, N. R., 1982, Plasma kinetics of aclacinomycin A and its major metabolites in man. *Cancer Chemother. Pharmacol.*, **8**, 41–46.

Egorin, M. J., Andrews, P. A., Nakazawa, H. and Bachur, N. R., 1983, Purification and characterization of aclacinomycin A and its metabolites from human urine. *Drug Metab. Disp.*, **11**, 167–171.

Eliot, H., Gianni, L. and Myers, C. E., 1983, Oxidative destruction of DNA by the adriamycin-iron complex. *Biochemistry*, **23**, 928–936.

Elstner, E., Osswald, W. F. and Konze, J. R., 1980, Reactive oxygen species: Electron donor-hydrogen peroxide complex instead of free OH radicals? *FEBS Lett.*, **121**, 219–221.

Felsted, R. L., Gee, M. and Bachur, N. R., 1974, Rat liver daunorubicin reductase. *J. Biol. Chem.*, **249**, 3672–3679.

Felsted, R. J., Richter, D. R. and Bachur, N. R., 1977, Rat liver aldehyde reductase. *Biochem. Pharmacol.*, **26**, 1117–1124.

Fiallo, M. M. L. and Garnier-Suillerot, A., 1985, Physicochemical studies of the iron(III)-carminomycin complex and evidence of the lack of stimulated superoxide production by NADH dehydrogenase. *Biochim. Biophys. Acta*, **840**, 91–98.

Folkers, K., Choe, J. Y. and Combs, A. B., 1978, Rescue by coenzyme Q10 from electrocardiographic abnormalities caused by the toxicity of adriamycin in the rat. *Proc. Natl. Acad. Sci.*, **75**, 5178–5180.

Freeman, R. W., MacDonald, J. S., Olson, R. D., Boerth, R. C., Oates, J. A. and Harbison, R. D., 1980, Effect of sulfhydryl-containing compounds on the antitumor effects of adriamycin. *Tox. Appl. Pharmacol.*, **54**, 168–175.

Fridovich, I., 1976, Oxygen radicals, hydrogen peroxide and oxygen toxicity. In *Free Radicals in Biology*, edited by W. A. Pryor (New York: Academic Press), Volume I, pp. 239–277.

Fujita, K., Shinpo, K., Yamada, K., Sato, T., Nimi, H., Shamoto, M., Nagatsu, T., Takeuhi, T. and Umezawa, H., 1982, Reduction of adriamycin toxicity by ascorbate in mice and guinea pigs. *Cancer Res.*, **42**, 309–316.

Gause, G. F., 1962, Biokhimicheskie mekhanizmy deistviga antibiotikov. *Antibiotiki*, **9**, 946–950.

Gianni, L., Zweir, J. L., Levy, A. and Myers, C. E., 1983 a, Characterization of the cycle of iron-mediated electron transfer from adriamycin to molecular oxygen. *J. Biol. Chem.*, **260**, 6820–6826.

Gianni, L., Corden, B. J. and Myers, C. E., 1983b. In *Reviews in Biochemical Toxicology*, edited by E. Hodgson, J. Bend and R. M. Philpot (New York: Elsevier/North Holland), pp. 1–82.

Gill, P., Favre, R., Durand, A., Iliadis, A., Cano, J. P. and Carcassone, Y., 1983, Time dependency of adriamycin and adriamycinol kinetics. *Cancer Chemother. Pharmacol.*, **10**, 120–124.

Gola, A., 1979, Daunorubicin reductase activity in leukemia leukocyte homogenates. *Arch. Immunol. Ther. Exp.*, **27**, 815–818.

Goodman, J. and Hochstein, P., 1977, Generation of free radicals and lipid peroxidation by redox cycling of adriamycin and daunomycin. *Biochem. Biophys. Res. Commun.*, **77**, 797–803.

Goormaghtigh, E., Pollakis, G. and Ruysschaert, J. M., 1983, Mitochondrial membrane modifications induced by adriamycin-mediated electron transport. *Biochem. Pharmacol.*, **32**, 889–893.

Goormaghtigh, E. and Ruysschaert, J. M., 1983, Evidence of a covalent linkage in the adriamycin-cardiolipid complex induced by adriamycin-mediated electron transport. *Res. Commun. Chem. Path. Pharmacol.*, **42**, 149–152.

Gosalvez, M., Blanco, M. F., Vivero, C. and Valles, F., 1978, Quelamycin, a new derivative of adriamycin with several possible therapeutic advantages. *Eur. J. Cancer*, **14**, 1185–1190.

Gutierrez, P. L., Gee, M. V. and Bachur, N. R., 1983, Kinetics of anthracycline antibiotic free radical formation and reductive glycosidase activity. *Arch. Biochem. Biophys.*, **223**, 68–75.

Gutteridge, J. M., 1983, Adriamycin-iron catalyzed phospholipid peroxidation: a reaction not involving reduced adriamycin or hydroxyl radicals. *Biochem. Pharmacol.*, **32**, 1949–1952.

Gutteridge, J. M., 1984, Lipid peroxidation and possible hydroxyl radical formation stimulated by the self-reduction of a doxorubicin–iron (III) complex. *Biochem. Pharmacol.*, **33**, 1725–1728.

Gutteridge, J. M. C. and Quinlan, G. J., 1985, Free radical damage to deoxyribose by anthracycline, aureolic acid and aminoquinone antitumor antibiotics. An essential requirement for iron, semiquinones and hydrogen peroxide. *Biochem. Pharmacol.*, **34**, 4099–4103.

Handa, K. and Sato, S., 1975, Generation of free radicals of quinone group containing anti-cancer chemicals in NADPH-microsome system as evidenced by initiation of sulfite oxidation. *Gann*, **66**, 43–47.

Handa, K. and Sato, S., 1976, Stimulation of microsomal NADPH oxidation by quinone group-containing anticancer chemicals. *Gann*, **67**, 523–528.

Halliwell, B. and Gutteridge, J. M., 1984, Oxygen toxicity, oxygen radicals, transition metals and disease. *Biochem. J.*, **219**, 1–14.

Harris, R. N. and Doroshow, J. H., 1985, Effect of doxorubicin-enhanced hydrogen peroxide and hydroxyl radical formation on calcium sequestration by cardiac sarcoplasmic reticulum. *Biochem. Biophys. Res. Commun.*, **130**, 739.

Hartman, N., Basseches, P. J. and Powis, G., 1982, Effect of cyclophosphamide pretreatment on the short-term disposition and biliary excretion of adriamycin and metabolites in rat. *Cancer Chemother. Pharmacol.*, **10**, 11–15.

Henry, D. W., 1979, Structure–activity relationships among daunorubicin and adriamycin analogs. *Cancer Treat. Rep.*, **63**, 845–854.

Herzog, V. and Fahimi, H. D., 1974, Microbodies (peroxisomes) containing catalase in myocardium: Morphologic and biochemical evidence. *Science*, **185**, 271–273.

Hickman, J., Chachwala, S. B. and Thompson, M. G., 1985, Interaction of the antibiotic adriamycin with the plasma membrane. *Adv. Enzym. Reg.*, **15**, 263–274.

Houée-Levin, C., Gardès-Albert, M. and Ferradini, C., 1984, Reduction of daunorubicin aqueous solutions by COO·-free radicals. Reactions of reduced transients with H_2O_2. *FEBS Lett.*, **173**, 27–30.

Houée-Levin, C., Gardès-Albert, M., Faraggi, M. and Klapper, M., 1985, Pulse radiolysis study of daunorubicin redox cycles, reduction of e_{aq}^- and $COO^{\cdot-}$ free radicals. *FEBS Lett.*, **179**, 46–50.

Hrushesky, W. J. M., Wood, P., Olshefski, R., Meshnick, S. and Eaton, J. W., 1985, Modifying intracellular redox balance: an approach to improving therapeutic index. *Lancet*, **1**, 565–566.

Huffman, D. H. and Bachur, N. R., 1972, Daunorubicin metabolism in acute myelocytic leukemia. *Blood*, **39**, 637–643.

Huffman, D. H., Benjamin, R. S. and Bachur, N. R., 1972, Daunorubicin metabolism in acute nonlymphocytic leukemia. *Clin. Pharmacol. Ther.*, **13**, 895–905.

Hutchinson, F., 1957, The distance that a radical formed by ionizing radiation can diffuse in a yeast cell. *Radiation Res.*, **7**, 473–483.

Israel, M., Pegg, W. J., Seshadri, R. and Parker, L. M., 1976. In *Abstracts Fifth Int. Symp. Med. Chem. Paris* (Paris: L'Imprimerie Levert), p. 63.

Israel, M., Wilkinson, P. M., Pegg, W. J. and Frei, E., 1978, Hepatobiliary metabolism and excretion of adriamycin and N-trifluoroacetyladriamycin-14-valerate in the rat. *Cancer Res.*, **38**, 365–370.

Israel, M., Karkowsky, A. M. and Khetarpal, V. K., 1981, Distribution of radioactivity and anthracycline-fluorescence in tissues of mice one hour after [^{14}C]-labeled AD 32 administration. *Cancer Chemother. Pharmacol.*, **6**, 25–30.

Iyanagi, T. and Yamazaki, T., 1969, One-electron-transfer reactions in biochemical systems. III. One-electron reduction of quinones by microsomal flavin enzymes. *Biochem. Biophys. Acta*, **172**, 370–381.

Iyanagi, T. and Yamazaki, I., 1970, One-electron reductions in biochemical systems. V. Difference in the mechanism of quinone reduction by the NADH dehydrogenase and the NAD(P)H dehydrogenase (DT-diaphorase). *Biochim. Biophys. Acta*, **216**, 282–294.

Jaenke, R. S., 1976, Delayed and progressive myocardial lesions after adriamycin administration in the rabbit. *Cancer Res.*, **36**, 2958–2966.

Johansen, P. B., Jensen, S. E., Rasmussen, S. N. and Dalmark, M., 1984, Pharmacokinetics of doxorubicin and its metabolite doxorubicinol in rabbits with induced acid and alkaline urine. *Cancer Chemother. Pharmacol.*, **13**, 5–8.

Johnston, J. B., Habernicht, B., Acton, E. M. and Glazer, R. I., 1983, 3′-(3-Cyano-4-morpholinyl)-3′-deaminoadriamycin: a new anthracycline with potency. *Biochem. Pharmacol.*, **32**, 3255–3258.

Kalyanaraman, B., Perez-Reyes, E. and Mason, R. P., 1980, Spin-trapping and direct electron spin resonance investigations of the redox metabolism of quinone anticancer drugs. *Biochim. Biophys. Acta*, **630**, 119–130.

Kalyanaraman, B., Sealy, R. C. and Sinha, B. K., 1984, An electron spin resonance study of the reduction of peroxides by anthracycline semiquinones. *Biochim. Biophys. Acta*, **799**, 270–275.

Kanter, P. M. and Schwartz, H. S., 1979, Quantitative models for growth inhibition of human leukemia cells by antitumor anthracycline derivatives. *Cancer Res.*, **39**, 3661–3672.

Kodama, M., Aida, M., Nagata, C., Oki, T. and Matsuzawa, Y., 1983, An electron spin resonance study on the free radicals produced from aclacinomycin A and its derivatives: analysis of hyperfine structure of the spectra by means of molecular orbital method. *Cancer Biochem. Biophys.*, **6**, 243–247.

Komiyama, T., Oki, T., Inui, T., Takeuchi, T. and Umezawa, H., 1978, NADH-dependent cinerulose reductase in rat liver microsomes. *Biochem. Biophys. Res. Commun.*, **82**, 188–195.

Komiyama, T., Oki, T. and Inui, T., 1979 a, A proposed reaction mechanism for the enzymatic reductive cleavage of glycosidic bond in anthracycline antibiotics. *Gann*, **32**, 1219–1222.

Komiyama, T., Oki, T., Inui, T., Takeuchi, T. and Umezawa, H., 1979 b, Reduction of cinerulose in aclacinomycin-A by soluble and microsomal cinerulose reductases. *Gann*, **70**, 395–401.

Komiyama, T., Kikuchi, T. and Sugiura, Y., 1982, Generation of hydroxyl radical by anticancer quinone drugs, carbazilquinone, mitomycin C, aclacinomycin A and adriamycin, in the presence of NADPH-cytochrome P-450 reductase. *Biochem. Pharmacol.*, **31**, 3651–3656.

Komiyama, T., Sawada, M. T., Kobayashi, K. and Yoshimoto, A., 1985, Enhanced production of ethylene from methional by iron chelates and heme containing proteins in the system consisting of quinone compounds and NADPH-cytochrome P-450 reductase. *Biochem. Pharmacol.*, **34**, 977–983.

Land, E. J., Mukherjee, T., Swallow, A. J. and Bruce, J. M., 1983, One-electron reduction of adriamycin: properties of the semiquinone. *Arch. Biochem. Biophys.*, **255**, 116–121.

Land, E. J., Mukherjee, T., Swallow, A. J. and Bruce, J. M., 1985, Possible intermediates in the action of adriamycin—A pulse radiolysis study. *Br. J. Cancer*, **51**, 515–523.

Legha, S. S., Benjamin, R. S., McKay, B., Ewer, M., Wallace, S., Valdivieso, M., Rasmussen, S. L., Blumenschein, G. R., Freireich, E. J., 1982, Reduction of doxorubicin cardiotoxicity by prolonged continuous intravenous infusion. *Ann. Int. Med.*, **96**, 133–139.

Lenzhofer, R., Magometschnigg, R., Dudczak, C., Cerni, C., Bolebruch, C. and Moser, K., 1983, Indication of reduced doxorubicin-induced cardiac toxicity by additional treatment with antioxidative substances. *Experientia*, **39**, 62–64.

Levin, M., Silber, R., Israel, M., Goldfeder, A., Khetarpel, V. K. and Potmesil, M., 1981, Protein-associated DNA breaks and DNA-protein cross-links caused by DNA nonbinding derivatives of adriamycin in L1210 cells. *Cancer Res.*, **41**, 1006–1010.

Londos-Gagliardi, D., Baurain, R., Robert, J. and Aubel-Sadron, G., 1982, Metabolism of daunorubicin in sensitive and resistant Ehrlich ascites tumor cells. Determination by high pressure liquid chromatography. *Cancer Chemother. Pharmacol.*, **9**, 45–48.

Lown, J. W., Chen, H. H., Plambeck, J. A. and Acton, E. M., 1979, Diminished superoxide anion generation by reduced 5-iminodaunorubicin relative to daunorubicin and the relationship to cardiotoxicity of the anthracycline antitumor agents. *Biochem. Pharmacol.*, **28**, 2563–2568.

Lown, J. W., Chen, H. H., Plambeck, J. A. and Acton, E. M., 1982, Further studies on the generation of reactive oxygen species from activated anthracyclines and the relationships to cytotoxic action and cardiotoxic effects. *Biochem. Pharmacol.*, **31**, 575–581.

Malatesta, V., Penco, S., Sacchi, N., Valentini, L., Vigevani, A. and Arcamone, F., 1984, Electrochemical deglycosidation of anthracyclines: stereoelectronic requirements. *Can. J. Chem.*, **62**, 2845–2850.

Mason, R. P., 1979, Free radical metabolites of foreign compounds and their toxicological significance. In *Reviews in Biochemical Toxicology*, Part 1, edited by E. Hodgson, J. R. Bend and R. M. Philpot (New York: Elsevier/North-Holland), pp. 151–200.

McGovren, J. P., Nelson, K. G., Lassus, M., Cradock, J. C., Plowman, J. and Christopher, J. P., 1984, Menogaril: a new anthracycline agent entering clinical trials. *Inv. New Drugs*, **2**, 359–367.

Mhatre, R. M., Herman, E. H., Waravdekar, V. S. and Lee, I. P., 1972, Distribution and metabolism of daunomycin, adriamycin and N-acetyldaunomycin in the Syrian golden hamster. *Biochem. Med.*, **6**, 445–453.

Michaelis, L., 1946. *Currents in Biochemistry Research*, edited by D. Greed (New York: Wiley), p. 207.

Mimnaugh, E. G., Siddik, Z. H., Drew, R., Sikic, B. I. and Gram, T., 1979, The effects of alpha-tocopherol on the toxicity, disposition, and metabolism of adriamycin in mice. *Tox. Appl. Pharmacol.*, **49**, 119–126.

Mimnaugh, E. G., Trush, M. A. and Gram, T. E., 1981, Stimulation of adriamycin of rat heart and liver microsomal NADPH-dependent lipid peroxidation. *Biochem. Pharmacol.*, **30**, 2797–2804.

Mimnaugh, E. G., Trush, M. A., Ginsburg, E. and Gram, T. E., 1982, Differential effects of anthracycline drugs on rat heart and liver microsomal reduced nicotinamide adenine dinucleotide phosphate-dependent lipid peroxidation. *Cancer Res.*, **42**, 3574–3582.

Mimnaugh, E. G., Gram, E. G. and Trush, M. A., 1983, Stimulation of mouse heart and liver microsomal lipid peroxidation by anthracycline anticancer drugs: characterization and effects of reactive oxygen scavengers. *J. Pharmacol. Exp. Ther.*, **226**, 806–816.

Mimnaugh, E. G., Kennedy, K. A., Trush, M. A. and Sinha, B. K., 1985, Adriamycin-enhanced membrane lipid peroxidation in isolated rat nuclei. *Cancer Res.*, **45**, 3296–3304.

Moore, H. W., 1977, Bioactivation as a model for drug design. Bioreductive alkylation. *Science*, **527–532**.

Muindi, J. R., Sinha, B. K., Gianni, L. and Myers, C. E., 1984, Hydroxyl radical production and DNA damage induced by anthracycline–iron complexes. *FEBS Lett.*, **172**, 226–230.

Muindi, J. R. F., Katki, A. G. and Myers, C. E., 1985 a, Role of membrane protein sulfhydryl groups in adriamycin-iron complex dependent membrane destruction. *Proc. Am. Ass. Cancer Res.*, **26**, 222.

Muindi, J., Sinha, B., Gianni, L. and Myers, C., 1985 b, Thiol-dependent DNA damage produced by anthracycline–iron complexes. The structure–activity relationships and molecular mechanisms. *Mol. Pharmacol.*, **27**, 356–365.

Muliawan, H., Scheulen, M. E. and Kappus, H., 1980, Acute adriamycin treatment of rats does not increase ethane expiration. *Res. Commun. Chem. Path. Pharmacol.*, **30**, 509–519.

Myers, C. E., 1982, In *Pharmacologic Principles of Cancer Treatment*, edited by B. Chabner (Philadelphia: W. B. Saunders), pp. 416–434.

Myers, C. E., McGuire, W. P,. and Young, R., 1976, Adriamycin: amelioration of toxicity by alpha-tocopherol. *Cancer Treat. Rep.*, **60**, 961–962.

Myers, C. E., McGuire, W. P., Liss, R. H., Ifrim, I., Grotzinger, K. and Young, R. C., 1977, Adriamycin: the role of lipid peroxidation in cardiac toxicity and tumor response. *Science*, **197**, 165–167.

Myers, C. E., Gianni, L., Simone, C. B., Klecker, R. and Greene, R., 1982, Oxidative destruction of erythrocyte ghost membranes catalyzed by the doxorubicin–iron complex. *Biochemistry*, **21**, 1707–1712.

Naff, M. B., Plowman, J. and Naryanan, V. L., 1982. In *Anthracycline Antibiotics*, edited by H. S. El Khadem (New York: Academic Press), pp. 1–57.

Nakazawa, H., Andrews, P. A., Callery, P. S. and Bachur, N. R., 1985, Superoxide radical reactions with anthracycline antibiotics. *Biochem. Pharmacol.*, **34**, 481–490.

Nettleton, D. E., Bradner, W. T., Bush, J. A., Coon, A. B., Moseley, J. E., Myllmaki, R. W., O'Herron, F. A., Schreiber, R. H. and Vulcano, A. L., 1977, New antitumor antibiotics: musettamycin and marcellomycin from bohemic acid complex. *J. Antibiot.*, **30**, 525–529.

Nobbs, P. and Barr, R. D., 1983, Soft-tissue injury caused by antineoplastic drugs is inhibited by topical dimethyl sulphoxide and alpha tocopherol. *Br. J. Cancer*, **48**, 873–876.

Nohl, H. and Jordan, W., 1983, OH·-generation by adriamycin semiquinone and H_2O_2: an explanation for the cardiotoxicity of anthracycline antibiotics. *Biochem. Biophys. Res. Commun.*, **114**, 197–205.

Oki, T., 1977, New anthracycline antibiotics. *Jap. J. Antibiot.*, **30**(Suppl.), S70–S84.

Oki, T., Matsuzawa, Y., Yoshimoto, A., Numata, K., Kitamura, I., Hori, S., Takamatsu, A., Umezawa, H., Ishizuka, M., Naganawa, H., Suda, H., Hamada, M. and Takeuchi, T., 1975, New antitumor antibiotics, aclacinomycin A and B. *J. Antibiot.*, **28**, 830–834.

Oki, T., Komiyama, T., Tone, H., Inui, T., Takeuchi, T. and Umezawa, H., 1977, Reductive cleavage of anthracycline glycosides by microsomal NADPH-cytochrome c reductase. *J. Antibiot. Tokyo*, **30**, 613–615.

Oki, T., Takeuchi, T., Oka, S. and Umezawa, H., 1981, New anthracycline antibiotic aclacinomycin A: Experimental studies and correlations with clinical trials. *Recent Res. Cancer Res.*, **76**, 21–40.

Olsen, R. D., MacDonald, J. S., Van Boxtel, C. J., Boerth, R. C., Harbison, R. D., Slonim, A. E., Freeman, R. W. and Oates, J. A., 1983, Regulatory role of glutathione and soluble sulfhydryl groups in the toxicity of adriamycin. *J. Pharmacol. Exp. Ther.*, **215**, 450–454.

Olson, H. M., Young, D. M., Prieun, D. J., Leroy, A. F. and Regan, R. L., 1974, Electrolyte and morphologic alterations of myocardium in adriamycin treated rabbits. *Am. J. Path.*, **77**, 439.

Olver, I. N. and Schwarz, M. A., 1983, Use of dimethyl sulfoxide in limiting tissue damage caused by extravasation of doxorubicin. *Cancer Treat. Rep.*, **67**, 407–408.

Oosterbaan, M. J. M., Dirks, R. J. M., Vree, T. B. and van der Kleijn, E., 1984, Pharmacokinetics of anthracyclines in dogs: Evidence for structure-related body distribution and reduction to their hydroxy metabolites. *Pharmaceut. Res.*, 33–38.

Painter, R. B., 1978, Inhibition of DNA replicon initiation by 4-nitroquinoline 1-oxide, adriamycin, and ethyleneimine. *Cancer Res.*, **38**, 4445–4449.

Pan, S.-S. and Bachur, N. R., 1980, Xanthine oxidase catalyzed reduced cleavage of anthracycline antibiotics and free radical formation. *Mol. Pharmacol.*, **17**, 95–99.

Pan, S., Gutierrez, P. and Bachur, N. R., 1980, Flavo-protein catalysis of anthracycline antibiotic reductive cleavage, free radical formation and free radical interconversions. *Fed. Proc.*, **39**, 310.

Pan, S.-S., Pedersen, L. and Bachur, N. R., 1981 a, Comparative flavoprotein catalysis of anthracycline antibiotic. Reductive cleavage and oxygen consumption. *Mol. Pharmacol.*, **19**, 184–186.

Pan, S., Gutierrez, P., Nakazawa, H. and Bachur, N. R., 1981 b, Formation of kinetics and interconversion of anthracycline free radicals catalyzed by flavoenzymes. *Proc. Am. Ass. Cancer Res.*, **22**, 265.

Pierce, R. N. and Jatlow, P. I., 1979, Measurement of adriamycin (doxorubicin) and its metabolites in human plasma using reversed-phase high-performance liquid chromatography and fluorescence detection. *J. Chromatogr.*, **164**, 471–478.

Pietronigro, D. D., McGinness, J. E., Koren, M. J., Crippa, R., Seligman, M. L. and Demopoulos, H. B., 1979, Spontaneous generation of adriamycin semiquinone radicals at physiologic pH. *Physiol. Chem. Phys.*, **11**, 405–413.

Pietronigro, D. D., Mignano, J. E. and Demopoulos, H. B., 1983, Direct quenching of adriamycin radicals by coenzyme Q10 and tetrazolium salts. *Biochem. Pharmacol.*, **32**, 1441–1444.

Pigram, W. J., Fuller, W. and Hamilton, L. D., 1972, Stereochemistry of intercalation: interaction of daunomycin with DNA. *Nature*, **235**, 17–19.

Pollakis, G., Goormaghtigh, E. and Ruysschaert, J. M., 1983, Role of the quinone structure in the mitochondrial damage induced by antitumor anthracyclines. Comparison of adriamycin and 5-iminodaunorubicin. *FEBS Lett.*, **155**, 267–272.

Pollakis, G., Goormaghtigh, E., Delmelle, M., Lion, Y. and Ruysschaert, J. M., 1984, Adriamycin and derivatives interaction with the mitochondrial membrane: O_2 consumption and free radicals formation. *Res. Commun. Chem. Path. Pharmacol.*, **44**, 445–459.

Pommier, Y., Schwartz, R. E., Zwelling, L. A. and Kohn, K. W., 1985, Effects of DNA intercalating agents on topoisomerase II induced DNA strand cleavage in isolated mammalian cell nuclei. *Biochemistry*, **24**, 6406–6410.

Potmesil, M., Kirschenbaum, S., Israel, M., Levin, M., Khetarpal, V. K. and Silber, R., 1983, Relationship of adriamycin concentrations to the DNA lesions induced in hypoxic and euoxic L1210 cells. *Cancer Res.*, **43**, 3528–3533.

Potmesil, M., Israel, M. and Silber, R., 1984, Two mechanisms of adriamycin-DNA interaction in L1210 cells. *Biochem. Pharmacol.*, **33**, 3137–3140.

Powis, G. and Appel, P. L., 1980, Relationship of the single-electron reduction potential of quinones to their reduction by flavoproteins. *Biochem. Pharmacol.*, **29**, 2567–2572.

Powis, G. and Svingen, B. A., 1981, pulse radiolysis measurement of one-electron reduction potential (E^1_7) of adriamycin derivatives. *Pharmacologist*, **23**, 181.

Powis, G., Svingen, B. A. and Appel, P. L., 1981, Quinone stimulated superoxide formation by subcellular fractions, isolated hepatocytes and other cells. *Mol. Pharmacol.*, **20**, 387–394.

Pratt, C. B., Ransom, J. L. and Evans, W. E., 1978, Age-related adriamycin cardiotoxicity in children. *Cancer Treat. Rep.*, **62**, 1381–1385.

Revis, N. W. and Marusic, N., 1978, Glutathione peroxidase activity and selenium concentration in the hearts of doxorubicin-treated rabbits. *J. Mol. Cell Cardiol.*, **10**, 945–951.

Reich, S. D. and Gordon, S., 1977, Pharmacology of adriamycin and ferric ion–adriamycin complex. *Proc. Am. Ass. Cancer Res.*, **18**, 72.

Riggs, C. E. and Schrader, S. L., 1985, Reduction in aglycone production from the anthracycline analogs, epirubicin esorubicin, and idarubicin, in vitro. *Proc. Am. Ass. Cancer Res.*, **26**, 219.

Robert, J., Vrignaud, P., Nguyen-Ngoc, T., Illiadis, A., Mauriac, L. and Hurteloup, P., 1985, Comparative pharmacokinetics and metabolism of doxorubicin and epirubicin in patients with metastatic breast cancer. *Cancer Treat. Rep.*, **69**, 633–640.

Rosso, R., Ravazzoni, C., Esposito, M., Sala, R. and Santi, L., 1972, Plasma and urinary levels of adriamycin in man. *Eur. J. Cancer*, **8**, 455–459.

Rowley, D. A. and Halliwell, B., 1983, DNA damage by superoxide-generating systems in relation to the mechanism of action of the anti-tumor antibiotic adriamycin. *Biochim. Biophys. Acta.*, **761**, 86–93.

Santone, K. S., Oakes, S. G., Taylor, S. R. and Powis, G., 1986, Anthracycline-induced inhibition of a calcium action potential in differentiated neuroblastoma cells. *Cancer Res.*, **46**, 2659–2664.

Sato, S., Iwaizumi, M., Handa, K. and Tamura, Y., 1977, Electron spin resonance study on the mode of generation of free radicals of daunomycin, adriamycin, and carboquone in NAD(P)H-microsome system. *Gann*, **68**, 603–608.

Sawyer, D. T., Roberts, J. L., Calderwood, T. S., Tsuchiya, T. and Stamp, J. J., 1983. In *Oxygen Radicals and Their Scavenger Systems*, edited by G. Cohen and R. A. Greenwald (New York: Elsevier Science), Volume 1, p. 8.

Scheulen, M. E., Kappus, H., Nienhaus, A. and Schmidt, C. G., 1982, Covalent protein binding of reactive adriamycin metabolites in rat liver and rat heart microsomes. *J. Cancer Res. Clin. Oncol.*, **103**, 39–48.

Schwartz, H. S., 1975, DNA breaks in P288 tumor cells in mice after treatment with daunorubicin and adriamycin. *Res. Commun. Chem. Path. Pharmacol.*, **10**, 51–64.

Schwartz, H. S., 1983, Enhanced antitumor activity of adriamycin in combination with allopurinol. *Cancer Lett.*, **20**, 69–74.

Schwartz, H. S. and Parker, N. B., 1981, Initial biotransformations of daunorubicin to aglycones by rat liver microsomes. *Cancer Res.*, **41**, 2343–2348.

Schwartz, H. S. and Paul, B., 1984, Biotransformation of daunorubicin aglycones by rat liver microsomes. *Cancer Res.*, **44**, 2480–2484.

Shinozawa, S. and Oda, I., 1981, Determination of adriamycin (doxorubicin) and related fluorescent compounds in rat lymph and gall by high-performance liquid chromatography. *J. Chromatogr.*, **212**, 323–330.

Siegfried, J. M., Sartorelli, A. C. and Tritton, T. R., 1983, Evidence for the lack of relationship between inhibition of nucleic acid synthesis and cytotoxicity of adriamycin. *Cancer Biochem. Biophys.*, **6**, 137–142.

Sinha, B. K., 1980, Binding specificity of chemically and enzymatically activated anthracycline anticancer agents to nucleic acids. *Chem.-Biol. Interactions.*, **30**, 67–77.

Sinha, B. K. and Chignell, C. F., 1979, Binding mode of chemically activated semiquinone free radicals from quinone anticancer agents to DNA. *Chem.-Biol. Interactions*, **28**, 301–308.

Sinha, B. K. and Gregory, J. L., 1981, Role of one-electron and two-electron reduction products of adriamycin and daunomycin in deoxyribonucleic acid binding. *Biochem. Pharmacol.*, **30**, 2626–2629.

Sinha, B. K., Trush, M. A., Kennedy, K. A. and Mimnaugh, E. G., 1984, Enzymatic activation and binding of adriamycin to nuclear DNA. *Cancer Res.*, **44**, 2892–2896.

Sinha, B. K., Muindi, J. R., Batist, G. and Myers, C. E., 1985, Hydroxyl radical formation and DNA damage by anthracycline antitumor drugs. *Proc. Am. Ass. Cancer Res.*, **26**, 225.

Skovsgaard, T., 1977, Transport and binding of daunorubicin, adriamycin, and rubidazone in Ehrlich ascites tumour cells. *Biochem. Pharmacol.*, **26**, 215–222.

Solie, T. N. and Yuncker, C., 1978, Adriamycin induced changes in translocation of sodium ions in transporting epithelial cells. *Life Sci.*, **22**, 1907–1910.

Speyer, J. L., Green, M. D., Israel, M., Sweatman, T. W. and Muggia, F., 1982, The clinical pharmacology of 4′-epiadriamycin (4′EPI) administered as a 6 hour (hr) infusion. *Proc. Am. Ass. Cancer Res.*, **23**, 129.

Sterrenberg, L., Julicher, R. H. M., Bast, A. and Noordhoek, J., 1984, Adriamycin stimulates NADPH-dependent lipid peroxidation in liver microsomes not only by enhancing the production of O_2 and H_2O_2, but also by potentiating the catalytic activity of ferrous ions. *Toxicol. Lett.*, **22**, 153–159.

Stuart, M. J., deAlarcon, P. A. and Barvinchak, M. K., 1978, Inhibition of adriamycin-induced human platelet lipid peroxidation by vitamin E. *Am. J. Hematol.*, **5**, 297–303.

Sugioka, K. and Nakano, M., 1982, Mechanism of phospholipid peroxidation induced by ferric ion-ADP-adriamycin-co-ordination complex. *Biochim. Biophys. Acta*, **713**, 333–343.

Sugioka, K., Nakano, H., Noguchi, T., Tsuchiya, J. and Nakano, M., 1981, Decomposition of unsaturated phospholipids by iron-ADP-adriamycin coordination complex. *Biochem. Biophys. Res. Commun.*, **100**, 1251–1258.

Sugioka, K., Nakano, H., Tsuchiya, J., Nakano, M., Sugioka, Y., Tero-Kubota, S. and Ikegami, V., 1984, Clear evidence for the participation of ·OH in gamma DNA breakage induced by the enzymatic reduction of adriamycin in the presence of iron-ADP. Importance of local ·OH concentration for DNA strand cleavage. *Biochem. Int.*, **9**, 237–242.

Svingen, B. A. and Powis, G., 1981, Pulse radiolysis studies on antitumor quinones: radical lifetimes, reactive with oxygen and one-electron reduction potentials. *Arch. Biochem. Biophys.*, **209**, 119–126.

Svingen, B. A., Powis, G., Appel, P. L. and Scott, M., 1981, Protection against adriamycin induced skin necrosis in the rat by dimethylsulfoxide and α-tocopherol. *Cancer Res.*, **41**, 3395–3399.

Takanashi, S. and Bachur, N. R., 1975, Daunorubicin metabolites in human urine. *J. Pharmacol. Exp. Ther.*, **195**, 41–49.

Takanashi, S. and Bachur, N. R., 1976, Adriamycin metabolism in man—evidence from urinary metabolites. *Drug Metab. Disp.*, **4**, 79–87.

Tewey, K. M., Rowe, T. C., Yang, L., Halligan, B. D. and Liu, L. F., 1984, Adriamycin-induced DNA damage mediated by mammalian DNA topoisomerase II. *Science*, **226**, 466–468.

Thayer, W. S., 1977, Adriamycin stimulated superoxide formation in submitochondrial particles. *Chem.-Biol. Interactions*, **19**, 265–278.

Thornalley, P. J. and Dodd, N. J. F., 1985, Free radical formation from normal and adriamycin-treated rat cardiac sarcomas. *Biochem. Pharmacol.*, **34**, 669–674.

Tobia, A. J., Couri, D. and Sagone, A., 1985, The effects of the quinone type drugs on hydroxyl radical (OH·) production by rat liver microsomes. *J. Tox. Envir. Hlth.*, **15**, 265–277.

Tong, G. L., Henry, D. W. and Acton, E. M., 1979, 5-Iminodaunorubicin, Reduced cardiotoxic properties in an antitumor anthracycline. *J. Med. Chem.*, **22**, 36–44.

Tritton, T. R., Murphree, S. A. and Sartorelli, A. C., 1978, Adriamycin: a proposal on the specificity of drug action. *Biochem. Biophys. Res. Commun.*, **84**, 802–808.

Turner, A. J. and Hick, P. E., 1976, Metabolism of daunorubicin by a barbiturate-sensitive aldehyde reductase from rat liver. *Biochem. J.*, **159**, 819–882.

Unverferth, D. V., Leier, C. V., Balcerzak, S. P. and Hamlin, R. C., 1985, Usefulness of a free radical scavenger in preventing doxorubicin-induced heart failure in dogs. *Am. J. Cardiol.*, **56**, 157–161.

Van Vleet, J. F., Ferrans, V. J. and Weirich, W. E., 1980, Cardiac disease induced by chronic adriamycin administration in dogs and an evaluation of vitamin E and selenium as cardioprotectants. *Am. J. Path.*, **99**, 13–42.

Vasanthakumar, G. and Ahmed, N. K., 1985, Uptake and metabolism of daunorubicin by human myelocytic cells. *Cancer Chemother. Rep.*, **15**, 35–39.

Weenen, H., Lankelma, J., Penders, P. A. M., McVie, J. G., Ten Bokkel Huinink, W. A., de Planque, M. M. and Pinedo, H. M., 1983, Pharmacokinetics of 4′-epi-doxorubicin in man. *Invest. New Drugs*, **1**, 59–61.

Weenen, H., Van Maanen, J. M. S. and DePlanque, M. M., 1984, Metabolism of 4′-modified analogs of doxorubicin. Unique glucuronidation pathway for 4′-epidoxorubicin. *Eur. J. Clin. Oncol.*, **20**, 919–926.

Weiss, A. J. and Manthel, R. W., 1977, Experience with the use of adriamycin in combination with other anticancer agents using a weekly schedule, with particular reference to lack of cardiac toxicity. *Cancer*, **40**, 2046–2052.

Winterbourn, C. C., 1981, Evidence for the production of hydroxyl radicals from the adriamycin semiquinone and H_2O_2. *FEBS Lett.*, **136**, 89–94.

Winterbourn, C. C., French, J. K. and Claridge, R. F. C., 1978, Superoxide dismutase as an inhibitor of reactions of semiquinone radicals. *FEBS Lett.*, **94**, 269–272.

Winterbourn, C. C. and Sutton, H. C., 1984, Hydroxyl radical production from hydrogen peroxide and enzymatically generated paraquat radicals: Catalytic requirements and oxygen dependence. *Arch. Biochem. Biophys.*, **235**, 116–126.

Yamanaka, N., Kato, T., Nishida, K., Fujikawa, T., Fukushima, M. and Ota, K., 1979, Elevation of serum lipid peroxide level associated with doxorubicin toxicity and its amelioration by [*dl*]-α-tocopheryl acetate or coenzyme Q10 in mouse (doxorubicin, toxicity, lipid peroxide, tocopherol, coenzyme Q10). *Cancer Chemother. Pharmacol.*, **3**, 223–227.

Yesair, D. W., Schwartzbach, E., Shuck, D., Denine, E. P. and Asbell, M. A., 1972, Comparative pharmacokinetics of daunomycin and adriamycin in several animal species. *Cancer Res.*, **32**, 1177–1183.

Yesair, D. W., Thayer, P. S., McNitt, S. and Teague, K., 1980, Comparative uptake, metabolism and retention of anthracyclines by tumors growing in vitro and in vivo. *Eur. J. Cancer*, **16**, 901–907.

Younes, M., Cornelius, S. and Siegers, C. P., 1985, Fe^{2+}-supported in vivo lipid peroxidation induced by compounds undergoing redox cycling. *Chem.-Biol. Interactions*, **54**, 97–103.

Young, R. C., Ozols, R. F. and Myers, C. E., 1981, Medical progress. The anthracycline antineoplastic drugs. *New Engl. J. Med.*, **305**, 139–153.

Youngman, R. J. and Elstner, E. F., 1981, Oxygen species in paraquat toxicity: the crypto-OH radical. *FEBS Lett.*, **129**, 265–268.

Youngman, R. J., Osswald, W. F. and Elstner, E. F., 1982 a, Crypto-OH· radical production by nitrofurantoin. *Biochem. Pharmacol.*, **31**, 603–606.

Youngman, R. J., Osswald, W. F. and Elstner, E. F., 1982 b, Mechanisms of oxygen activation by nitrofurantoin and relevance to its toxicity. *Biochem. Pharmacol.*, **31**, 3723–3729.

Zbinden, G., Bachmann, E. and Holnegger, C., 1978, Model systems for cardiotoxic effects of anthracyclines. *Antibiot. Chemother.*, **23**, 255–270.

Zenebergh, A., Baurain, R. and Trouet, A., 1984, Cellular pharmacology of detorubicin and doxorubicin in L1210 cells. *Eur. J. Cancer Clin. Oncol.*, **20**, 115–121.

Zini, G., Vicario, G. P., Lazzati, M. and Arcamone, F., 1984, Radioactive species in rat urines and tissues after [^{14}C] AD 32 administration. *Cancer Chemother. Pharmacol.*, **12**, 154–156.

Zweier, J. L., 1983, Reduction of O_2 by iron-adriamycin. *J. Biol. Chem.*, **259**, 6056–6058.

Zweier, J. L., 1985, Iron-mediated formation of an oxidized adriamcyin free radical. *Biochim. Biophys. Acta*, **839**, 209–213.

Zwelling, L. A., Kerrigan, D. and Michaels, S., 1982, Cytotoxicity and DNA strand breaks by 5-iminodaunorubicin and mouse leukemia L1210 cells: Comparison with adriamycin and 4′-(9-acridinylamino)methanesulfon-*m*-anisidide. *Cancer Res.*, **42**, 2687–2691.

9. Anti-steroidal agents

Simon P. Robinson and V. Craig Jordan

Historical introduction

Breast and prostate cancers are leading causes of cancer deaths in women and men throughout the world. Great efforts have been made to understand the causes of these diseases and to develop successful treatments.

Steroid hormones

More than 30 years before the first steroid hormone was isolated (Marrion, 1930), a supportive role in tumour growth had been indicated for an ovarian product (Beatson, 1896). Following the isolation of oestrone, intensive research was directed to identify steroidal hormones and to elucidate their metabolic pathways. These studies involved the development and application of chromatographic and column methods to separate steroids and physical methods such as X-ray crystallography, infra-red spectroscopy, mass spectroscopy and nuclear magnetic resonance to identify them. These techniques allowed some steps in hormone biosynthesis to be determined, but one of the crucial advances came with the use of radioactive compounds (deuterium, ^{14}C or tritium labelled). The use of radiolabelled compounds *in vivo* and the perfusion of isolated glands with media containing agents to be examined enabled the identification of specific biosynthetic pathways (for detailed reviews, see Dorfman and Ungar, 1965; Samuels and Eik-Nes, 1968; Briggs and Brotherton, 1970).

The information gathered from the biochemical investigations has been used to describe the biosynthesis of steroid hormones in the ovary, testis and adrenal gland. The synthetic pathway through to progesterone is common to all three glands. Enzyme differences after this point determine the nature of the major end product (see Figure 1).

Ablative and additive therapy

During the years when the steroid biosynthetic pathways were being elucidated, the treatment of cancer by surgery or hormone therapy was being developed and refined.

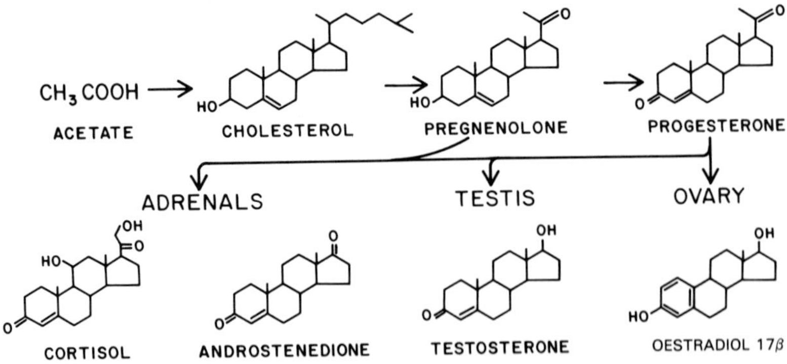

Figure 1. Biosynthetic pathway of steroid hormones.

When castration was first used, the reason for the success of the therapy in the treatment of breast or prostate cancer was obscure. The discovery of steroidal hormone synthesis in the ovary and testis presented a potential link with tumour growth and paved the way for experimentation with additive therapies. Haddow and co-workers (Haddow, 1938; Haddow *et al.*, 1944) showed that large doses of oestradiol benzoate retard breast tumour growth and they suggested that suppression of pituitary function was partially responsible for the growth inhibitory effect. High-dose oestrogen therapy was also found to be effective in the treatment of prostatic cancer and has been widely used up to the present day.

In 1952, Huggins and Bergenstal described the use of adrenalectomy as a further ablative therapy following castration for the treatment of both breast and prostate cancer. Adrenalectomy was made possible by replacement therapy using cortisone acetate to maintain salt balance. Huggins and Bergenstal (1952) speculated that the mechanism behind the anti-tumour action involved oestrogenic and/or androgenic changes, but at the time, details of hormone biosynthesis in the adrenals had not been elucidated.

Later the effect of hypophysectomy was examined on the basis of producing a "super castration" status in the patient. Some remissions were seen following this procedure (Luft and Olivecrona, 1953).

Steroid hormone receptor sites

A crucial step forward in understanding the interaction between hormone-producing glands and the growth of breast and prostate cancers was made when specific binding sites for oestrogens and androgens were identified in the steroid target tissues. The binding of the appropriate ligand to its receptor in the tumour cell was demonstrated to produce a cascade of biochemical events which initiates cell division. The availability of the ligand and the presence of receptor are, therefore, important in determining the tumour response.

Prediction of tumour response to endocrine therapy on the basis of presence or absence of oestrogen receptors in breast cancer biopsy specimens has been used to help select treatment regimes. This is recommended for breast cancer patients, as only 30–40% of an unselected patient population will respond to endocrine therapy. Preselection of patients who are oestrogen-receptor positive or are oestrogen- and progesterone-receptor positive increases the response rate to endocrine therapy to 60% and 80% respectively (McGuire, 1980).

Although androgen receptors have been determined in prostate cancer tissue, the 60–80% response rate to hormonal therapy makes selection unnecessary.

Clinical application of antisteroidal agents

Based on our current understanding of hormonal regulation of tumour growth, various medical strategies have been developed to treat hormone-dependent cancers (see Figures 2 and 3).

One in eleven women will experience breast cancer in their lifetime and the risk increases with age. Oestrogen will support the growth of approximately a third of these tumours. The oestrogen is produced predominantly in the

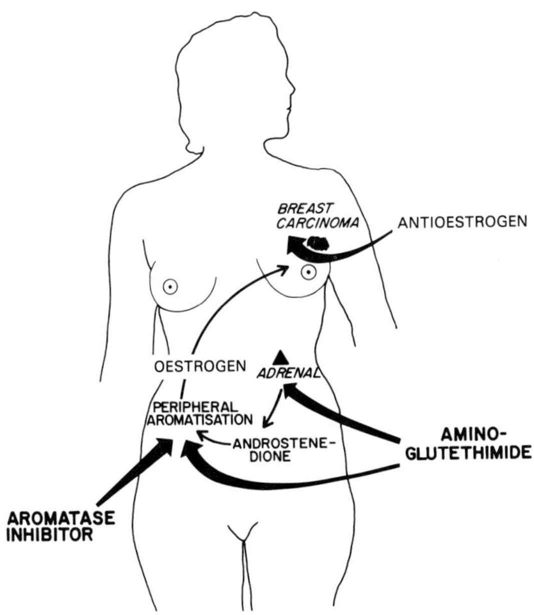

Figure 2. Sites of antisteroid hormone therapy of postmenopausal breast cancer.

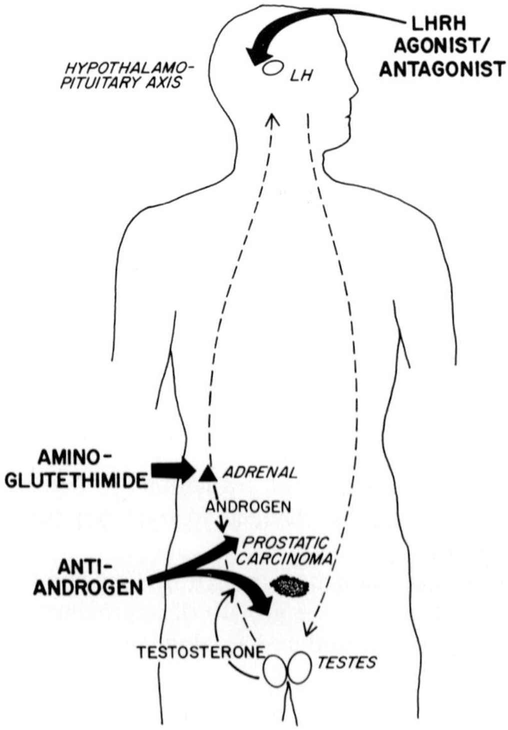

Figure 3. Sites of antisteroid hormone therapy of prostatic cancer.

ovary in premenopausal women or via peripheral aromatization of adrenal derived androstenedione in the postmenopausal women. However, even the low circulating levels observed in the postmenopausal women are sufficient to support tumour growth through oestrogen-receptor activation.

Anti-oestrogens

The non-steroidal anti-oestrogen tamoxifen is used extensively for the treatment of breast cancer (see Furr and Jordan, 1984, for review). Tamoxifen binds to the oestrogen receptor (to block oestrogen binding) and can initiate some oestrogen-like actions but is unable to promote cell division. This result in a blockage at the G_1/S interface of the breast cancer cell cycle (Osborne *et al.*, 1983; Sutherland *et al.*, 1983). The biochemical pharmacology of anti-oestrogens is extremely complex and no satisfactory theory for their mechanism of actions is applicable for all systems or species (Jordan, 1984).

Tamoxifen is initially effective for the treatment of breast cancer, in premenopausal patients (Furr and Jordan, 1984). Unfortunately, the anti-oestrogen inhibits the negative feedback mechanism for oestrogens to regulate the release of follicle-stimulating hormone (FSH) from the pituitary gland. An increase in the level of FSH occurs and, as a result, an increase in oestrogen biosynthesis. Clearly, this is not optimal for the control of oestrogen-dependent disease with a competitive oestrogen antagonist. The best application of tamoxifen is for the treatment of postmenopausal breast cancer in a low-oestrogen environment.

Tamoxifen is a tumouristatic agent and must be given for prolonged periods (Jordan, 1983). Fortunately, the drug has a low incidence of side-effects (Furr and Jordan, 1984) and several years of tamoxifen adjuvant therapy can be considered in order to prevent disease recurrence following mastectomy. Tamoxifen, either alone (Baum *et al.*, 1985) or in combination with chemotherapy (Fisher *et al.*, 1983) can significantly improve the disease-free interval. In fact, one study has shown that tamoxifen alone can improve the overall survival of node-positive patients (Baum *et al.*, 1985) and also prevent the development of a second primary breast cancer (Cuzick and Baum, 1985). Clinical trials are currently evaluating the long-term (greater than 5 years) use of tamoxifen as an adjuvant therapy to determine the optimal application of the drug in a low-oestrogen environment (Tormey and Jordan, 1984).

Inhibitors of steroid synthesis

Another approach to the treatment of breast cancer in postmenopausal women is to reduce the level of circulating oestrogen. This can be achieved with aminoglutethimide, which inhibits conversion of cholesterol into pregnenolone in the adrenals (Cash *et al.*, 1967) and the aromatization of androstenedione into oestrone in peripheral tissues (Santen *et al.*, 1978). However, aminoglutethimide is unable to control oestrogen production in the ovary (Santen *et al.*, 1980) and is, therefore, unsuitable for use in premenopausal women with breast cancer.

Inhibition of steroid metabolism in the adrenal gland by aminoglutethimide also affects glucocorticoid synthesis. If a glucocorticoid is not administered with this agent, a reflex rise in the secretion of adrenocorticotrophic hormone (ACTH) by the pituitary will ensue and the blockade of pregnenolone synthesis will be overcome. Hence, hydrocortisone is usually co-administered in order to prevent this reflex response.

Clinical trials have indicated a similar response rate for aminoglutethimide therapy to that for other forms of endocrine manipulation, but often a better control of bone pain is observed. Combined therapy with tamoxifen does not appear to be advantageous, but some patients who failed on tamoxifen alone have been found to respond to aminoglutethimide (Murray and Pitt, 1982).

The high frequency of dose-related side-effects with aminoglutethimide treatment is a major disadvantage with the agent. Interest has therefore been focused on the application of low-dose aminoglutethimide therapy aimed at inhibiting only peripheral aromatase enzymes. Similarly, new drugs are being developed which will only inhibit peripheral aromatization without affecting adrenal steroidogenesis.

LHRH analogues

The successful application of drugs to control adrenal steroidogenesis has focused attention upon medical methods to produce chemical castration. The repeated administration of superactive luteinizing hormone releasing hormone (LHRH) analogues has, somewhat paradoxically, been shown to achieve this effect (Klijn and Dejong, 1982). The castration-like response is produced by a desensitization of the pituitary gland which results in a reduced LH secretion and decreased stimulation of the gonads. The effect, however, occurs after an initial stimulation of the pituitary gland with an increased LH secretion for several days (Nicholson *et al.*, 1984).

LHRH agonist analogues have been used successfully in the treatment of breast cancer in premenopausal women and in the therapy of prostate cancer (see Schally *et al.*, 1984, for review). The side-effects of these agents are minimal. However, a tumour flare is sometimes seen in both breast and prostate cancer patients as a result of the initial stimulation of LH secretion.

Inhibition of the synthesis of androgens in the testis removes one of the major sources of male hormone. However, the prostate cancer cells may receive almost half of their androgenic stimulation from the adrenal glands (Labrie *et al.*, 1984).

Anti-androgens

A series of steroidal and non-steroidal anti-androgens have been developed and shown to be effective in the treatment of prostate cancer (Neri, 1976).

Cyproterone acetate was originally developed as a synthetic progestational agent and possesses substantial progestational activity as well as anti-androgenic properties. Cyproterone acetate does not produce a rise in LH secretion through the inhibition of the negative feedback produced by endogenous androgens on the hypothalamic pituitary axis. The difference between the gonadotrophin response to cyproterone acetate and the pure anti-androgens is probably a consequence of the progestational activity of cyproterone acetate producing an inhibition of LH secretion (Neumann and Schenck, 1976).

Unlike cyproterone acetate, the pure anti-androgens flutamide and RU 23908 inhibit the negative feedback on gonadotrophins by androgen. This makes the use of these agents inappropriate for the prolonged treatment of prostate cancer, as raised LH levels will result in an increased synthesis of testosterone by the Leydig cells of the testis. The combination of LHRH analogues and pure anti-androgens has recently been used on the basis that desensitization of the pituitary by the LHRH analogue will prevent any negative feedback on LH secretion. Dual therapy has the advantages over the LHRH analogue alone in that not only is there chemical castration but any remaining endogenous androgen (e.g., adrenal) will be prevented from stimulating tumour growth by competition for the androgen receptor with the anti-androgen (for review, see Labrie *et al.*, 1984).

The following sections of this chapter will consider the metabolism and pharmacokinetics of the antisteroidal agents currently being used or evaluated for the treatment of hormone-dependent breast and prostate cancer.

Tamoxifen: a non-steroidal anti-oestrogen

Structural features

The important structural features of the tamoxifen molecule (Figure 4) can be divided into two main categories: substitution in the phenyl equivalent to the A ring of the steroid nucleus, and alteration or removal of the dimethylaminoethoxy side-chain. Most of the important changes are observed with tamoxifen's different metabolites.

Introduction of a single *para*-hydroxyl into tamoxifen to produce Metabolite B (4-hydroxytamoxifen) markedly increases the affinity of the ligand for the oestrogen receptor (Jordan *et al.*, 1977) and the anti-oestrogenic

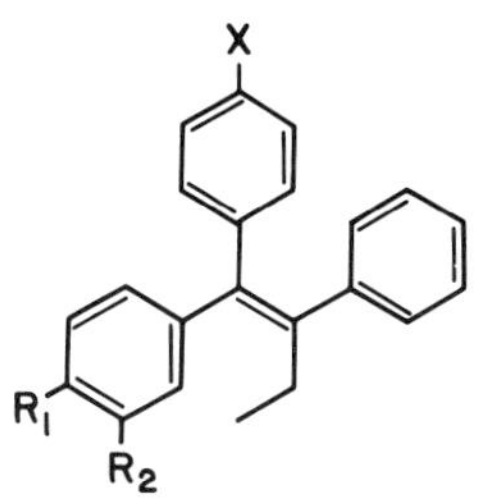

	R_1	R_2	X
Tamoxifen	H	H	$OCH_2CH_2N(CH_3)_2$
Metabolite B	OH	H	$OCH_2CH_2N(CH_3)_2$
Metabolite D	OH	OH	$OCH_2CH_2N(CH_3)_2$
Metabolite X	H	H	$OCH_2CH_2NHCH_3$
Metabolite Z	H	H	$OCH_2CH_2NH_2$
Metabolite Y	H	H	OCH_2CH_2OH
Metabolite E	H	H	OH

Figure 4. Metabolites of the anti-oestrogen tamoxifen.

potency. The introduction of two hydroxyls, one in the *para* and one in the *meta* position of tamoxifen to produce metabolite D again increases ligand affinity when compared to tamoxifen, but the anti-oestrogenic activity *in vivo* is low (Jordan *et al.*, 1977). This may be because the catechol derivative of tamoxifen is very unstable (Jordan *et al.*, 1984).

Modification of the side-chain of tamoxifen by removal of one methyl group (Metabolite X), two methyl groups (Metabolite Z) or replacement of the dimethylamine by hydroxyl (Metabolite Y) produces metabolites with low binding affinity for the oestrogen receptor and weak anti-oestrogenic activity (Jordan *et al.*, 1983; Kemp *et al.*, 1983). In contrast removal of the dimethylaminoethane side-chain to form Metabolite E produces a metabolite with a low binding affinity for the oestrogen receptor but oestrogenic properties (Jordan and Gosden, 1982).

Animal metabolism

The pharmacokinetics of tamoxifen have been studied extensively in laboratory animals. After i.v. injection of spayed female mice with [^{14}C]-tamoxifen, concentrations are higher after 5 min and 4 h in lung, liver, adrenal, kidney, pancreas, uterus, salivary glands and mammary tissue than in blood (Wilking *et al.*, 1981, 1982). Although high concentrations of drug would be predictable in the mammary glands and in the organs of metabolism and excretion, the high concentrations of tamoxifen in the pancreas and lung were not expected. There is, however, the possibility of binding to anti-oestrogen binding components in tissues which are not true oestrogen target tissues (Sutherland *et al.*, 1980; Sudo *et al.*, 1983).

Using [^{3}H]tamoxifen, Major *et al.* (1976) showed that radioactivity was concentrated and retained by the reproductive tract and pituitary gland of female rats. This was later confirmed by direct measurement when higher uterine, compared with blood, concentrations of both tamoxifen and *N*-desmethyltamoxifen were found (Adam, 1981 b). It was also shown in this study that tamoxifen was the predominant species in subcellular fractions of rat uterus. After administration of [^{14}C]tamoxifen to patients before hysterectomy, Fromson and Sharp (1974) found, perhaps predictably, radioactivity to be 2–3 times higher in uterus than in blood.

The distribution of [^{3}H]4-hydroxytamoxifen has been reported in the immature rat (Jordan and Bowser-Finn, 1982). This anti-oestrogen has a longer biological half-life than [^{3}H]oestradiol. However, like oestradiol, 4-hydroxytamoxifen binds (with oestrogen specificity) in the uterus and vagina. 4-Hydroxytamoxifen also accumulates in the liver, but this binding is not oestrogen-specific. The binding of 4-hydroxytamoxifen in the liver is, however, inhibited by the co-administration of other anti-oestrogens. This result demonstrates the ability of anti-oestrogens to bind to sites other than the oestrogen receptor.

The metabolism of ^{14}C-labelled tamoxifen in rat, mouse, rhesus monkey and dog was first reported by Fromson and co-workers (1973 a). Conversion of tamoxifen to 4-hydroxytamoxifen was observed in all species. However, several other metabolites have been identified (Figure 4). The catechol, metabolite D, is present as a glucuronide in the faeces of all species studied and Metabolite E, tamoxifen without the dimethylaminoethane side-chain, is found as a minor metabolite in dog bile.

4-Hydroxytamoxifen is the major metabolite of tamoxifen in the chicken (Borgna and Rochefort, 1981; Lazier and Jordan, 1982; Lyman and Jordan 1985 a) and *Xenopus* (Reigel *et al.*, 1986). Similarly, large doses of tamoxifen have been used to demonstrate metabolism to 4-hydroxytamoxifen in the ovariectomized rat (Bowman *et al.*, 1982). Nevertheless, several different polar metabolites have been observed but not characterized. Borgna and Rochefort (1981) described a polar metabolite, M2, which accumulates in the nucleus of rat uteri following [^{3}H]tamoxifen administration. Robertson and co-workers (1982) have also observed several polar metabolites of tamoxifen in rat uterus.

Borgna and Rochefort (1981) found that tamoxifen is converted to 4-hydroxytamoxifen by liver, chicken oviduct and lamb uterus, but not by rat uterus and MCF-7 breast cancer cells. Indeed, chick liver was used to produce the first quantity of [^{3}H]4-hydroxytamoxifen from [^{3}H]tamoxifen (Borgna and Rochefort, 1980). Rat liver microsomes convert tamoxifen to 4-hydroxytamoxifen and *N*-desmethyltamoxifen (Foster *et al.*, 1980). The *N*-oxide of tamoxifen has been identified as a metabolite of tamoxifen when microsomes from phenobarbital-treated rats are used (Foster *et al.*, 1980).

Ruenitz and co-workers (1984) have studied the effects of phenobarbital pretreatment on tamoxifen metabolism by rat liver microsomes. Barbiturate treatment caused an increase in *N*-demethylation and a decrease in 4-hydroxylation. The enzyme inhibitor metyrapone had no effect on tamoxifen metabolism by rabbit microsomes but decreased *N*-demethylation by rat microsomes. In contrast, SKF 525A inhibited microsomal metabolism in both species, although *N*-oxidation of tamoxifen was unaffected in either species. Two novel metabolites have also been observed: 4′-hydroxytamoxifen and tamoxifen epoxide (Ruenitz *et al.*, 1984). The epoxide may be a precursor of Metabolite A, a triphenylethanol reported originally by Fromson, Pearson and Bramah (1973 a) (Figure 5). There are no biological data about Metabolite A but the structurally related compound MER 25 is an anti-oestrogen in all species (Lerner *et al.*, 1958; Lyman and Jordan, 1985 b). The metabolite 4′-hydroxytamoxifen has a higher binding affinity for the oestrogen receptor than tamoxifen and is an anti-oestrogen *in vitro* (Jordan *et al.*, 1984) and *in vivo* (Ruenitz *et al.*, 1982).

Tamoxifen and its metabolites might also be able to alter the metabolism of other agents. Meltzer and co-workers (1984) have demonstrated that tamoxifen, *N*-desmethyltamoxifen and 4-hydroxytamoxifen are potent inhibitors of hepatic cytochrome P-450-dependent mixed-function oxidases. This finding

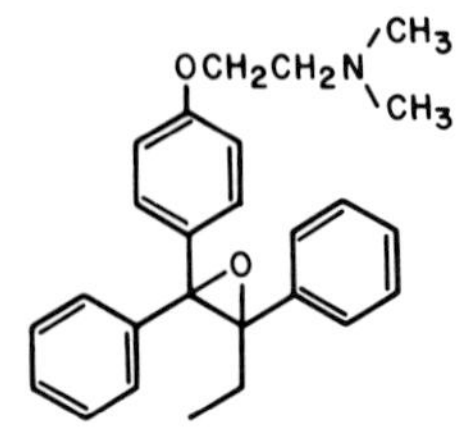

Tamoxifen epoxide

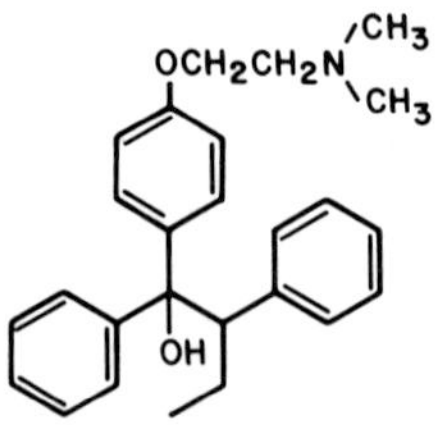

Metabolite A

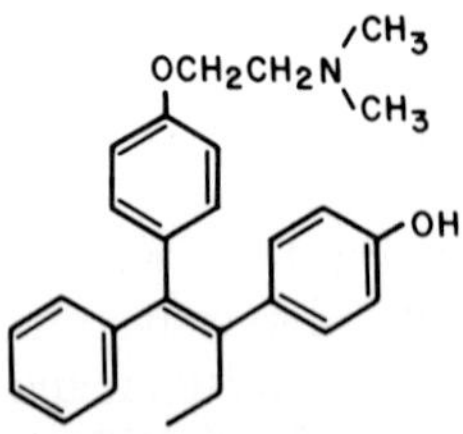

4' hydroxytamoxifen

Figure 5. Putative tamoxifen metabolites.

raises the question of whether tamoxifen can adversely affect the metabolism and excretion of cytotoxic cancer chemotherapeutic agents.

Human metabolism

Using [^{14}C]tamoxifen it has been shown that the drug is well absorbed and extensively metabolized after oral administration. The major metabolites are shown in Figure 4. Metabolites are excreted chiefly as conjugates in the bile and little or no tamoxifen is eliminated as unchanged drug. Urinary excretion appears to be greater in primates, including man, than in rodents but is still only a minor route of elimination of the drug.

A similar pattern of metabolites was found in animals and patient serum by thin-layer chromatography which led Fromson *et al.* (1973 b) to conclude, erroneously, that 4-hydroxytamoxifen was present in human serum at higher concentrations than the parent drug. It is now clear, however, that the chromatographic peak designated as 4-hydroxytamoxifen is, in fact, Metabolite X (*N*-desmethyltamoxifen). In serum from women treated with tamoxifen, 4-hydroxytamoxifen is only present at very low concentrations (Daniel *et al.*, 1979).

Recently Metabolite Y, a side-chain primary alcohol, has been identified in serum from women treated with tamoxifen (Bain and Jordan, 1983) and Metabolite Z (*N*-didesmethyltamoxifen) has been tentatively identified (Kemp *et al.*, 1983). In addition, using a combination of thin-layer chromatography (TLC) and a high-pressure liquid chromatography (HPLC) system (Brown *et al.*, 1983), Metabolite Y has been measured in patients on high dose (150 mg b.i.d.) tamoxifen therapy (Jordan *et al.*, 1983).

Assay methods have been developed for tamoxifen, 4-hydroxytamoxifen and *N*-desmethyltamoxifen, using either TLC, HPLC or gas chromatography–mass spectrometry (GC–MS). The assays used and their sensitivities are shown in Table 1. The compounds are estimated in TLC or HPLC assays by fluorescence detection after UV conversion to the phenanthrene derivatives. Alternatively, the ratio of peak heights of the molecular ion of a tamoxifen derivative and an internal standard are used to determine tamoxifen concentrations by high-resolution mass spectrometry after gas-liquid chromatography. These methods have been used to study the pharmacokinetics of tamoxifen in breast cancer patients.

Mendenhall *et al.* (1978) showed that after a single oral dose of 10 mg m^{-2} a peak serum value of 30 ng ml^{-1} was obtained after 3 h. This preliminary work was extended by Fabian and Sternson (1979) who found a median blood concentration of 16 ng ml^{-1} between 3 and 6 h after administration of the drug. After a single dose to patients with breast cancer, there is, however, a wide spread in serum concentrations; the differences between the highest and lowest values are around 20-fold at 3 h and 7-fold at 6 h after dosing (Fabian

Table 1. Assay methods available to measure the concentration of tamoxifen and metabolites

Assay procedure	Compound measured	Sensitivity	Reference
Thin-layer chromatography	Tamoxifen	2·5 ng	Adam *et al.* (1980 a)
	N-Desmethyltamoxifen	2·5 ng	Adam *et al.* (1980 b)
High-performance liquid chromatography	Tamoxifen	1 ng	Mendenhall *et al.* (1978)
	4-Hydroxytamoxifen	1 ng	Mendenhall *et al.* (1978)
	Tamoxifen	100 pg	Golander and Sternson (1980)
	N-Desmethyltamoxifen	100 pg	Golander and Sternson (1980)
	4-Hydroxytamoxifen	100 pg	Golander and Sternson (1980)
	Tamoxifen	2 ng	Brown *et al.* (1983)
	N-Desmethyltamoxifen	2 ng	Brown *et al.* (1983)
	Metabolite Y	1 ng	Brown *et al.* (1983)
	Tamoxifen	100 pg	Camaggi *et al.* (1983)
	N-Desmethyltamoxifen	100 pg	Camaggi *et al.* (1983)
	4-Hydroxytamoxifen	100 pg	Camaggi *et al.* (1983)
Gas chromatography –mass spectrometry	Tamoxifen	—	Gaskell *et al.* (1978)
	Tamoxifen	1 ng	Daniel *et al.* (1979)
	4-Hydroxytamoxifen	1 ng	Daniel *et al.* (1979)
	Tamoxifen	—	Daniel *et al.* (1981)
	N-Desmethyltamoxifen	—	Daniel *et al.* (1981)
	4-Hydroxytamoxifen	—	Daniel *et al.* (1981)
Gas chromatography	Tamoxifen	—	Sane *et al.* (1985)

et al., 1980). Similarly, Wilkinson *et al.* (1980) found mean peak serum concentrations of 17·4 ng ml^{-1}, ranging between 15 and 25 ng ml^{-1} at 3 h after a single oral dose of 10 mg tamoxifen, which is roughly equivalent to 15 mg m^{-2}. *N*-Desmethyltamoxifen was undetectable (<2·5 ng ml^{-1}) in this study.

In a detailed study in healthy male volunteers given a single oral dose of 20 mg tamoxifen, mean peak serum concentrations of tamoxifen and *N*-desmethyltamoxifen were 42 (range 35–45) and 12 (range 10–20) ng ml^{-1}, respectively (Adam *et al.*, 1980 a).

A number of studies have described the serum concentrations of tamoxifen, *N*-desmethyltamoxifen, 4-hydroxytamoxifen and Metabolite Y under steady-state conditions in women with breast cancer. The results of these studies, which show excellent agreement, are summarized in Table 2. Tamoxifen concentrations in blood are approximately 300 ng ml^{-1} after chronic doses of

Table 2. Concentrations of tamoxifen, *N*-desmethyltamoxifen, 4-hydroxytamoxifen and metabolite Y in blood from patients with breast cancer. The values shown are the mean with the range in parentheses. Drug administration in these studies was chronic.

Dose of tamoxifen	Compound measured	Concentration (ng ml^{-1})	Reference
10 mg b.i.d.	Tamoxifen	167 (143–197)	Daniel *et al.* (1979)
	4-HO-Tam	3·4 (2–5)	
10 mg m^{-2} b.i.d.	Tamoxifen	260	Fabian *et al.* (1980)
20 mg b.i.d.	Tamoxifen	285 (153–494)	Patterson *et al.* (1980)
	N-Desmethyl-Tam	477 (189–202)	
10 mg b.i.d.	Tamoxifen	125	Wilkinson *et al.* (1980)
	N-Desmethyl-Tam	160	
20 mg b.i.d.	Tamoxifen	300 (270–520)	Daniel *et al.* (1981)
	N-Desmethyl-Tam	462 (210–761)	
	4-HO-Tam	6·7 (2·8–11·4)	
20 mg m^{-2} after loading doses	Tamoxifen	163 (95–240)	Fabian *et al.* (1981); Fabian and Sternson (1981)
	N-Desmethyl-Tam	289 (187–325)	
	4-HO-Tam	10 (4–21)	
10 mg b.i.d.	Tamoxifen	165 (89–274)	Jordan (1982)
	N-Desmethyl-Tam	294 (208–452)	
10 mg b.i.d.	Tamoxifen	113 (77–189)	Jordan *et al.* (1983)
	N-Desmethyl-Tam	214 (163–265)	
	Metabolite Y	18 (5–49)	
20 mg b.i.d.	Tamoxifen	310 (164–494)	Kemp *et al.* (1983)
	N-Desmethyl-Tam	481 (300–851)	
	Metabolite Y	49 (22–136)	

4-HO-Tam is 4-hydroxytamoxifen and *N*-desmethyl-Tam is *N*-desmethyltamoxifen.

20 mg b.i.d. In all of the studies, concentrations of *N*-desmethyltamoxifen are about 50% higher than those of tamoxifen, while those of 4-hydroxytamoxifen are very low (approx. 3 ng ml^{-1} at 10 mg b.i.d. and approx. 6 ng ml^{-1} at 20 mg b.i.d.). In women, peak ^{14}C levels in serum were found 4–7 h after a single oral dose, but at the time only 20–30% of the radioactive material was tamoxifen. After an initial blood half-life of 7–14 h, serum concentrations of total radioactivity decayed with a secondary half-life of more than seven days. Using direct assay methods initial reports described the elimination half-life of tamoxifen in patients to be between 5 and 44 h (Fabian and Sternson, 1979; Wilkinson *et al.* 1980). However, when the duration of the study was extended, it became clear that the true half-life was around seven days for tamoxifen (Adam, 1981 b). This concurs with Patterson *et al.* (1980), who showed serum tamoxifen concentrations to be maximal 3 h after oral administration and that steady-state serum concentrations are achieved only after four weeks' treatment. Steady-state serum *N*-desmethyltamoxifen concentrations are reached after eight weeks, indicating a likely biological half-life for the metabolite of 14 days (Patterson *et al.*, 1980). In healthy males, half-lives of four and seven days for tamoxifen and *N*-desmethyltamoxifen, respectively, have been reported (Adam, 1981 a).

Relationship between metabolism and biological activity

One goal of the study of tamoxifen's metabolism in different species is to identify potentially oestrogenic metabolites which might explain the disparate pharmacology of the drug. Tamoxifen is a full oestrogen in the mouse, a partial oestrogen/anti-oestrogen in rats and humans, and in anti-oestrogen in chicks. The pharmacology of tamoxifen has recently been reviewed (Furr and Jordan, 1984; Jordan, 1984). As yet, however, no significant differences in the metabolism of tamoxifen in different species have been noted (Lyman and Jordan, 1985 a). In fact, there are some interesting biological models that argue against the idea that differential metabolism or the production of oestrogenic metabolites from tamoxifen is responsible for oestrogenic actions in the mouse. The breast cancer cell line MCF-7 will only grow into solid tumours in athymic mice if the animals are implanted with slow-release oestrogen pellets. Growth is dependent upon oestrogen stimulation. In contrast, tamoxifen causes an increase in the uterine weight of athymic mice but does not cause growth of implanted MCF-7 breast cancer cells (Gottardis *et al.*, 1985). Tamoxifen inhibits oestrogen-stimulated growth of MCF-7 breast cancer cells *in vivo* (Osborne *et al.*, 1985). The metabolism of tamoxifen in the athymic mouse is currently under investigation and 4-hydroxytamoxifen has been identified as the primary metabolite which binds to both the uterine and human tumour oestrogen receptor (S. P. Robinson and V. C. Jordan, unpublished observations). Since the same metabolites are sequestered in different tissues, the ligand–receptor complex must be interpreted differentially to act as either a growth promoter or a growth inhibitor.

The administration of [^{3}H]tamoxifen to immature rats results in the binding of polar metabolites in the uterus (Borgna and Rochefort, 1981). However, this should not imply that metabolic activation is required for the anti-oestrogen action of tamoxifen, because the pharmacokinetics of a single injection do not correspond to the steady-state conditions observed during continuous therapy. An extremely complex interaction of parent compound and metabolites with the oestrogen receptor will occur during the therapeutic use of anti-oestrogens.

If tamoxifen has to be converted to 4-hydroxytamoxifen before receptor binding in target tissues *in vivo*, then perhaps an inhibition of this metabolic step would yield compounds without activity. A series of 4 fluoro-, chloro- and methyl-derivatives of tamoxifen that cannot be converted to 4-hydroxytamoxifen have been shown to be weakly anti-oestrogenic in immature rat uterine weight tests (Allen *et al.*, 1980). Similarly, all the substituted derivatives of tamoxifen are partial oestrogen agonists in the rat uterus, but are less potent than tamoxifen. 4-Hydroxytamoxifen is, however, at least as potent as tamoxifen, suggesting that the effect of tamoxifen is probably the combined effect of the parent compound and this hydroxylated metabolite. In man, where *N*-desmethyltamoxifen is present at higher concentrations than tamoxifen and there are negligible concentrations of 4-hydroxytamoxifen present under steady-state conditions, *N*-desmethyltamoxifen may also contribute to the pharmacological activity observed (Reddel *et al.*, 1983).

Overall, these results suggest that conversion of tamoxifen to 4-hydroxytamoxifen and *N*-desmethyltamoxifen may be an advantage but is not a requirement for the inhibition of oestrogen action. This conclusion is consistent with the observed activity of tamoxifen *in vitro* where metabolism cannot be detected (Horwitz *et al.*, 1978). Furthermore, tamoxifen and 4-methyltamoxifen have a similar ability to inhibit the binding of [^{3}H]oestradiol to oestrogen receptors from rat pituitary glands and to inhibit oestradiol-stimulated increases in prolactin synthesis in cultures (Lieberman *et al.*, 1983).

Aminoglutethimide: an inhibitor of steroid synthesis

Structural features

Aminoglutethimide (Orimeten®) is the *p*-amino derivative of the hypnotic glutethimide (see Figure 6). *p*-Aminoglutethimide blocks the cholesterol side-chain cleaving enzyme desmolase, which converts cholesterol to pregnenolone, and the aromatase enzyme which converts androstenedione and testosterone to oestrone and oestradiol respectively (for review see Stuart-Harris and Smith, 1984). Structure–activity relationship studies have shown that the position of the amino group will markedly influence the degree and type of

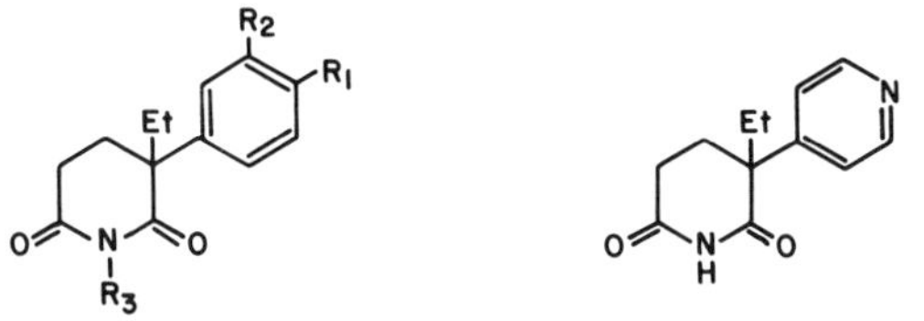

glutethimide = no substitutions
p-aminoglutethimide = NH_2 at R_1
m-aminoglutethimide = NH_2 at R_2
N-aminoglutethimide = NH_2 at R_3

4-pyridyl analogue

Figure 6. Derivatives of glutethimide and a structural analogue examined for aromatase and desmolase inhibitory activity.

enzyme-inhibiting activity. The parent compound glutethimide, for example, has little desmolase or aromatase inhibitory action. On the other hand, the *m*-amino or the *N*-amino derivatives (see Figure 6) have equal or more desmolase inhibitory activities respectively than *p*-aminoglutethimide itself, but only weak or no inhibitory activity on the aromatase enzyme (Foster *et al.*, 1983).

Substitution of pyridine for the aniline constituent of glutethimide to give 4-pyridyl-glutethimide (see Figure 6) produces an agent with strong inhibitory action on the aromatase system but devoid of desmolase inhibitory activity. The 2- and 3-pyridyl derivatives, however, inhibit neither enzyme system (Foster *et al.*, 1985).

The primary aromatic amine makes aminoglutethimide metabolism substantially different to that of glutethimide, by making the agent susceptible to *N*-acetylation.

Animal metabolism

Studies in the rat have shown aminoglutethimide is mainly (65%) absorbed from the lower intestine following oral administration. The maximum plasma concentration is reached 1 h after dosing and an even distribution throughout the tissues of the body occurs (Douglas and Nicholls, 1965). In the rat, elimination of [^{14}C]aminoglutethimide is almost complete 48–96 h after oral administration. The proportion in the urine or faeces is dependent on the dose administered, more being found in the urine at higher doses (Egger *et al.*, 1982).

Nicholls (1982) reported that oral administration of [^{14}C]aminoglutethimide (60 mg/kg) to rats resulted in excretion of 10% in the faeces, 1% in expired air and the remainder in the urine. Similar administration to the guinea-pig resulted in 51% of the dose being eliminated in the urine and 40% in the faeces, whereas the rabbit excreted the whole dose in the urine.

Intravenous administration of [^{14}C]aminoglutethimide to rats results in a

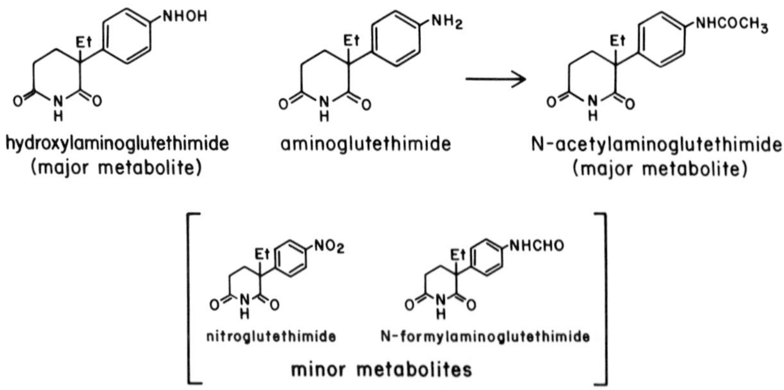

Figure 7. Aminoglutethimide and metabolites.

substantial amount of radioactivity in the faeces, suggesting biliary excretion. Studies using bile-duct-cannulated rats confirm this and indicate that entero-hepatic circulation is probable (Egger *et al.*, 1982; Nicholls, 1982).

The major urinary metabolite found in rats, guinea-pigs and rabbits is the *N*-acetyl derivative (Nicholls, 1982) (see Figure 7). In the rat this constitutes 37% of the urinary excretion. Detailed analysis using [^{14}C]aminoglutethimide has identified eight other minor metabolites, six of which have acetyl groups. The main metabolic reactions accounting for the metabolites are acetylation and hydroxylation with cleavage of the glutarimide ring.

Only about 4% of rat urinary excretion was in the form of amino-glutethimide itself. A small amount of *p*-nitroglutethimide has also been detected, but this may be the result of an impurity in the original agent administered, because aminoglutethimide is synthesized from *p*-nitroglutethimide.

Biliary excretion is less complex, with 22% being unchanged drug and 8% *N*-acetylaminoglutethimide and *p*-nitroglutethimide. However, the bulk of radioactivity (45%) from bile extracts was not separated in the TLC system used (Egger *et al.*, 1982).

Human metabolism

Plasma levels of aminoglutethimide reach a maximum (5·6–6·3 μg/ml) 0·7–1·5 h after oral administration of 2 × 250 mg tablets. Plasma proteins bind about 25% of aminoglutethimide and the plasma half-life is about 10–15 h (Thompson *et al.*, 1982; Nicholls, 1981). Blood cells *in vitro* have been found to contain 1·4–1·7 times the concentration of aminoglutethimide found in plasma.

The major urinary metabolite of aminoglutethimide in humans was first identified by Douglas and Nicholls (1965) as *N*-acetylaminoglutethimide (see Figure 7). Subsequent studies have examined the influence of acetylator phenotype on the ability to metabolize aminoglutethimide. In one study subjects characterized as slow acetylators excreted more aminoglutethimide (28% at 250 mg dose) than subjects characterized as rapid acetylators (12%), whereas the rapid acetylators excrete more *N*-acetylaminoglutethimide (8·8% at 250 mg dose) than slow acetylators (3·9%) (Coombes *et al.*, 1982). These findings were supported by similar studies performed by Adam *et al.* (1984). Paradoxically the latter authors found that the half-life of aminoglutethimide is longer in fast acetylators (19·5 h) than slow acetylators.

Analysis of urine has, as in the rat, identified the presence at low levels of nitroglutethimide (see Figure 7). These findings do not exclude the possibility that this precursor in the synthesis of aminoglutethimide was not administered as a contaminant. However, the difference in levels of this compound in urine between slow (0·1% of dose) and fast (0·047% of dose) acetylators suggests that metabolism has an influence on its abundance. *N*-Formylaminoglutethimide (see Figure 7) has also been identified as a further minor metabolite (Coombes *et al.*, 1982).

Following prolonged treatment with aminoglutethimide, the half-life is significantly reduced as a consequence of enzyme induction. The amount of *N*-acetylation decreases and a new derivative, hydroxylaminoglutethimide, becomes the major urinary metabolite (see Figure 7). Hydroxylaminoglutethimide is not detectable after a single dose and requires aminoglutethimide to induce oxidation pathways to cause its production (Gross *et al.*, 1985). The production of this derivative has not been observed in the rat even after 23 days of treatment. This suggests a difference in metabolic pathways between the species.

Activity of metabolites

Patients receiving aminoglutethimide initially experience many side-effects (e.g., rash, fever, lethargy, dizziness, ataxia), but these diminish after the first few weeks of treatment. During the initial period of medication, the half-life of aminoglutethimide is markedly reduced and the major metabolite changes from *N*-acetylaminoglutethimide to hydroxylaminoglutethimide. However, the severity of the side-effects has not been related to metabolite formation (Murray *et al.*, 1979).

The metabolites detected in human urine following single doses of aminoglutethimide do not appear to play a positive role in preventing steroid formation, as the major metabolite, *N*-acetylaminoglutethimide, has no aromatase or desmolase inhibitory action and the minor metabolites, *N*-formylaminoglutethimide and nitroglutethimide, are only weakly active (Foster *et al.*, 1983).

Hydroxylaminoglutethimide is pharmacologically less active than the parent compound (Chohan *et al.*, 1982) but is more active than *N*-acetylaminoglutethimide. The change in the major metabolite from the *N*-acetyl derivative to the hydroxyl derivative during prolonged therapy with aminoglutethimide represents a potential improvement in enzyme-inhibiting activity on the basis of *in vitro* studies. However, the shorter half-life for aminoglutethimide after enzyme induction would suggest an overall adverse influence through more rapid clearance and potentially decreased inhibitory activity.

The oxidative enzymes induced by aminoglutethimide not only influence its own half-life but also those of other drugs. This is illustrated by a decrease in the biological half-life of dexamethasone and warfarin during therapy with aminoglutethimide (Murray *et al.*, 1979).

Luteinizing hormone releasing hormone analogues

Structural features

LHRH is a decapeptide (see Figure 8) which has blocked N-(Pyro Glu) and C ($Gly\text{-}NH_2$) terminals, making it resistant to conventional amino or carboxy-peptidases. However, degradation of LHRH has been observed in several tissues and the circulating half-life is very short (for review see Griffiths and McDermott, 1983).

Stabilization of the LHRH peptide to give superactive agonists has been achieved by the substitution of Gly^6 and $Gly\text{-}NH_2{}^{10}$. Insertion of certain D-amino acids for Gly^6 and ethylamine or azo-Gly for $Gly\text{-}NH_2{}^{10}$ not only reduces enzymatic degradation by brain homogenates but also increases the binding affinity for the LHRH receptor (Griffith and Hopkinson, 1979;

1 2 3 4 5 6 7 8 9 10

Pyro Glu – His – Trp – Ser – Tyr – Gly – Leu – Arg – Pro – Gly NH_2

LHRH

Pyro Glu – His – Trp – Ser – Tyr – D-Ser (Bu^t) – Leu – Arg – Pro – NH ET

Hoe 766 (Buserelin)

Pyro Glu – His – Trp – Ser – Tyr – D-Leu – Leu – Arg – Pro – NH ET

A 43818 (Leuprolide)

Pyro Glu – His – Trp – Ser – Tyr – D-Ser (Bu^t) – Leu – Arg – Pro – Az Gly NH_2

ICI 118630 (Zoladex)

Pyro Glu – His – Trp – Ser – Tyr – D-Nal (2) – Leu – Arg – Pro – Gly NH_2

Nafarelin

Figure 8. The structures of luteinizing hormone releasing hormone and four agonist analogues undergoing clinical evaluation.

Loumaye *et al.*, 1982). Examples of some superactive agonist analogues currently in clinical trials are shown in Figure 8.

Substitutions in the 6 position with novel hydrophobic "amino acids" have been examined to increase binding to plasma membranes and hydrophobic carrier proteins in order to reduce renal clearance. Nafarelin (see Figure 8), for example, has a half-life of 2·4 h following s.c. administration, compared to 4–12 minutes for LHRH itself. The ratio of bound to free determined in plasma for Nafarelin, using equilibrium dialysis, is 80 : 20, whereas LHRH is only 25 : 75 (Nestor *et al.*, 1984). Buserelin (see Figure 8) on the other hand, is bound to serum proteins to about the same extent as LHRH and has a similar rate of elimination even though it is less susceptible to enzyme degradation.

Pyro Glu^1, His^2 and Trp^3 has been found to be a vital region in the maintenance of agonist activity. Removal of the His^2 produces a partial agonist. Replacement by D-Phe produces a weak antagonist. This finding has been used in the development of superactive antagonists (Horsthemke *et al.*, 1981).

Animal metabolism

Studies in the rat, dog, pig and ewe show that LHRH is rapidly cleared from the circulation (initial $t_{1/2} = 3–12$ min). The removal of the Gly-NH_2 terminal and introduction of ethylamide and substitution of D-Ser or D-Ser (Bu^t) for Gly^6 produce analogues with resistance to enzyme degradation, but these alterations do not prolong the circulating half-life (Swift and Crighton, 1979; Bennett and McMartin, 1979; Sandow *et al.*, 1984).

Studies examining the distribution of tritium-labelled LHRH in rats and mice show an accumulation in the anterior and posterior pituitary, pineal gland, kidney and liver (Redding and Schally, 1973; DuPont *et al.*, 1974). Accumulation of ^{125}I-labelled LHRH in the pituitary has been reported to last less than 10 minutes whereas ^{125}I-labelled Buserelin was still present in significant levels 60 minutes after injection (Sandow and Kong, 1979).

Analysis of tissue samples from male rats following injection of ^{125}I-labelled Buserelin showed metabolism in the liver and kidney was to the 4–9 hexapeptide and in the anterior pituitary to an unknown metabolite, possibly the 2–9 octapeptide (Sandow *et al.*, 1980).

Urinary excretion in the rat of immunoreactive Buserelin has been reported to be 30% of the dose administered, whereas the excretion of immunoreactive LHRH averaged only 0·23%. These findings are in keeping with the analogues having a greater stability to enzyme degradation than LHRH.

Detailed studies of renal metabolism of LHRH have been performed primarily on the rat and rabbit. Proximal tubule brush border metablism has been demonstrated to result in the formation from LHRH of Pyro Glu-His, Pyro Glu-His-Trp and Pyro Glu-His-Trp-Ser and additional intracellular metabolism to produce Pyro Glu (Carone *et al.*, 1982; Stetler-Stevenson *et al.*, 1981, 1983).

Studies in vitro

Synthetic LHRH is rapidly degraded when incubated with liver or kidney homogenate extracts from sheep, dogs and pigs (Bennett and McMartin, 1979; Swift and Crighton, 1979). However, plasma of rat, guinea-pig, chicken, dog or sheep origin has little if any degrading activity (for reviews see Bennett and McMartin, 1979; Griffiths and Kelly, 1979).

Both the supernatant and particulate fractions of rat hypothalamic and pituitary homogenates contain enzymes capable of degrading LHRH. The enzymes in these two tissues have been demonstrated to be very similar.

Changes in the LHRH-degrading activity in different regions of the hypothalamus has been described and an influence of hormonal treatment on this activity observed (for reviews, see Griffiths and Kelly, 1979; Griffiths and McDermott, 1983).

Since only a small fraction of the circulation passes through the pituitary and hypothalamus, little effect of these tissues would be expected on blood levels of LHRH or its analogues. However, the enzymes may influence intra-tissue concentrations of these peptides. The main enzymes involved in deactivation are an endopeptidase which cleaves between amino acids 5 and 6 of LHRH and a post-proline-cleaving enzyme acting on the Pro^9–Gly^{10}-NH_2 bond. The substitution of D-amino acids for Gly^6 and alteration by either deletion or substitution of the C terminal produces analogues protected from these enzymes (see analogues shown in Figure 8).

Human metabolism

The half-life of LHRH in humans is similar to that determined in laboratory animals (see Bennett and McMartin, 1979 for review). However, renal metabolism may differ slightly from the rat and rabbit, as Pyro Glu has been identified in the urine of subjects following [^3H]LHRH administration (Redding *et al.*, 1973).

In patients receiving high-dose Buserelin to treat prostate cancer, only the parent compound was identified in plasma but a second non-biologically active metabolite was observed in urine samples (Sandow *et al.*, 1984).

Activity of peptide fragments

The replacement of the C-terminal glycinamide of LHRH with ethylamide stabilizes the peptide to degradation without loss of biological activity (Griffiths and Hopkinson, 1979; Horsthemke *et al.*, 1981). However, removal of the C-terminal glycinamide from LHRH substantially reduces its ability to cause LH release *in vivo* (Griffiths *et al.*, 1975). Removal of Pro^9-Gly-NH_2^{10} leaving the LHRH (1–8) octapeptide decreases the biological activity to 0·01% of the complete LHRH decapeptide (Monaham *et al.*, 1972).

Studies performed on Buserelin indicate not only a reduced susceptibility to metabolism but also activity of some of the metabolites. Buserelin has been demonstrated to be metabolized to the 4–9 hexapeptide and perhaps the 2–9 octapeptide (Sandow *et al.*, 1980). Sandow and Konig (1979) showed the induction of ovulation in phenobarbitone-blocked rats can be achieved by Buserelin fragments 3–9, 4–9, 5–9 and even 6–9, although more compound is required as the peptide is shortened.

The removal of the comparable N-terminal amino acids of LHRH leaving the 3–10 octapeptide results in an almost complete loss of activity in a test comparable to that used for Buserelin fragments (Sandow *et al.*, 1976). The loss of activity with N-terminal deletions in LHRH but only partial loss with similar deletions in Buserelin may be the consequence of a resistance to further degradation arising from the D-Ser $(Bu^t)^6$ or Des-Gly-NH_2^{10} ethylamide alterations. The relevance of this to the prolonged activity of the analogues of LHRH is uncertain.

Steroidal and non-steroidal anti-androgens

Structural features

The anti-androgens can be divided into two groups on the basis of structure. The first group to be developed was based on the steroid nucleus. The most clinically useful agent in the steroidal anti-androgens is cyproterone acetate. This drug is a hydroxyprogesterone derivative (see Figure 9) and was initially examined as a potential orally active progestogen (see Neumann *et al.*, 1979). Studies have demonstrated a high affinity for the progesterone receptor and the production of progestational responses. The progestational activity of cyproterone acetate prevents the rise in LH that is seen with other anti-androgens. In contrast, cyproterone (the free alcohol) has a much lower

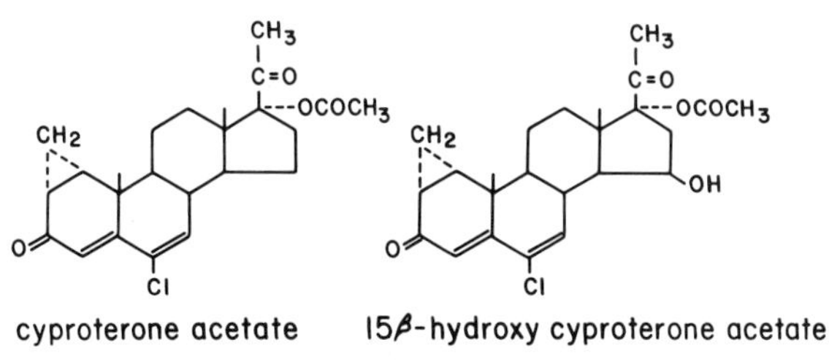

Figure 9. Cyproterone acetate and its major metabolite.

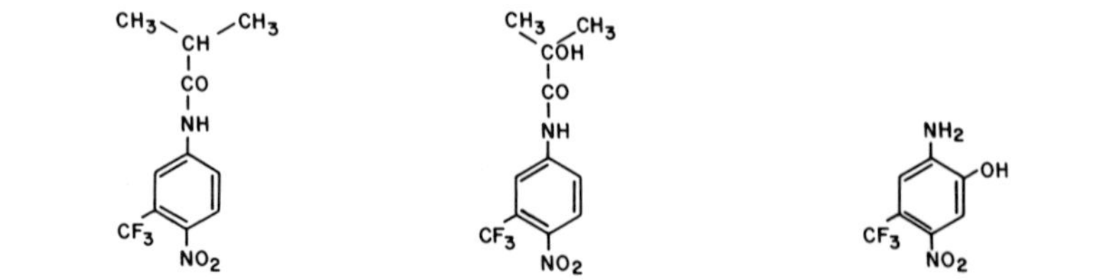

Figure 10. Metabolites of flutamide.

affinity for the progesterone receptor and little progestational activity (Grill *et al.*, 1985).

The second group of anti-androgens are non-steroidal compounds. Until recently, flutamide was accepted as the major clinically useful non-steroidal anti-androgen (see Figure 10). The drug appears to be specific for androgen receptors and does not interact with other steroid systems. The selectivity of action has given rise to the term "pure anti-androgen".

RU 23908 was developed from flutamide and has recently been introduced into clinical trials. This agent, like flutamide, is a pure anti-androgen (see Raynaud *et al.*, 1984 for review) and causes a rise in LH in men because it blocks the negative feedback mechanism by testosterone in the hypothalamo-pituitary axis. The increase in testosterone that results makes the pure anti-androgens poor candidates for the treatment of prostate cancer. Although this is a rapidly expanding area of research, it should be pointed out that very little has been published about the structure–activity relationships of anti-androgens.

Animal metabolism

Cyproterone acetate

The systemic absorption of cyproterone acretate is extensive following oral administration to rats, dogs and monkeys. The circulating half-life, as determined by radioimmunoassay of plasma following an intravenous injection of cyproterone acetate, is similar for the rat (26·3 h) and rhesus monkey (25·3 h) but considerably longer in the dog (109 h) (Düsterberg *et al.*, 1981).

Schulz (1976) found, using radiolabelled cyproterone acetate, an average of 81% absorption of an oral dose in the monkey and a circulating half-life of 1·6–1·8 days. Radioactivity in the urine and faeces was in the ratio of 0·7 : 1·0 respectively.

Shortly (30 min) after intravenous administration of [^{3}H]cyproterone acetate to male rats, a large amount of radioactivity accumulates in the liver.

The radioactivity is, however, predominantly associated with a metabolite rather than the parent compound. Similarly, analysis of plasma demonstrates that the principal peak of radioactivity is also associated with a metabolite. Nevertheless, cyproterone acetate is the predominant compound identified in androgen target tissues such as the prostate, seminal vesicles and bulbo-cavernosus and levator ani muscle (Szalay *et al.*, 1975).

Analysis of dog plasma following long-term (4 weeks) oral treatment (100 mg/kg/day) with cyproterone acetate has identified a 15β-hydroxy derivative (11 μg/ml) as well as the parent (4 μg/ml) (see Figure 9). In plasma samples from rhesus monkey following long-term (12 weeks) oral treatment (40 mg/kg/day) with cyproterone acetate, only minimal amounts of unconjugated 15β-hydroxycyproterone acetate and cyproterone acetate were detected (0·5 μg/ml plasma). The major metabolite found in the urine of these monkeys was the 15β-hydroxy derivative. Additional undetermined minor metabolites were also observed (Bhargava *et al.*, 1977).

In the female rat, cyproterone acetate has been shown to cause considerable enlargement of the liver and to be a potent inducer of hepatic microsomal mono-oxygenase activity. This effect is less pronounced in the male rat and has been attributed to the inhibition of endogenous androgens which are known to induce certain pathways of drug metabolism (Schulte-Hermann and Parzefall, 1980; Schulte-Hermann *et al.*, 1980).

Flutamide and RU 23908

Few studies have been published on the metabolism of these agents in animals.

From studies performed with flutamide on rat prostate tissue *in vivo* and on tissue *in vitro*, a disparity was observed between the activities in the two systems. It was hypothesized that a metabolite of flutamide may be the active agent. A study in humans was used to identify the metabolic pathway (see following section) and a hydroxy derivative was identified as the major plasma metabolite (see Figure 10). A similar metabolic pathway has been indicated for the rat (see review by Neri, 1976).

The metabolism and excretion of [^{14}C]RU 23908 by the rat has been studied and reported by Raynaud and co-workers (1985). Absorption following oral administration of [^{14}C]RU 23908 (10 mg/kg) to rats is rapid and radioactivity in the plasma reaches a peak equivalent to 5–6 μg/ml of drug. The major proportion of plasma radioactivity observed is related to unchanged compound. The terminal half-life reported in the rat is 11 h.

The major route of excretion of [^{14}C]RU 23908 in the rat (two thirds of the radioactivity) is via the kidneys after either oral or intravenous administration. The majority (94%) of the urinary excretion takes place in the first two days. Analysis of rat urine following enzyme hydrolysis has identified the metabolites shown in Figure 11 as the major contributors to the radioactivity found in urine. Only very small quantities of the parent compound is excreted.

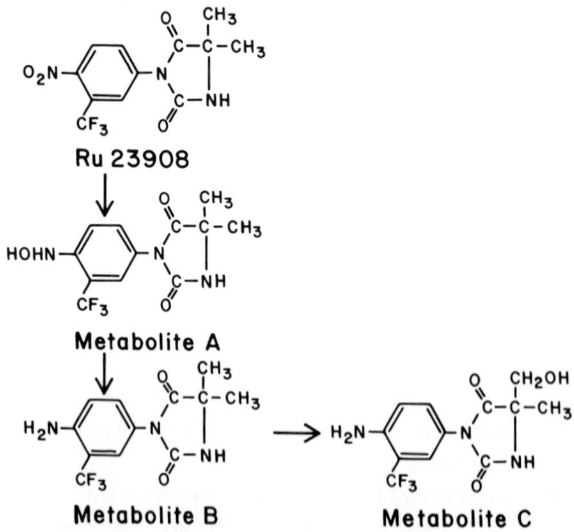

Figure 11. Major route of metabolism of RU 23908.

The major metabolites are compounds resulting from partial (metabolite A) and full (metabolite B) reduction of the nitro group or the primary alcohol of metabolite B (metabolite C).

Human metabolism

Cyproterone acetate

Cyproterone acetate is almost completely absorbed following oral dosing (2 mg) and plasma levels are maximum by 1–4 h. Plasma half-life of cyproterone acetate is 1·5–2 days. About 30–35% of the total dose administered is excreted in the urine and about 50–60% in the faeces within 8–10 days (Speck *et al.*, 1976; Humpel *et al.*, 1977).

Repeated doses of cyproterone acetate (2 mg/day) result in increasing circulating levels of this agent. This accumulation reaches steady-state levels after 5–8 days of treatment which is 2–3 times that observed after a single administration. The apparent volume of distribution for cyproterone acetate is larger than that of body fluids, indicating a distribution into body fats (Humpel *et al.*, 1979).

The major metabolite of cyproterone acetate in man is the 15β-hydroxy derivative. Plasma levels of this metabolite reach about twice the levels of cyproterone acetate itself (Frith and Phillipou, 1985). This more polar metabolite has a much smaller apparent volume of distribution than cyproterone acetate and is the predominant urinary product. Hence overall, there appears to be a steady state reached between re-transfer of cyproterone acetate from tissue, metabolism to 15β-hydroxy cyproterone acetate and/or elimination. The lipophilic nature of cyproterone acetate may be the determining factor in its long half-life.

Predominantly free metabolite and parent compound are excreted in the urine. About 30% of the metabolites in the urine and 50–60% in the bile are conjugated with glucuronic acid and 10% in both as sulphates (see Hümpel *et al.*, 1979, for detailed studies of pharmacokinetics).

Flutamide and RU 23908

Flutamide is rapidly and extensively absorbed following oral administration to humans and significant absorption has been reported following topical application (Katchen *et al.*, 1976; Katchen and Buxbaum, 1975). Extensive metabolism of flutamide occurs. Just one hour after oral administration, levels of hydroxyflutamide (see Figure 10), the major plasma metabolite, were 10 times that of flutamide itself. The rapid appearance of this metabolite suggests a first pass metabolism. The metabolic pathway for flutamide has been proposed as removal, by stepwise oxidation, of the isobutyryl side-chain followed by hydroxylation of the resulting nitroaniline or phenylenediamine (Katchen and Buxbaum, 1975).

Excretion of tritium-labelled flutamide has been observed to be mainly through the kidney. Glusulase hydrolysis of urine samples results in an increase of extractable tritium from 44·7% to 77·5%. The major urinary metabolite has been identified as ααα-trifluoro-2-amino-5-nitro-*p*-cresol, which constitutes 32% of the extractable radioactivity (see Figure 10) (Katchen and Buxbaum, 1975).

Activity of metabolites

Cyproterone acetate

The 15β-hydroxy derivative of cyproterone acetate has been observed to have a greater inhibitory action of the sebaceous gland function than the parent compound following systemic administration. The activity of this major metabolite in the classical target organs is, however, less than that of cyproterone acetate (Neumann *et al.*, 1979).

15β-Hydroxycyproterone acetate has a much lower binding affinity for the progesterone receptor than cyproterone acetate and has considerably less progestational activity (Frith and Phillipou, 1985; Grill *et al.*, 1985).

In vitro studies indicate the formation of the 15β-hydroxy derivative is not required for anti-androgen activity.

Flutamide

Hydroxyflutamide has been observed to be capable of inhibitory testosterone propionate stimulation of prostate and seminal vesicles in castrate rats. This major metabolite was about 1·5 times as active as flutamide in this test. Both flutamide and its hydroxy derivative inhibit the uptake of radiolabelled androgen into rat prostate tissue *in vivo*. However, *in vitro* flutamide is considerably less effective than its metabolites in inhibiting the uptake of androgen (Neri *et al.*, 1979). The higher binding affinity of hydroxyflutamide than flutamide for the androgen receptor supports the suggestion that this metabolite is the active form *in vivo*.

Other metabolites of flutamide possess little or no anti-androgenic activity (Neri, 1976).

RU 23908

The binding affinity of RU 23908 for the androgen receptor is similar to that of hydroxyflutamide (Wakeling *et al.*, 1981). A study *in vitro* designed to examine possible activation to a more potent agent found no evidence for this (Brown *et al.*, 1981). Investigations using metabolites A and B of RU 23908 (see Figure 11) indicate that these compounds are unable to bind to the androgen receptor (Raynaud *et al.*, 1985).

Future directions

Tamoxifen and the LHRH analogue Leuprolide are the only drugs of the anti-steroidal agents discussed to have been passed by the FDA for clinical use in the treatment of hormone-dependent cancer; the other agents are under investigation in clinical trials. Clearly more of these agents will become available for clinical application in the future.

From the promising reports from trials using aminoglutethimide, increased interest is focused to find new treatment regimens and therapeutic agents which produce fewer side-effects but are equally or more effective in suppressing oestrogen production.

Trials are being performed using low-dose (125 mg twice daily) aminoglutethimide therapy (Stuart-Harris *et al.*, 1984). Although the dose is lower than usually used to cause adrenal inhibition through desmolase blockade, effective aromatase inhibition is still achieved and a suppression of oestrogen levels produced (Harris *et al.*, 1983). In these recent studies some objective response has been reported with this regimen (Stuart-Harris and Smith, 1984). The number and degree of severity of side-effects have been reduced with low-dose therapy (Cantwell *et al.*, 1984). However, care is needed to ensure that the auto-induction of metabolic enzymes by repeated administration does not reduce circulating levels of aminoglutethimide to ineffective levels.

Studies have started on the novel compounds trilostane and ketoconazole, which have been found to inhibit steroid biosynthetic pathways. In the case of ketoconazole, interaction with the cytochrome P-450 enzyme complex involved with C_{17-20} lyase has been indicated (Vanden Bossche *et al.*, 1985). Studies with ketoconazole have so far been concentrated on the inhibition of testosterone synthesis (Pont *et al.*, 1982). Prolonged treatment with low doses of ketoconazole results in a compensating rise in LH levels, which overcomes the blockade of steroid synthesis. High-dose therapy, however, may not be overcome in this manner (Santen *et al.*, 1983). Some suppression of cortisol synthesis has also been reported.

Trilostane has been shown to inhibit adrenal steroid biosynthesis and has been successfully used in the treatment of some cases of Cushing's Syndrome (Komanicky *et al.*, 1978). The use of this agent in breast cancer therapy without combination with corticosteroid supplement has been reported to be ineffective (Coombes *et al.*, 1985), whereas with corticosteroid replacement, a more favourable response was observed (Beardwell *et al.*, 1983).

Work in the LHRH analogue field has resulted in the production of LHRH antagonists with high affinity for the LHRH receptor and a prolonged duration of action (Nestor *et al.*, 1984; Geiger, 1984). LHRH analogue antagonists have yet to be tested clinically but the application of these analogues may avoid the problems of flare often seen with agonists.

As briefly mentioned previously, the combination of LHRH analogues and pure anti-androgens theoretically is more effective for the treatment of prostate cancer than either given alone. Clinical trials have indicated a very high response rate with this type of combination (Labrie *et al.*, 1984). The use of other dual or triple combinations to ensure total suppression of endocrine stimulation are also possible. The use of LHRH analogues in combination with anti-oestrogen would be a possible approach to treating premenopausal breast cancer. The addition of an adrenal or aromatase inhibitory agent to ensure complete suppression is logical on the basis of our current understanding of steroid biosynthesis. However, none of these agents have been demonstrated to be tumouricidal and therefore continuous therapy for many years may be needed to prevent relapse. The metabolism, toxicity and side-effects of these agents when administered for extended periods may therefore be an important factor in agent suitability. Tamoxifen is the only agent so far to be tested over long periods (5 years) in therapeutic studies (Tormey and Jordan, 1984).

References

Adam, H. K., 1981 a, What we know and don't know about the pharmacokinetics of tamoxifen. In *Chemotherapeutic Effects of 'Nolvadex'* (*Tamoxifen Citrate*). Customer Communications in Postgraduate Medicine (New York: McGraw Hill), pp. 29–34.

Adam, H. K., 1981 b, Pharmacokinetic studies with 'Nolvadex'. *Reviews of Endocrine-Related Cancer*, Suppl. 9, 131–143.

Adam, H. K., Gay, M. A. and Moore, R. H., 1980 a, Measurement of tamoxifen in serum by thin layer densitometry. *J. Endocrinol.*, **84**, 35–41.

Adam, H. K., Patterson, J. S. and Kemp, J. V., 1980 b, Studies on the metabolism and pharmacokinetics of tamoxifen in normal volunteers. *Cancer Treat. Rep.*, **64**, 761–764.

Adam, A. M., Rogers, H. J., Amiel, S. A. and Rubens, R. D., 1984, The effect of acetylator phenotype on the disposition of aminoglutethimide. *Br. J. Clin. Pharmacol.*, **18**, 495–505.

Allen, K. E., Clark, E. R. and Jordan, V. C., 1980, Evidence for the metabolic activation of non-steroidal antioestrogens: A study of structure-activity relationships. *Br. J. Pharmacol.*, **16**, 1007–1015.

Bain, R. and Jordan, V. C., 1983, Identification of a new metabolite of tamoxifen in patient serum during breast cancer therapy. *Biochem. Pharmacol.*, **32**, 373–375.

Baum, M. and other members of the Nolvadex Adjuvant Trials Organization, 1985, Controlled trial of tamoxifen as single adjuvant agent in management of early breast cancer. *Lancet*, **1**, 836–840.

Beardwell, C. G., Hindley, A. C., Wilkinson, P. M., Todd, I. D., Ribeiro, G. G. and Bu'Lock, D., 1983, Trilostane in the treatment of advanced breast cancer. *Cancer Chemother. Pharmacol.*, **10**, 158–160.

Beatson, G. T., 1896, On the treatment of inoperable cases of carcinoma of the mamma. Suggestions for a new method of treatment with illustrative cases. *Lancet*, **2**, 104–107.

Bennett, H. P. J. and McMartin, C., 1979, Peptide hormones and their analogues: Distribution, clearance from the circulation, and inactivation *in vivo*. *Pharmacol. Rev.*, **30**, 247–292.

Bhargava, A. S., Seeger, A. and Günzel, P., 1977, Isolation and identification of 15β-hydroxy cyproterone acetate as a new metabolite of cyproterone acetate in dog, monkey and man. *Steroids*, **30**, 407–418.

Borgna, J. L. and Rochefort, H., 1980, High affinity binding to the estrogen receptor of [^{3}H]4-hydroxytamoxifen, an active antiestrogen metabolite. *Mol. Cell. Endocrinol.*, **20**, 71–85.

Borgna, J. L. and Rochefort, H., 1981, Hydroxylated metabolites of tamoxifen are formed *in vivo* and bound to estrogen receptor in target tissues. *J. Biol. Chem.*, **256**, 859–868.

Bowman, S. P., Leake, A. and Morris, I. D., 1982, Hypothalamic, pituitary and uterine cytoplasmic and nuclear oestrogen receptors and their relationship to the serum concentration of tamoxifen and its metabolite, 4-hydroxytamoxifen, in the ovariectomized rat. *J. Endocrinol.*, **94**, 167–175.

Briggs, M. H. and Brotherton, J., 1970, *Steroid Biochemistry and Pharmacology* (New York: Academic Press).

Brown, T. R., Rothwell, S. W., Sultan, C. and Migeon, C. J., 1981, Inhibition of androgen binding in human foreskin fibroblasts by antiandrogens. *Steroids*, **37**, 635–648.

Brown, R. R., Bain, R. and Jordan, V. C., 1983, Determination of tamoxifen and metabolites in human serum by high performance liquid chromatography with post-column-fluorescence activation. *J. Chromatogr.*, **272**, 351–358.

Camaggi, C. M., Strocchi, E. and Canova, N., 1983, High performance liquid chromatographic analysis of tamoxifen and major metabolites in human plasma. *J. Chromatogr.*, **275**, 436–442.

Cantwell, B. M. J., Sainsbury, R., Harris, A. L., Wilson, R. G., Farndon, J., Dawes, P., Evans, R. G. B. and Dowsett, M., 1984, Low dose aminoglutethimide for advanced postmenopausal breast cancer. *Br. J. Cancer*, **50**, 252.

Carone, F. A., Peterson, D. R. and Flouret, G., 1982, Renal tubular processing of small peptide hormones. *J. Lab. Clin. Med.*, **100**, 1–14.

Cash, R., Brough, A. J., Cohen, M. N. P. and Satoh, P. S., 1967, Aminoglutethimide (Elipten-Ciba) as an inhibitor of adrenal steroidogenesis: Mechanism of action on therapeutic trial. *J. Clin. Endocrinol.*, **27**, 1239.

Chohan, P. B., Coombes, R. C., Foster, A. B., Harland, S. J., Jarman, M., Leung, C. S., Rowland, M. G. and Taylor, G. N., 1982, Metabolism of aminoglutethimide in man: desmolase and aromatase inhibition studies. In *Aminoglutethimide—An Alternative Therapy for Breast Carcinoma.* Royal Society of Medicine International Congress and Symposium, Series No. 53, edited by R. W. Elsdon-Dew, I. M. Jackson and G. F. B. Birdwood (London: Academic Press and the Royal Society of Medicine), pp. 19–21.

Coombes, R. C., Foster, A. B., Harland, S. J., Jarman, M. and Nice, E. C., 1982, Polymorphically acetylated aminoglutethimide in humans. *Br. J. Cancer*, **46**, 340–345.

Coombes, R. C., Powles, T. J., Muindi, J., Hunt, J., Ward, M., Perez, D. and Neville, A. M., 1985, Trilostane therapy for advanced breast cancer. *Cancer Treat. Rep.*, **69**, 351–354.

Cuzick, J. and Baum, M., 1985, Tamoxifen and contralateral breast cancer. *Lancet*, **1**, 282.

Daniel, C. P., Gaskell, S. J., Bishop, H. and Nicholson, R. I., 1979, Determination of tamoxifen and an hydroxylated metabolite in plasma from patients with advanced breast cancer using gas chromatography-mass spectrometry. *J. Endocrinol.*, **83**, 401–408.

Daniel, C. P., Gaskell, S. J., Bishop, H., Campbell, C. and Nicholson, R. I., 1981, Determination of tamoxifen and biologically active metabolites in human breast tumours and plasma. *Eur. J. Cancer Clin. Oncol.*, **17**, 1183–1189.

Dorfman, R. J. and Ungar, F., 1965, *Metabolism of Steroid Hormones* (New York: Academic Press).

Douglas, J. S. and Nicholls, P. J., 1965, The urinary excretion of aminoglutethimide in man. *J. Pharm. Pharmacol.*, **17** Suppl., 1155.

Dupont, A., Labrie, F., Pelletier, G., Puviani, R., Coy, D., Coy, E. and Schally, A., 1974, Organ distribution of radioactivity and disappearance of radioactivity from plasma after administration of [^{3}H]-luteinizing hormone releasing hormone to mice and rats. *Neuroendocrinology*, **16**, 65–73.

Düsterberg, B., Humel, M. and Speck, U., 1981, Terminal half lives in plasma and bioavailability of Norethisterone, Levonorgestrel, cyproterone acetate and gestodene in rats, beagles and rhesus monkey. *Contraception*, **24**, 673–683.

Egger, H., Bartlett, F., Itterly, W., Rodebaugh, R. and Shimanskas, C., 1982, Metabolism of aminoglutethimide in the rat. *Drug Metab. Disp.*, **10**, 405–412.

Fabian, C. and Sternson, L., 1979, Tamoxifen (TAM). Blood levels following initial and chronic dosing in patients with breast cancer: correlation with clinical data. *Proc. Am. Soc. Clin. Oncol.*, Abstract C-145.

Fabian, C. and Sternson, L. A., 1981, Tamoxifen pharmacokinetics in patients with breast cancer: comparison of traditional and loading dose schedules. *Reviews of Endocrine-Related Cancer*, Suppl. 9, 155–168.

Fabian, C., Sternson, L. and Barnett, M., 1980, Clinical pharmacology of tamoxifen in patients with breast cancer: comparison of traditional and loading dose schedules. *Cancer Treat. Rep.*, **64**, 765–773.

Fabian, C., Tilzer, L. and Sternson, L., 1981, Comparative binding affinities of tamoxifen, 4-hydroxytamoxifen, and desmethyltamoxifen for estrogen receptors isolated from human breast carcinoma: correlation with blood levels in patients with metastatic breast cancer. *Biopharm. Drug Disp.*, **2**, 381–390.

Fisher, B., Redmond, C., Brown, A., Wickerman, D. L., Wolmark, N., Allegra, J.,

Escher, G., Lippman, M., Savlov, E., Wittliff, J. L. and Fisher, E. R., 1983, Influence of tumor estrogen and progesterone receptor levels on the response to tamoxifen and chemotherapy in primary breast cancer. *J. Clin. Oncol.*, **1**, 227–241.

Foster, A. B., Griggs, L. J., Jarman, M. and Van Maanen, J. M. S., 1980, Metabolism of tamoxifen by rat liver microsomes: formation of the *N*-oxide, a new metabolite. *Biochem. Pharmacol.*, **29**, 1977–1979.

Foster, A., Jarman, M., Leung, C., Rowlands, M. and Taylor, G., 1983, Analogues of aminoglutethimide: selective inhibition of cholesterol side chain cleavage. *J. Med. Chem.*, **26**, 50–54.

Foster, A., Jarman, M., Leung, C., Rowlands, M., Taylor, G., Plevey, R. and Sampson, P., 1985, Analogues of aminoglutethimide: selective inhibition of aromatase. *J. Med. Chem.*, **28**, 200–204.

Frith, R. C. and Phillipou, G., 1985, 15-Hydroxycyproterone acetate and cyproterone acetate levels in plasma and urine. *J. Chromatogr.*, **338**, 179–186.

Fromson, J. M. and Sharp, D. S., 1974, The selective uptake of tamoxifen by human uterine tissue. *J. Obst. Gynaecol. Br. Commonw.*, **81**, 321–323.

Fromson, J. M., Pearson, S. and Bramah, S., 1973 a, The metabolism of tamoxifen (ICI 46474) Part I. In laboratory animals. *Xenobiotica*, **3**, 693–709.

Fromson, J. M., Pearson, S. and Bramah, S., 1973 b, The metabolism of tamoxifen (ICI 46474) Part II. In female patients. *Xenobiotica*, **3**, 711–714.

Furr, B. J. A. and Jordan, V. C., 1984, The pharmacology and clinical uses of tamoxifen. *Pharmacol. Ther.*, **25**, 127–205.

Gaskell, S. J., Daniel, C. P. and Nicholson, R. I., 1978, Determination of tamoxifen in rat plasma by gas chromatography–mass spectrometry. *J. Endocrinol.*, **78**, 2983–2994.

Geiger, R., 1984, Design and synthesis of LH-RH agonists and antagonists. In *LHRH and its Analogues*, edited by F. Labrie, A. Belanger and A. Dupont (Amsterdam: Elsevier), pp. 36–49.

Golander, Y. and Sternson, L. A., 1980, Paired-ion chromatographic analysis of tamoxifen and two major metabolites in plasma. *J. Chromatogr.*, **181**, 41–49.

Gottardis, M. M., Robinson, S. P. and Jordan, V. C., 1985, Control of estrogen-responsive human breast cancer cell lines in athymic mice by long-term tamoxifen therapy. *Breast Cancer Res. Treat.*, **6**, Abstract 38.

Griffiths, E. and Hopkinson, C., 1979, Inactivation of two hyperactive LH-RH analogues by rat hypothalamic peptidases. *Hormone Res.*, **10**, 233–242.

Griffiths, E. and Kelly, J., 1979, Mechanisms of inactivation of hypothalamic regulatory hormones. *Mol. Cell. Endocrinol.*, **14**, 3–17.

Griffiths, E. and McDermott, J., 1983, Enzymic inactivation of hypothalamic regulatory hormones. *Mol. Cell. Endocrinol.*, **33**, 1—25.

Griffiths, E., Hooper, K. and Hopkinson, C., 1975, Further studies on enzymic inactivation of luteinizing hormone-releasing hormone (LH-RH) by peptidases in the rat hypothalamus. *Acta Endocrinol.*, **79**, 7–15.

Grill, H. J., Manz, B., Elger, W. and Pollow, K., 1985, ^{3}H-Cyproterone acetate: binding characteristics to human uterine progestagen receptors. *J. Endocrinol. Invest.*, **8**, 135–141.

Gross, P. E., Jarman, M. and Griggs, L. J., 1985, Metabolism of aminoglutethimide in humans: quantification and clinical relevance of induced metabolism. *Br. J. Cancer*, **51**, 259–262.

Haddow, A., 1938, Influence of carcinogenic compounds and related substances on rate of growth of spontaneous tumours of mouse. *J. Pathol. Bacteriol.*, **47**, 567–579.

Haddow, A., Watkinson, J. M. and Paterson, E., 1944, Influence of synthetic oestrogens upon advanced malignant disease. *Br. Med. J.*, **2**, 393–398.

Harris, A. L., Dowsett, M., Smith, I. E. and Jeffcoate, S. L., 1983, Endocrine effects of low dose aminoglutethimide in advanced postmenopausal breast cancer. *Br. J. Cancer*, **47**, 621–627.

Horsthemke, B., Knisatschek, H., Rivier, J., Sandow, J. and Bauer, K., 1981, Degradation of luteinizing hormone-releasing hormone and analogs by adeno-hypophyseal peptidases. *Biochem. Biophys. Res. Commun.*, **100**, 753–759.

Horwitz, K. B., Koseki, Y. and McGuire, W. L., 1978, Estrogen control of progesterone receptor in human breast cancer: role of estradiol and anti-estrogen. *Endocrinology*, **103**, 1742–1751.

Huggins, C. and Bergenstal, D. M., 1952, Inhibition of human mammary and prostate cancers by adrenalectomy. *Cancer Res.*, **12**, 134–141.

Humpel, M., Wendt, H., Dogs, G., Weib, Chr., Rietz, S. and Speck, U., 1977, Intra-individual comparison of pharmacokinetic parameters of *d*-Norgestrel, Lynestrenol and cyproterone acetate in 6 women. *Contraception*, **16**, 199–215.

Humpel, M., Nieuweboer, B., Düsterberg, B. and Wendt, H., 1979, Pharmacokinetics of cyproterone acetate in man. In *Androgenization in Women*, edited by J. Hammerstein, U. Lachnit-Fixson, F. Neumann and G. Plewig (Amsterdam: Excerpta Medica), pp. 209–217.

Jordan, V. C., 1982, Metabolites of tamoxifen in animals and man: identification, pharmacology and significance. *Breast Cancer Res. Treat.*, **3**, 123–138.

Jordan, V. C., 1983, Laboratory studies to develop general principles for the adjuvant treatment of breast cancer with antiestrogens: problems and potential for future clinical applications. *Breast Cancer Res. Treat.*, **3**(Suppl), 73–86.

Jordan, V. C., 1984, Biochemical pharmacology of antiestrogen action. *Pharmacol. Rev.*, **36**, 245–276.

Jordan, V. C. and Bowser-Finn, R. A., 1982, Binding of [^{3}H]-monohydroxytamoxifen by immature rat tissues *in vivo*. *Endocrinology*, **110**, 1281–1291.

Jordan, V. C. and Gosden, B., 1982, Importance of the alkylaminoethoxy side-chain for the estrogenic antiestrogen actions of tamoxifen and trioxifene in the immature rat uterus. *Mol. Cell. Endocrinol.*, **7**, 291–306.

Jordan, V. C., Bain, R. R., Brown, R. R., Gosden, B. and Santos, M. A., 1983, Determination and pharmacology of a new hydroxylated metabolite of tamoxifen observed in patient sera during therapy for advanced breast cancer. *Cancer Res.*, **43**, 1446–1450.

Jordan, V. C., Lieberman, M. E., Cormier, E., Koch, R., Bagley, J. R. and Ruenitz, P. C., 1984, Structural requirements for the pharmacological activity of non-steroidal antiestrogens *in vitro*. *Mol. Pharmacol.*, **26**, 272–278.

Katchen, B. and Buxbaum, S., 1975, Dispostion of a new, non-steroidal, antiandrogen, $\alpha\alpha\alpha$-trifluoro-2-methyl-4′-nitro-*m*-propionotoluidide (flutamide), in men following a single oral 200 mg dose. *J. Clin. Endocrinol. Metab.*, **41**, 373.

Katchen, B., Dancik, S. and Millington, G., 1976, Percutaneous penetration and metabolism of topical [^{14}C]-flutamide in men. *J. Invest. Dermatol.*, **66**, 379–382.

Kemp, J. V., Adam, H. K., Wakeling, A. E. and Slater, R., 1983, Identification and biological activity of tamoxifen metabolites in human serum. *Biochem. Pharmacol.*, **32**, 2045–2052.

Klijn, J. G. M. and Dejong, F. H., 1982, Treatment with luteinizing-hormone releasing hormone analogue (buserelin) in premenopausal patients with metastatic breast cancer. *Lancet*, **1**, 1213–1216.

Komanicky, P., Spark, R. F. and Melby, J. C., 1978, Treatment of Cushing's Syndrome with trilostane (WIN 24,540), in inhibitor of adrenal steroid biosynthesis. *J. Clin. Endocrinol. Metab.*, **47**, 1042–1051.

Labrie, F., Dupont, A., Belanger, A. and members of Laval University Prostate Cancer Program, 1984, Spectacular response to combined antihormonal treatment in advanced prostate cancer. *Endocrinology*, edited by F. Labrie and L. Proulx (Amsterdam: Elsevier).

Lazier, C. B. and Jordan, V. C., 1982, High affinity binding of anti-oestrogen to the chick liver nuclear oestrogen receptor. *Biochem. J.*, **206**, 387–394.

Lerner, L. J., Holthaus, J. F. and Thompson, C. R., 1958, A non-steroidal estrogen antagonist (1-(*p*-2-diethylaminoethoxyphenyl)-1-phenyl-2-*p*-methoxyphenylethanol. *Endocrinology*, **63**, 295–318.

Lieberman, M. E., Jordan, V. C., Fritsch, M., Santos, M. A. and Gorski, J., 1983, Direct and reversible inhibition of estradiol-stimulated prolactin synthesis by antiestrogen *in vitro*. *J. Biol. Chem.*, **258**, 4734–4740.

Loumaye, E., Naor, Z. and Catt, K., 1982, Binding affinity and biological activity of gonadotrophin-releasing hormone agonists in isolated pituitary cells. *Endocrinology*, **111**, 730–736.

Luft, R. and Olivecrona, H., 1953, Experiences with hypophysectomy in man. *J. Neurosurg.*, **10**, 301–316.

Lyman, S. D. and Jordan, V. C., 1985 a, Metabolism of tamoxifen and its uterotrophic activity. *Biochem. Pharmacol.*, **34**, 2787–2794.

Lyman, S. D. and Jordan, V. C., 1985 b, Possible mechanisms for the agonist actions of tamoxifen and the antagonist actions of MER25 (ethamoxytriphetol) in the mouse uterus. *Biochem. Pharmacol.*, **34**, 2795–2806.

Major, J. S., Green, B. and Heald, P. J., 1976, Interactions of oestradiol-17β and tamoxifen in the uterus of the pregnant rat. *J. Endocrinol.*, **71**, 315–324.

Marrion, G. F., 1930, The chemistry of oestrin III. An improved method of preparation and the isolation of active crystalline material. *Biochem. J.*, **24**, 435–445.

McGuire, W. L., 1980, Steroid hormone receptors in breast cancer treatment strategy. *Recent Prog. Hormone Res.*, **36**, 135–146.

Meltzer, N. M., Stang, P. and Sternson, L. A., 1984, Influence of tamoxifen and its N-desmethyl and 4-hydroxy metabolites on rat liver microsomal enzymes. *Biochem. Pharmacol.*, **33**, 115–123.

Mendenhall, D. W., Kobayashi, H., Shih, F. M. L., Sternson, L. A., Higuchi, T. and Fabian, C., 1978, Clinical analysis of tamoxifen, an anti-neoplastic agent, in plasma. *Clin. Chem.*, **24**, 1518–1524.

Monaham, M., Rivier, J., Vale, W., Ling, N., Grant G., Amoss, M., Guillemin, R., Burgus, R., Nicholaides, L., and Rebstock, M., 1972, Structure–biological activity relationships on thyrotropin and luteinizing hormone releasing factor analogues. In *Chemistry and Biology of Peptides*, edited by J. Meinhofer (Ann Arbor Science), p. 601.

Murray, R. M. and Pitt, P., 1982, Aminoglutethimide in tamoxifen resistant patients: The Melbourne experience. *Cancer Res.*, **42**(Suppl.), 3437s–3441s.

Murray, F., Santner, S., Samojlik, E. and Santen, R. J., 1979, Serum aminoglutethimide levels: Studies of serum half-life, clearance, and patient compliance. *J. Clin. Pharmacol.*, **19**, 704–711.

Neri, R. O., 1976, Antiandrogens. *Adv. Sexual Hormone Res.*, **2**, 233–262.

Neri, R., Peets, E. and Watnick, A., 1979, Anti-androgenicity of flutamide and its metabolite Sch 16423. *Biochem. Soc. Transact.*, **7**, 565–569.

Nestor, J., Ho, T., Tahilramani, R., McRae, G. and Vickery, B., 1984, Long acting LH-RH agonists and antagonists. In *LH-RH and its Analogues*, edited by F. Labrie, A. Belanger and A. Dupont (Amsterdam: Elsevier), pp. 24–35.

Neumann, F. and Schenck, B., 1976, New antiandrogens and their mode of action. *J. Reprod. Fert.*, **24**(Suppl.), 129–145.

Neumann, F., Schleusener, A. and Albring, M., 1979, Pharmacology of anti-androgens. In *Androgenization in Women*, edited by J. Hammerstein, U. Lachnit-Fixson, F. Neumann and G. Plewig (Amsterdam: Excerpta Medica), pp. 147–190.

Nicholls, P. J., 1982, Pharmacokinetic and balance studies of aminoglutethimide in animals and man. In *Aminoglutethimide—An Alternative Endocrine Therapy for Breast Carcinoma*, edited by R. W. Elsdon-Dew, I. M. Jackson and G. F. B. Birdwood. Royal Society of Medicine International Congress and Symposium, Series No. 53 (London: Academic Press and the Royal Society of Medicine).

Nicholson, R. I., Walker, K. J., Turkes, A., Turkes, A. O., Dyas, J., Blamey, R. W., Cambell, F. C., Robinson, M. R. G. and Griffiths, K., 1984, Therapeutic significance and the mechanism of action of the LH-RH agonist ICI 118630 in breast cancer and prostate cancer. *J. Steroid Biochem.*, **20**, 129–135.

Osborne, C. K., Boldt, D. H., Clark, G. M. and Trent, J. M., 1983, Effects of tamoxifen in human breast cancer cell cycle kinetics: Accumulation of cells in early G1 phase. *Cancer Res.*, 3583–3585.

Osborne, C. K., Hobbs, K. and Clark, G. M., 1985, Effect of estrogens and antiestrogens on growth of human breast cancer cells in athymic nude mice. *Cancer Res.*, **45**, 584–590.

Patterson, J. S., Settatree, R. S., Adam, H. K. and Kemp, J. V., 1980, Serum concentrations of tamoxifen and major metabolite during long-term Nolvadex therapy, correlated with clinical response. In *Breast Cancer—Experimental and Clinical Aspects*, edited by H. T. Mouridsen and T. Palshof (Oxford: Pergamon Press), pp. 89–92.

Pont, A., Williams, P. C., Azhar, S., Reitz, R. E., Bochra, C., Smith, E. R. and Stevens, D. A., 1982, Ketoconazole blocks testosterone synthesis. *Arch. Int. Med.*, **142**, 2137–2140.

Raynaud, J. P., Bonnie, C., Moguilewsky, M., Lefebvre, F. A., Belanger, A. and Labrie, F., 1984, The pure antiandrogen RU 23908 (Anandron®), a candidate of choice for the combined antihormone treatment of prostate cancer. A review. *The Prostate*, **5**, 299–311.

Raynaud, J. P., Moguilewsky, M., Tournemine, C., Pottier, J., Coussediere, D., Salmon, J., Husson, J. M., Beertagna, C., Tremblay, D., Pendyala, L., Brisset, J. M., Vallancien, G., Serment, G., Navratit, N., Dupont, A. and Labrie, F., 1985, Pharmacology and clinical studies with RU 23908 (Anandron®). EORTC Genitourinary Group Monograph 2, Part A: *Therapeutic Principles in Metastatic Prostatic Cancer* (New York: Alan R. Liss), pp. 99–120.

Reddel, R. R., Murphy, L. C. and Sutherland, R. L., 1983, Effects of biologically active metabolites of tamoxifen on the proliferation kenetics of MCF-7 human breast cancer cells *in vitro*. *Cancer Res.*, **43**, 4618–4624.

Redding, T. and Schally, A., 1973, The distribution, half-life and excretion of tritiated luteinizing hormone releasing hormone (LH-RH) in rats. *Life Sci.*, **12**, 23–32.

Redding, T., Kastin, A., Gonzalez-Barcena, D., Coy, D., Coy, E., Schalch, D. and Schally, A., 1973, The half-life, metabolism and excretion of tritiated luteinizing hormone-releasing hormone (LH-RH) in man. *J. Clin. Endocrinol. Metab.*, **37**, 626.

Reigel, A. T., Jordan, V. C., Bain, R. R. and Schoenberg, D. R., 1986, The effects of tamoxifen and 4-hydroxytamoxifen on vitellogenin gene expression in *Xenopus laevis* liver. *J. Steroid Biochem* (in the press).

Robertson, D. W., Katzenellenbogen, J. A., Long, D. J., Rorke, E. A. and Katzenellenbogen, B. S., 1982, Tamoxifen antiestrogens. A comparison of the activity, pharmacokinetics and metabolic activation of the *cis* and *trans* isomers of tamoxifen. *J. Steroid Biochem.*, **16**, 1–13.

Ruenitz, P. C., Bagley, J. R. and Mokler, C. M., 1982, Estrogenic and antiestrogenic activity of monophenolic analogues of tamoxifen (2)-2-[*p*(1,2-diphenyl-1-butenyl)phenoxy]-*N*,*N*-dimethylethylamine. *J. Med. Chem.*, **25**, 1056–1060.

Ruenitz, P. C., Bagley, J. R. and Pape, C. W., 1984, Some chemical and biochemical aspects of liver microsomal metabolism of tamoxifen. *Drug Metab. Disp.*, **12**, 478–483.

Samuels, L. T. and Eik-Nes, K. B., 1968, In *Metabolic Pathways*, Vol. II, edited by D. M. Greenberg (New York: Academic Press), pp. 169–220.

Sandow, J. and Konig, W., 1979, Studies with fragments of a highly active analogue of luteinizing hormone releasing hormone. *J. Endocrinol.*, **81**, 175–182.

Sandow, J., Von Rechenberg, W. and Jerzabek, G., 1976, The effect of LH-RH prostaglandins and synthetic analogues of LH-RH on ovarian metabolism. *Eur. J. Obst., Gynaecol. Reprod. Biol.*, **6**, 185–190.

Sandow, J., Jerzabek, G., Stoll, W. and Kuhl, H., 1980, Metabolism, of ^{125}I luteinizing hormone releasing hormone analogue (buserelin) in rats *in vivo* and *in vitro*. *J. Endocrinol.* (proceedings), **85**, 11.

Sandow, J., Jerzabek-Sandow, G., Krauss, B. and Schmidt-Gollwitzer, M., 1984, Pharmacokinetics and metabolism of LH-RH agonists, clinical aspects. In *LH-RH and Its Analogues*, edited by F. Labie, A. Belanger and A. Dupont (Amsterdam: Elsevier), pp. 123–132.

Sane, R. T., Desai, S. V., Sonawne, K. K. and Nagak, V. G., 1985, Quantitative gas chromatographic determination of tamoxifen citrate in pharmaceuticals. *J. Chromatogr.*, **331**, 432–436.

Santen, R. J., Santner, S., Davis, B., Veldhuis, J., Samojlik, E. and Ruby, E., 1978, Aminoglutethimide inhibits extraglandular estrogen production in postmenopausal women with breast carcinoma. *J. Clin. Endocrinol. Metab.*, **47**, 1257–1265.

Santen, R. J., Samojlik, E. and Wells, S. A., 1980, Resistance of the ovary to blockage of aromatization with aminoglutethimide. *J. Clin. Endocrinol. Metab.*, **51**, 473–477.

Santen, R. J., Vanden Bossche, H., Symoens, J., Brugmans, J. and Decoster, R., 1983, Site of action of low dose ketoconazole on androgen biosynthesis in men. *J. Clin. Endocrinol. Metab.*, **57**, 732–736.

Schally, A. V., Redding, T. W. and Comaru-Schally, A. M., 1984, Potential use of analogues of luteinizing hormone-releasing hormones in the treatment of hormone-sensitive neoplasms. *Cancer Treat. Rep.*, **68**, 281–289.

Schulte-Hermann, R. and Parzefall, W., 1980, Adaptive responses of rat liver to the gestagen and anti-androgen cyproterone acetate and other inducers. I. Induction of drug-metabolism enzymes. *Chem.-Biol. Interactions*, **31**, 279–286.

Schulte-Hermann, R., Hoffman, V., Parzefall, W., Kallenbach, M., Gerhardt, A. and Schuppler, J., 1980, Adaptive responses of rat liver to the gestagen and anti-androgen cyproterone acetate and other inducers. II. Induction of growth. *Chem.-Biol. Interactions*, **31**, 287–300.

Schulz, V. V., 1976, Distribution, absorption and elimination of radioactivity following oral and intravennous application of 2-^{14}C-labelled cyproterone acetate to Rhesus monkey. *Arzneimittel-Forsch.*, **26**, 544–546.

Speck, V. U., Jentsch, D., Kuhne, G., Schulze, E. and Wendt, H., 1976, Bioverfügbarkeit und Pharmakokinetik von ^{14}C-cyproteronacetat nach Applikation als 50-mg-Tablette. *Arzneimittel-Forsch.*, **26**(a), 1717–1720.

Stetler-Stevenson, M., Flouret, G. and Peterson, D., 1981, Handling of luteinizing hormone-releasing hormone by renal proximal tubular segments *in vitro*. *Am. J. Physiol.*, **241**, F117—F122.

Stetler-Stevenson, M., Flouret, G., Wakamura, S., Gulcyzynski, B. and Carone, F.,

1983, *In vivo* metabolism of tritiated LH-RH by the whole kidney and individual tubules of rats. *Am. J. Physiol.*, **244**, F628—F632.

Stuart-Harris, R. and Smith, I., 1984, Aminoglutethimide in the treatment of advanced breast cancer. *Cancer Treat. Rep.*, **11**, 189–204.

Stuart-Harris, R., Dowsett, M., Bozek, T., McKinna, J. A., Gazet, J-C., Jeffcoate, S. L., Kurkure, A. and Carr, L., 1984, Low-dose aminoglutethimide in treatment of advanced breast cancer. *Lancet*, **ii**, 604–606.

Sudo, K., Monsma, F. J. and Katzenellenbogen, B. S., 1983, Antiestrogen binding sites distinct from the estrogen receptor: subcellular localization, ligand specificity and distribution in tissues of the rat. *Endocrinology*, **112**, 425–434.

Sutherland, R. L., Murphy, L. C., Foo, M. S., Green, M. D., Whybourne, A. M. and Krozowski, Z. S., 1980, High affinity antioestrogen binding site distinct from the oestrogen receptor. *Nature* (*Lond*), **288**, 273–275.

Sutherland, R. L., Green, M. D., Hall, R. E., Reddel, R. R. and Taylor, S. W., 1983, Tamoxifen induces accumulation of MCF-7 human mammary carcinoma cells in the G_0/G_1 phase of the cell cycle *Eur. J. Cancer Clin. Oncol.*, **19**, 615–621.

Swift, A. and Crighton, D., 1979, Relative activity, plasma elimination and tissue degradation of synthetic luteinizing hormone releasing hormone and certain of its analogues. *J. Endocrinol.*, **80**, 141–152.

Szalay, B., Krieg, M., Schmidt, H. and Voigt, K. D., 1975, Metabolism and mode of action of androgens in target tissues of male rats. *Acta Endocrinol.*, **80**, 592–602.

Thompson, T. A., Vermeulen, J. D., Wagner, W. and Lesher, A. R., 1981, Aminoglutethimide bioavailability, pharmacokinetics, and binding to blood constituents. *J. Pharm. Sci.*, **70**, 1040–1043.

Tormey, D. C. and Jordan, V. C., 1984, Long-term tamoxifen adjuvant therapy in node positive breast: a metabolic and pilot clinical study. *Breast Cancer Res. Treat.*, **4**, 297–302.

Vanden Bossche, H., Lauwers, W., Willemsens, G. and Cools, W., 1985, Ketoconazole, an inhibitor of the cytochrome P450 dependent testosterone biosynthesis. In *Therapeutic Principles in Metastatic Prostatic Cancer*, EORTC Genitourinary Group Monograph 2, Part A (New York: Alan R. Liss), pp. 187–196.

Wakeling, A. E., Furr, B. J. A., Glen, A. T. and Hughes, L. R., 1981, Receptor binding and biological activity of steroidal and non-steroidal antiandrogens. *J. Steroid Biochem.*, **15**, 355–359.

Wilking, N., Applegren, L. E., Carstrom, K., Nordgren, T. and Theve, N. O., 1981, The distribution and metabolism of ^{14}C-labelled tamoxifen in spayed female mice. *Rev. Endocrine-Related Cancer*, Suppl. 9, 223–239.

Wilking, N., Applegren, L. E., Carlstrom, K., Pousette, A. and Theve, N. O., 1982, The distribution and metabolism of ^{14}C-labelled tamoxifen in spayed female mice. *Acta Pharmacol. Toxicol.*, **50**, 161–168.

Wilkinson, P., Ribiero, G., Adam, H. and Patterson, J., 1980, Clinical pharmacology of tamoxifen and *N*-desmethyltamoxifen in patients with advanced breast cancer. *Cancer Chemother. Pharmacol.*, **5**, 109–111.

10. Metabolism of anti-cancer drugs in development

Matthew M. Ames

Introduction

Metabolism is the major route of elimination for most drugs (Rowland and Tozer, 1980), and can also give rise to species responsible for some or all of the activity and toxicity of a drug. Distribution and elimination studies (including metabolism) are important elements in the development of new therapeutic agents. Results from these collective studies provide a pharmacological characterization of new drugs and are often of immediate value in the clinical application of new agents. Optimal routes of administration, relationships between blood concentrations of drug (and metabolites) and pharmacological activity, and schedules required to maintain optimal blood concentrations can often be determined on the basis of pharmacological studies.

Historically, relatively little information on distribution, excretion and metabolism has accompanied the development of new anti-cancer agents. This is due in part to the fact that many well-defined relationships between drug disposition and clinical effects are not readily applicable to anti-cancer agents. The long time after drug administration before appearance of many toxicities and certainly response, the often irreversible nature of interaction of drug or metabolites with target molecules (in contrast to well-defined rapid and reversible interactions of most drugs with receptors), and the multiple and frequently ill-defined mechanisms of action are some of the factors which make it difficult to apply anti-cancer agent pharmacology studies to clinical settings. In addition, the relatively rapid pace of new agent development combined with the limited potential for ultimate clinical utility of new anti-cancer agents have served to restrain enthusiasm for detailed pharmacology studies which must be carried out over relatively short periods of time. In contrast, a modest degree of clinical success tended (and tends) to spawn detailed disposition, elimination, pharmacokinetic and, when possible, cellular pharmacological studies.

In recent years there have been changes in the approach to development of new anti-cancer agents. In the United States, the National Cancer Institute (NCI) requires more detailed information with regard to the preclinical pharmacology of new agents before clinical trials begin, and supports preclinical pharmacology and toxicology studies in hopes of developing more rational approaches to early clinical trials (Collins *et al.*, 1986; Grieshaber and Marsoni, 1986). Clinical pharmacology studies are regularly conducted in conjunction with Phase I clinical trials. Increased participation in drug development by industry has also begun to yield more pharmacological data on new agents prepared and/or studied by pharmaceutical firms. Finally, new and more elegant methods have begun to provide information about the action and metabolism of agents at the cellular level, such as for cytosine arabinoside (Ara-C) in patient leukaemic cells (Plunkett *et al.*, 1985; Preisler *et al.*, 1985) and 5-fluorouracil (FUra) in patient colon carcinoma and normal tissues (Kovach *et al.*, 1986). The increased availability of better pharmacological data at earlier stages of anti-cancer drug development combined with a more sophisticated analysis of data have begun to yield productive integration of data from preclinical and clinical pharmacological studies into the design and analysis of clinical trials, and to yield a better understanding of the pharmacology of new agents.

Among the many pharmacological studies of anti-cancer agents currently under development are a number which include substantial data on metabolism. Agents to be discussed in this chapter were selected only on the basis that metabolism played a role in the pharmacology of that agent. In some instances that role was of consequence for better appreciation or use of the drug in clinical trials, while in others it simply constituted an interesting aspect of new agent pharmacology.

Diaziquone (Aziridinylbenzoquinone, AZQ, NSC 182986)

Diaziquone (Figure 1) is one of a family of aziridinylbenzoquinone analogues synthesized by Driscoll and his colleagues at the National Cancer Institute (Chou *et al.*, 1976; Khan and Driscoll, 1976). In an evaluation of many quinone-containing agents for anti-tumour activity, *para*-benzoquinone analogues containing aziridinyl moieties were found to be among the most active (Driscoll *et al.*, 1974). Those analogues possessed characteristics associated with penetration of drugs into the central nervous system (CNS), such as lipid solubility and minimal ionization at physiological pH values.

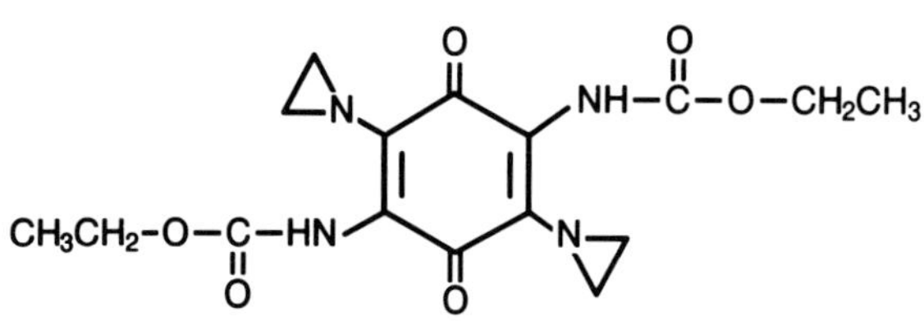

Figure 1. Structure of diaziquone.

Diaziquone was prepared in an effort to develop an aziridinylbenzoquinone analogue which would penetrate the CNS and have activity against intracerebrally implanted murine tumour systems, and yet retain adequate water solubility for parenteral administration (Khan and Driscoll, 1976; Chou *et al.*, 1976). Diaziquone had activity against a variety of murine tumours, including intracerebrally implanted L1210, P388 and ependymoblastoma (Driscoll *et al.*, 1979). Major toxicities observed in preclinical studies were associated with bone marrow, lymphoid tissues and the gastrointestinal tract (Diaziquone Clinical Brochure, National Cancer Institute, 1979). The dose-limiting toxicity in all Phase I trials was myelosuppression, most notably thrombocytopenia (Bender *et al.*, 1983; Griffin *et al.*, 1982; Schilsky *et al.*, 1982). Diaziquone was evaluated against a variety of diseases in Phase II clinical trials. The results of several trials were summarized by Bender *et al.* (1983). Activity was observed in the treatment of primary brain tumours and other solid neoplasms.

Preclinical pharmacology studies provided evidence that diaziquone was converted to unidentified products, presumably by enzymatic metabolism, and that diaziquone did in fact cross the blood–brain barrier. Following intravenous administration of ^{14}C-labelled diaziquone to mice, chloroform-extractable radioactivity in plasma, all of which co-chromatographed with parent drug by thin-layer chromatographic analysis, declined rapidly as non-chloroform extractable radioactivity appeared which was also rapidly cleared from plasma (Spiegel *et al.*, 1982). Recovery of total radioactivity in urine was not reported in this study. Both chloroform extractable and non-extractable radioactivity were found in most tissues, including the brain, after intravenous administration of labelled drug (Spiegel *et al.*, 1982). Metabolites were also detected in plasma following intravenous administration of drug to beagles, based on total radioactivity compared to radioactivity associated with diaziquone as determined by high-performance liquid chromatography (Feun *et al.*, 1983). Recoveries of total radioactivity and parent drug in 90-hour urine were approximately 40% and 5%, respectively. Diaziquone and unidentified metabolites were observed in cerebrospinal fluid within one hour of intravenous administration to beagles (Feun *et al.*, 1983) and rhesus monkeys (Gormley *et al.*, 1981; Zimm *et al.*, 1984). Higher cerebrospinal fluid concentrations were observed following intracarotid or intraventricular administration of drug to beagles and monkeys, respectively, as compared to intravenous drug administration (Feun *et al.*, 1983; Zimm *et al.*, 1984). Diaziquone was converted to non-chloroform-extractable metabolites (not identified) by mouse liver homogenates in a temperature-dependent reaction (Spiegel *et al.*, 1982).

A number of clinical pharmacology studies of diaziquone have been reported, most employing reversed-phase high-performance liquid chromatography (HPLC) assays similar to those published by Kelley and Siu Chong (1981) and Allen *et al.* (1981). Plasma elimination of diaziquone following intravenous administration appears to be best fit by a two-compartment open model with terminal phase half-life values of 25–35 minutes and total body clearance values of approximately 500 ml/min/m^2 (Bachur *et al.*, 1982; Curt *et al.*, 1983; Frytak *et al.*, 1984; Griffin *et al.*, 1982; Schilsky *et al.*, 1982). When determined, 24 hour urinary recovery of parent drug was less than 1%, consistent with the extensive metabolism of parent drug observed in animals. Diaziquone was found in cerebrospinal fluid, cyst fluid of glioma tumours, and in tumour tissue following intravenous administration of drug to patients (Bachur *et al.*, 1982; Curt *et al.*, 1983). The area under the curve (AUC) for cerebrospinal fluid was 20–40% of that for plasma (Bachur *et al.*, 1982). Thus, preclinical and clinical pharmacology studies were consistent with rapid clearance of diaziquone from the blood, penetration of parent drug and metabolites into a variety of tissues including brain, and extensive metabolism of parent drug. To date, there are no published data on the identity of diaziquone metabolites.

Based on the chemistry of appropriately related molecules, two structural features of diaziquone should play an important role in the biological effects of this agent. The first structural feature is the presence of two aziridine moieties in the molecule. Aziridines are reactive species which can react covalently with nucleophiles of small molecules as well as with protein and DNA. Indeed, diaziquone was designed to have bifunctional alkylating activity via the two aziridine moieties, and this has been demonstrated with DNA alkaline elution methods. DNA–protein cross-links and DNA–DNA inter-strand cross-links were detected following incubation of diaziquone with Chinese hamster ovary cells (King *et al.*, 1984 a) and with several human tumour cell lines (Szmigiero *et al.*, 1984). Cell killing among cell lines was correlated with DNA–DNA inter-strand cross-link, but not DNA–protein cross-link formation.

The second important structural feature of diaziquone is the presence of the quinone moiety. A variety of quinone anti-tumour agents including many anthracyclines and mitomycin C, are reduced by microsomal preparations to free radical semiquinone species (Bachur *et al.*, 1978; Sato *et al.*, 1977). Such reductions have been shown to be catalysed by NADPH-dependent cytochrome P-450 reductase (Komiyama *et al.*, 1982). As might be expected, diaziquone was converted to a free radical intermediate species by rat liver microsomes, rat liver nuclei and purified NADPH–cytochrome P-450 reductase when incubations contained NADPH (Gutierrez *et al.*, 1982; Svingen *et al.*, 1980). Electron spin resonance (ESR) signals were observed in the presence or absence of oxygen, in contrast to most examples of quinone reduction catalysed by NADPH-dependent cytochrome P-450 reductase in which oxygen inhibits ESR radical signal formation. Electrochemical reduction of diaziquone generated an ESR spectrum similar to that obtained in microsomal studies, provided the drug solutions contained water as did the microsomal incubation mixtures (Gutierrez *et al.*, 1984). Free radicals have also been detected when diaziquone was incubated with human and murine tumour cell lines (Gutierrez *et al.*, 1985; Svingen *et al.*, 1980; G. Powis, personal communication). Cell lines varied significantly in their ability to generate the free radical species. For example, the human myelogenous leukaemia line K562 produced more free radicals than did the human peripheral blood leukocyte line HL-60 (Gutierrez *et al.*, 1985). The time-dependent increase in rate of ESR signal was much greater for a renal cell carcinoma cell line (A498) than for a rhabdomyosarcoma cell line A204 (Svingen *et al.*, 1980; G. Powis, personal communication). Radical formation was reported under both anaerobic and aerobic conditions by Gutierrez *et al.* (1985), while Svingen *et al.* (1980) and Powis (personal communication) found that oxygen inhibited radical formation in their studies.

Efforts have been made to delineate the relative importance of DNA alkylation (via the aziridine moieties) and free radical generation (via reductive metabolism) in the cytotoxicity of diaziquone. Exposure of diaziquone to human tumour cell lines followed by alkaline elution results in significant numbers of DNA single-strand breaks as well as DNA–DNA inter-strand cross-links (King *et al.*, 1984 a; Szmigiero *et al.*, 1984). Agents which form free radicals are known to introduce DNA single-strand breaks. However, diaziquone cytotoxicity against the tumour cell lines correlated with DNA–DNA inter-strand cross-links, but not with DNA strand scission (Szmigiero *et al.*, 1984). Svingen *et al.* (1980) found that while diaziquone radical formation in human tumour cells was inhibited in the presence of oxygen, cytotoxicity was not. These studies suggest that cytotoxicity may be primarily dependent on DNA alkylation rather than on radical formation via reductive metabolism.

There are data which suggest that metabolism (conversion to radical species) and alkylation of DNA may be related, and that both may be involved in the cytotoxicity of this agent. DNA single-strand break formation and DNA–DNA inter-strand cross-link formation were detected following incubation of diaziquone with nuclei isolated from tumour cells (Szmigiero and Kohn, 1984). DNA single-strand breaks (readily observed when diaziquone was incubated with whole cell preparations) were detected only in the presence of a reducing cofactor such as NADPH, consistent with the known presence of NADPH-dependent cytochrome P-450 reductase in the nucleus and the absence of significant quantities of NADPH in such preparations. Metabolism proceeds in the nucleus in the presence of added drug and cofactors necessary for enzymatic reduction of diaziquone to the radical species which introduce DNA single-strand breaks. Unexpectedly, DNA–DNA inter-strand cross-links were also detected only when NADPH was added to incubation mixtures of diaziquone and isolated nuclei (Szmigiero and Kohn, 1984). In addition, alkylating activity as determined by reaction with 4-(*p*-nitrobenzyl)pyridine was stimulated in the presence of NADPH (Szmigiero and Kohn, 1984). Studies with rat liver microsomes, NADPH and sodium borohydride suggested that reduction may precede nucleophilic attack of the aziridine moieties as required for alkylation (King *et al.*, 1984 b). Similarly, we found that NADPH stimulated covalent binding of radiolabelled diaziquone to microsomal protein suggesting that alkylating activity of diaziquone was dependent on NADPH (M. M. Ames, unpublished data). Taken together these data suggest that bifunctional alkylation of DNA and protein by diaziquone may be influenced by reductive metabolism of the molecule. From a chemical standpoint, one might predict that the parent drug (e.g., the *para*-quinone) would promote alkylation through the aziridine moieties, while reduction to the semiquinone or hydroquinone (contributing increased electron density to the molecule) would reduce reactivity of the aziridine moieties. However, as noted by Szmigiero and Kohn (1984), the quinone might not be able to effectively activate the aziridines, because significant electron withdrawal from the aziridine nitrogen would require the aziridine ring to be coplanar with the quinone, a very strained geometry. In addition, the reduced molecule might increase alkylation by hydrogen bonding between the hydroxyl proton and the aziridine nitrogen. While these are all clearly speculations, metabolism and related studies raise the possibility that diaziquone is a bioreductive alkylating agent.

Fludarabine phosphate (9-β-D-arabinofuranosyl-2-fluoroadenine-5′-monophosphate, F-ara-AMP, NSC 312887)

Fludarabine phosphate or F-ara-AMP (Figure 2) is a purine antimetabolite currently being evaluated in the treatment of haematological malignancies. Metabolism plays an important role in virtually all aspects of F-ara-AMP pharmacology, including uptake into normal and tumour cells, conversion to active and toxic species, and elimination of the drug. In addition, species differences in F-ara-AMP metabolism are relevant in the consideration of preclinical and clinical toxicology data, and metabolism of F-ara-AMP in tumour cells may be of value in predicting toxicity and/or efficacy for individual patients. Finally, consideration of F-ara-AMP metabolism focuses on enzymes involved in activation and degradation of purines and pyrimidines

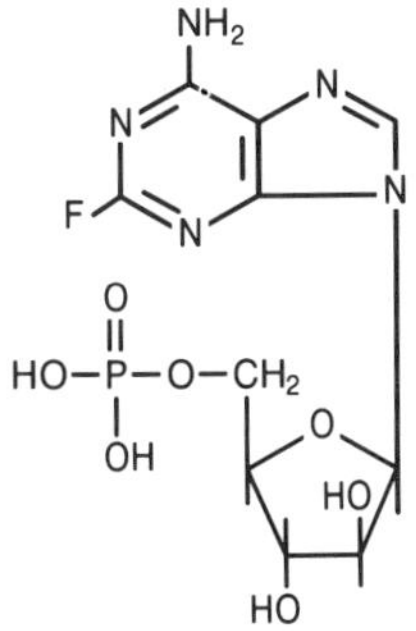

Figure 2. Structure of fludarabine phosphate.

rather than enzymes more commonly associated with drug metabolism such as mono-oxygenases and conjugating enzymes.

F-ara-AMP was synthesized as one approach to overcoming difficulties associated with the development of adenosine analogues such as 9-β-D-arabinofuranosyladenine (ara-A). Therapeutic activity of ara-A was limited by rapid deamination via adenosine deaminase and poor water solubility (Brink and LePage, 1984; LePage *et al.*, 1973). To prevent the rapid deamination, adenosine deaminase inhibitors were studied for use in combination therapy with ara-A. 2′-Deoxycoformycin, an adenosine deaminase inhibitor which produces lymphopenia when administered to humans (due to increased intracellular concentrations of purine deoxynucleotides achieved by inhibition of adenosine deaminase), does increase intracellular concentrations of ara-A (Plunkett *et al.*, 1984). Therapeutic potency and therapeutic index of ara-A were increased in animal model systems when the two drugs were administered as a combination (LePage *et al.*, 1976). There were indications of clinical anti-tumour activity for the combination in limited studies (Grever *et al.*, 1984; Kufe, 1984).

Another approach to further study of adenosine analogues has been the development of compounds resistant to deamination by adenosine deaminase. Based on information that 2-fluoroadenosine was resistant to adenosine deaminase, 9-β-D-arabinofuranosyl-2-fluoroadenine (F-ara-A, the nucleoside precursor of F-ara-AMP) was prepared (Montgomery and Hewson, 1969) and found to be resistant to deamination and to have activity against model tumour systems (Brockman *et al.*, 1977; Montgomery and Hewson, 1969). F-ara-AMP was developed as a more water-soluble analogue of F-ara-A and had activity against a variety of model tumour systems (Avramis and Plunkett, 1983; Brockman *et al.*, 1980). Toxicity at the maximally tolerated dose (MTD) in Phase I trials (approx. 160 and 20 mg/m^2 daily on the single dose and daily ×5 schedules, respectively) was myelosuppression (Hutton *et al.*, 1984). Phase II trials are currently under way. The mechanism of F-ara-AMP anti-tumour activity appears to involve its ultimate conversion to the triphosphate F-ara-ATP (described below) which inhibits both ribonucleotide reductase and DNA polymerase alpha (Tseng *et al.*, 1982).

F-ara-AMP was rapidly hydrolysed to F-ara-A following administration to mice, dogs and humans (Avramis and Plunkett, 1983; Danhauser *et al.*, 1986; DeSouza *et al.*, 1984; Malspeis *et al.*, 1984; Noker *et al.*, 1983). Plasma elimination of parent drug was very rapid (20–30 min) following intravenous administration to mice and dogs (Noker *et al.*, 1983), and F-ara-AMP was detected for only several minutes in plasma following intravenous administration to patients (DeSouza *et al.*, 1984; Malspeis *et al.*, 1984). Intracellular activation of F-ara-AMP can occur only following hydrolysis of parent drug and uptake of the nucleoside, F-ara-A, by normal and tumour cells. Following administration of F-ara-AMP to mice bearing P388 leukaemia, the monophosphate F-ara-AMP, the triphosphate F-ara-ATP and smaller quantities of the diphosphate F-ara-ADP were found in tumour cells as well as host tissue cells such as bone marrow and gastrointestinal mucosa (Avramis and Plunkett, 1983). These phosphates are formed intracellularly following uptake of the nucleoside, F-ara-A. Unlike ara-A, which is phosphorylated by adenosine kinase, F-ara-A is converted to F-ara-AMP by the pyrimidine salvage enzyme deoxycytidine kinase (Brockman *et al.*, 1980; Tseng *et al.*, 1982), thus distinguishing the intracellular activation pathway of F-ara-A from that of non-halogenated adenosine analogues. The triphosphate was detected in tumour cells and marrow cells from patients with relapsed leukaemia and lymphoma following administration of F-ara-AMP (Danhauser *et al.*, 1986). These investigators found that F-ara-ATP concentrations in peripheral blood leukaemic cells correlated with F-ara-ATP levels in bone marrow blasts when measured as trough levels during five-day therapy. In addition, there was a correlation between DNA synthetic capacity in circulating leukaemic blasts and F-ara-ATP concentrations. It may therefore be possible to relate F-ara-ATP concentrations in tumour cells to clinical responses and biochemical effects of fludarabine phosphate as has been previously done with Ara-C (Plunkett *et al.*, 1985; Preisler *et al.*, 1985). Studies on the correlation of F-ara-ATP in tumour cells with clinical and biochemical parameters will undoubtedly continue in conjunction with clinical trials.

Following dephosphorylation of F-ara-AMP, the nucleoside undergoes degradative metabolism in all species studied to date. In addition to parent drug (as previously noted), F-ara-A and the deaminated product F-ara-hypoxanthine (F-ara-Hyp) were detected in plasma following administration of F-ara-AMP to mice, dogs and humans. F-ara-AMP and F-ara-A pharmacokinetic parameters for mice, dogs and humans are summarized in Table 1. There appear to be species differences in metabolism related to the extent of F-ara-A deamination. In a study comparing the disposition of F-ara-AMP in mice and dogs, parent drug was detected briefly in plasma and the total body clearance (Cl_{TB}) of F-ara-A was somewhat greater in the dog than in the mouse (Noker *et al.*, 1983, Table 1). Plasma concentrations of F-ara-Hyp were significantly greater relative to F-ara-A concentrations in the dog than in the mouse (Noker *et al.*, 1983). Twenty-four hour urinary recoveries of F-ara-A and F-ara-Hyp (as % of administered dose) were approximately 90% and 10%, respectively, for the mouse, and approximately 40% and 40%, respectively, for the dog (Noker *et al.*, 1983). The authors concluded that deamination was more rapid in the dog.

Similar results were found in a study on the disposition of F-ara-A (rather than F-ara-AMP) in mice, dogs, and monkeys (El Dareer *et al.*, 1980). While plasma elimination did not differ dramatically among the three species (elimination phase half-life ($t_{½}$) values derived from a two-compartment open model were 72, 112 and 125 minutes for mice, dogs and monkeys, respectively), there were greater quantities of "metabolites" in dog plasma than in the other two species. In follow-up studies (Struck *et al.*, 1982), these observations were confirmed by determining urinary recoveries of F-ara-A and F-ara-Hyp in the three species. Twenty-four hour urinary recovery of F-ara-A and

Table 1. F-ara-AMP and F-ara-A pharmacokinetics following intravenous administration of F-ara-AMP to mice, dogs and humans.

Dose	F-ara-AMP	F-ara-A			References
(mg/m^2)	$t_{1/2}$ (min)	$t_{1/2}$ (min)	Cl_{TB} ($ml/min/m^2$)[c]	V_d (l/m^2)[c]	
Mice					
40	21	114[a]	49	8[d]	Noker *et al.* (1983)
500	27	184[a]	44	12[d]	Noker *et al.* (1983)
Dogs					
40	30	97[a]	105	15[d]	Noker *et al.* (1983)
500	51	90[a]	85	11[d]	Noker *et al.* (1983)
260		96[a]	124	16[e]	DeSouza *et al.* (1984)
Humans					
260		592 (9·9 h)[b]	79	46[e]	DeSouza *et al.* (1984)

[a] β half-life derived from two-compartment model.
[b] γ half-life derived from three-compartment model.
[c] Converted to m^2 values using standard mouse, dog and human weight–surface area data.
[d] Total body volume of distribution.
[e] Steady-state volume of distribution.

F-ara-Hyp in mice, dogs and monkeys were 63% and 13%, 13% and 52%, and 58% and 25%, respectively. Clearly the dog more efficiently deaminates F-ara-A than does the mouse or the monkey.

In another comparative study, metabolism of F-ara-AMP in dogs and in patients participating in Phase I trials was compared at Ohio State University. Cl_{TB} was only moderately higher in dogs than in patients (DeSouza *et al.*, 1984, Table 1). However, comparison of urinary excretion patterns of F-ara-A and F-ara-Hyp in the two species revealed significant differences in degradative metabolism. Within 12 hours, 70% of the F-ara-AMP dose administered to dogs was recovered in the urine as F-ara-Hyp and an additional 20% was recovered as F-ara-A. In marked contrast, patients excreted less than 1% of the administered dose as F-ara-Hyp after 30 hours, but 40% as F-ara-A.

The disposition and metabolism of F-ara-AMP briefly reviewed above are of particular interest in relation to preclinical and clinical toxicity studies with this agent. The dose in mice which produces 10% lethality (LD_{10}) and the equivalent dose in the dog (the mouse equivalent LD_{10} or MELD-10) for a single dose of F-ara-AMP was 2623 mg/m^2, while the LD_{10} in mice and the MELD-10 in dogs for the daily times five schedule was 1118 mg/m^2/day (C. K. Grieshaber, personal communication). Little myelosuppression was observed at these doses in either species. In fact, 3–4 times the MELD-10 dose was required to produce significant marrow toxicity in the dog, i.e,. approximately 10 500 mg/m^2 for a single dose or 4500 mg/m^2/day for the daily times five schedule. As is usually the case, based on the mouse LD_{10} and dog MELD-10 toxicity studies, Phase I clinical trials were initiated at one tenth the LD_{10} or 260 mg/m^2 for the single-dose schedule (Phase I Working Group meeting minutes, National Cancer Institute, Bethesda, MD, 20–22 September 1983). However, unexpected and substantial myelosuppression was observed in patients at the first dose level. Following an initial dose reduction to 80 mg/m^2, the eventual MTD in patients was approximately 160 mg/m^2. A similar pattern of toxicity was observed for daily times five studies. The MTD at the University of Texas was 18 mg/m^2/day (Hutton *et al.*, 1984) as compared to the mouse daily times five LD_{10} dose of 117 mg/m^2/day. In recent reviews which include considerations of the relationship between preclinical toxicology mouse LD_{10} values and ultimate MTD values arising from Phase I trials, the "average" ratio of human MTD to mouse LD_{10} is 1–3 (Collins *et al.*, 1986; Grieshaber *et al.*, 1986). The ratios for the single dose and daily times five schedules for F-ara-AMP were approximately 0·10 and 0·03, respectively. In other words, F-ara-AMP was much more toxic to humans than predicted by either mouse or dog preclinical toxicology studies.

When considering F-ara-AMP pharmacokinetics, it is apparent that dogs deaminate F-ara-A derived from parent drug more rapidly than humans, as pointed out by investigators at Ohio State University (Desouza *et al.*, 1984). These workers suggested that this species difference in metabolism of F-ara-A, the dephosphorylated product of parent drug required for cellular uptake and intracellular activation, might play a role in the greater susceptibility of humans to F-ara-AMP toxicity. However, it should be recalled that both the dog and the mouse are relatively resistant to F-ara-AMP toxicity, and the mouse did not rapidly deaminate F-ara-A as did the dog. Furthermore, all three species have relatively similar total body clearance of F-ara-A derived from F-ara-AMP (Table 1). The modest differences could not account for the dramatically greater toxicity in humans. The only notable differences in pharmacokinetic parameters among the three species are the longer elimination $t_{1/2}$ values for humans (approximately 10 hours) compared to mice and dogs (approximately 2 hours), and the differences in the percentage of dose excreted as F-ara-Hyp over 12–30 hours (~10%, ~50%, ~1% for mice, dogs and humans, respectively). With regard to half-life values, since Cl_{TB} values differ only by a factor of 2–3 fold, the prolonged half-life of F-ara-A for patients does not translate into dramatically greater exposure to drug. With regard to deamination, while humans are much less efficient at converting F-ara-A to F-ara-Hyp than dogs, this does not result in greatly decreased clearance of F-ara-A which might account for the increased toxicity. These factors do not readily explain the much greater toxicity of F-ara-AMP in humans than in dogs or mice.

One possible explanation may be related to the importance of time of F-ara-A exposure to critical cells, rather than total AUC determined from plasma measurements. The longer plasma elimination phase half-life in humans may be important with regard to marrow exposure to threshold concentrations of toxic species. A more plausible explanation may involve the intracellular activation of F-ara-A derived from parent drug, particularly the initial phosphorylation catalysed by deoxycytidine kinase. It has been suggested that the greater than anticipated toxicity of F-ara-AMP in patients might be due to the markedly different tissue distributions of deoxyadenosine phosphorylating activities in mouse and man (Hutton *et al.*, 1984). However, this is very unlikely given observations that most if not all F-ara-A phosphorylation appears to be catalysed by deoxycytidine kinase (Brockman *et al.*, 1980). A more likely explanation can be found in consideration of differences in activity of deoxycytidine kinase among mice, dogs and humans. Marrow deoxycytidine kinase activity (measured as conversion of deoxycytidine to the phosphorylated nucleotide) for a group of six dogs ranged between 0·01 and 0·03 nmol/h/10^6 cells whereas the average value for nine cancer patients was approximately 0·20 nmol/h/10^6 cells (DeSouza *et al.*, 1985; L. Malspeis, personal communication). Investigators at NCI are evaluating deoxycytidine kinase activity and F-ara-A toxicity in human and mouse marrow cells. F-ara-A is more toxic to human marrow cells than to mouse marrow cells at equivalent concentrations. Deoxycytidine kinase activity studies with F-ara-A as substrate are currently under way (J. Collins, personal communication). Thus, the basis for increased marrow toxicity in humans relative to mice and dogs may reside more with intracellular activation of the nucleoside F-ara-A in marrow, while the reduced toxicity in the dog relative to the mouse may be due to accelerated deamination of F-ara-A formed from F-ara-AMP.

These interesting studies on F-ara-AMP metabolism will be of value in further investigations with F-ara-AMP and development of other new agents. The studies by Plunkett and his colleagues (Danhauser *et al.*, 1986) may provide methods to monitor effectiveness and/or toxicity of this drug in patients, based on blood and/or tumour cell metabolism of F-ara-AMP. The observations with regard to species differences in toxicity and deamination of F-ara-AMP and species differences in intracellular phosphorylation of F-ara-A may assist in analysing preclinical pharmacological and toxicological studies with other antimetabolites.

Menogaril (NSC 269148)

Menogaril is a semisynthetic anthracycline analogue derived from the antibiotic nogalamycin (Figure 3). The latter agent was studied some years ago, but produced unacceptable renal and pulmonary toxicity in animals (Bhuyan *et al.*, 1980). Subsequently, a number of nogalamycin analogues were synthesized and screened for anti-tumour activity. Of those, menogaril was selected for development based on its relatively broad spectrum activity against murine model systems including B16 melanoma, CD8F mammary, colon 26 and

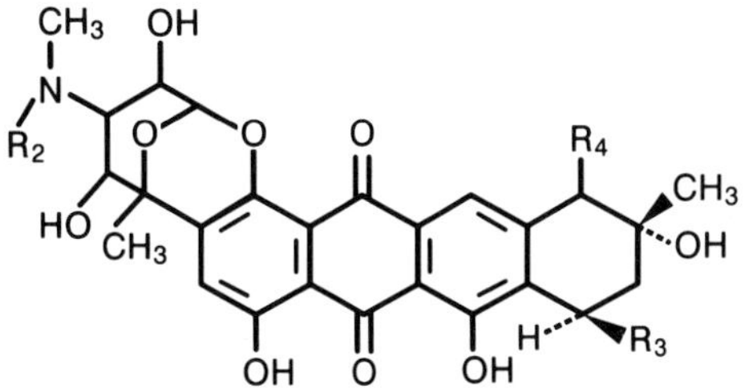

Compound	R_2	R_3	R_4
Nogalamycin	CH_3	Nogalose	$COOCH_3$
Menogaril	CH_3	OCH_3	H
N-Demethyl Menogaril	H	OCH_3	H
Nogarol	CH_3	OH	H
7-Deoxynogarol	CH_3	H	H
N-Demethyl-7-Deoxynogarol	H	H	H

Figure 3. Structure of menogaril and related compounds.

L1210 leukaemia (Neil *et al.*, 1979). Activity was also reported when menogaril was administered orally to tumour-bearing mice (McGovern, 1980). The major toxicity in animals (rats and dogs) was myelosuppression. Data obtained from rabbit toxicity studies suggested that menogaril may be less cardiotoxic than anthracyclines such as doxorubicin (McGovern *et al.*, 1979). Chronic anthracycline cardiomyopathy was not observed in rabbits until administration of cumulative doses of menogaril greater than 3000 mg/m^2 as compared to cumulative doses of doxorubicin greater than 200 mg/m^2 (McGovern *et al.*, 1979).

There is evidence that the mechanism of action of menogaril may differ from that of anthracyclines such as doxorubin. Thermal denaturation and absorption data suggested much reduced binding of menogaril to DNA as compared to doxorubicin (Richardson *et al.*, 1981). Menogaril did not inhibit RNA polymerase II transcription at concentrations which, for doxorubicin, produced greater than 90% inhibition (Richardson *et al.*, 1981). Cell cycle phase-specific lethality also differed for menogaril and doxorubicin. Menogaril was most toxic to Chinese hamster ovary cells in postmetaphase plus G_1 whereas doxorubicin was most toxic to cells during S-phase (Bhuyan *et al.*, 1980).

Several Phase I clinical trials have been completed with menogaril. Haematological toxicity (primarily leukopenia) was dose-limiting when menogaril was administered on one day every three weeks (Dorr *et al.*, 1985), on days one and eight every four weeks (Brown *et al.*, 1985), and for three days every three weeks (Zimet *et al.*, 1985). Dose-limiting toxicity in a 72-hour continuous infusion study was venous irritation including erythaema, burning pain, and oedema at the infusion site (Long *et al.*, 1985). Local reactions were reported in the other studies as well, and are consistent with observations in the preclinical toxicology studies. Currently, Phase II clinical trials are in progress in the United States, Europe and Canada in approximately 25 disease categories (P. J. McGovren, Upjohn Company, personal communication).

Based on preclinical and clinical pharmacology studies, menogaril appears to be metabolized and/or taken up extensively by tissues. There is limited information on the metabolic pathways. In mice, menogaril was eliminated with a terminal half-life of 10–12 h following intravenous administration (Dodion *et al.*, 1984; Pratt *et al.*, 1982). Using HPLC assay with fluorescence detection, two metabolites were observed in mouse plasma, one with a retention time identical to *N*-demethylmenogaril (Figure 3) (Dodion *et al.*, 1984; Pratt *et al.*, 1982). In accompanying studies *in vitro*, it was determined that NADPH fortified rat liver homogenates converted menogaril to two unidentified metabolites under anaerobic conditions, one with a retention time similar to that of the unidentified plasma metabolite (Dodion *et al.*, 1984). Under aerobic conditions the homogenates converted menogaril to *N*-demethylmenogaril (Dodion *et al.*, 1984). The *N*-demethylated metabolite had much reduced activity but greater potency at optimal doses against P388 and B16 melanoma murine tumours *in vivo* (Pratt *et al.*, 1982). Tissue distribution studies revealed that neither menogaril nor detected metabolites were found in brain to any significant extent, and menogaril appeared to be sequestered in the lungs rapidly after administration, a phenomenon observed with other anthracyclines. Following intravenous administration of menogaril to beagle dogs, plasma elimination was biphasic with an elimination $t_{1/2}$ of 3·3 h (Pratt and Adams, 1983). Three plasma metabolites were detected, one apparently *N*-demethylmenogaril.

More detailed metabolism studies of menogaril in the rabbit were reported by Dodion *et al.* (1985). Plasma elimination was biphasic in nature with a terminal $t_{1/2}$ of 2·7 h and (Cl_{TB} of 57·6 ml/min/kg. No metabolites were detected in plasma by HPLC with fluorescent detection. Four urinary metabolites were detected, one with a retention time identical to that of *N*-demethylmenogaril. The other three metabolites were not identified. Total urinary recovery of parent drug and metabolites, based on fluorescence of menogaril and metabolites, was less than 2% of the administered dose after 8 h. Parent drug and six metabolites were observed in the bile following administration of menogaril to rabbits (Dodion *et al.*, 1985). In addition to *N*-demethylmenogaril and the three unidentified metabolites also found in urine, two additional products were observed and tentatively identified by chromatographic retention times as 7-deoxynogarol and *N*-demethyl-7-deoxynogarol (Figure 3). Total biliary recovery of parent drug and metabolites, again based on fluorescence, was less than 4% over 8 h following drug administration.

Data on the fate of menogaril following intravenous administration to humans are available from several recent pharmacological studies. Employing

HPLC-fluorescence detection assays, plasma elimination of menogaril was most commonly fit to two-compartment models with terminal $t_{1/2}$ values of 10–20 h (Egorin *et al.*, 1986; Kuhn *et al.*, 1985; Grochow *et al.*, 1985). In a 72 hour continuous infusion Phase I study, the rise in plasma concentrations of menogaril was fit to a one-compartment model with a $t_{1/2}$ of 12 hours (Long *et al.*, 1985). Plasma elimination of drug was fit to a three-compartment model in a recent Phase I pharmacological study, with a terminal half-life value of 29·5 hours (Dodion *et al.*, 1986). Only one metabolite, *N*-demethylmenogaril, has been detected in human plasma (Dodion *et al.*, 1986; Egorin *et al.*, 1986; Grochow *et al.*, 1985) and urine (Egorin *et al.*, 1986). As in animal studies, urinary recovery of parent drug and metabolites based on fluorescence was very low, 5–15% (Egorin *et al.*, 1986; Grochow *et al.*, 1985; Long *et al.*, 1985). Egorin *et al.* (1986) analysed bile from two patients with biliary trace drains and detected only parent drug and *N*-demethylmenogaril (Egorin *et al.*, 1986).

Data from preclinical studies show that menogaril is metabolized to as many as six products in several animal species. *N*-Demethylation and reductive cleavage of the C-7 methoxy moiety (R_3 in Figure 3) have been identified as metabolic pathways. Using analytical methodologies similar to those utilized in animal studies, several groups found minimal amounts of *N*-demethylmenogaril as the only human metabolite. The low recoveries of parent drug and metabolites in urine and bile observed in preclinical and clinical pharmacology are similar to observations with agents such as adriamycin (<10% urinary recovery of parent drug plus metabolites over 3–7 days) (Riggs and Bachur, 1983). Additional metabolism may play a role in the disposition and elimination of menogaril. The low recovery of metabolites may be due to lack of detection (e.g., they may not fluoresce) or inappropriate chromatography and inappropriate isolation techniques developed for parent drug rather than metabolites. Alternatively, menogaril may be very effectively taken up and sequestered by tissues, as observed for other anthracycline-like drugs. Metabolism of menogaril may be reduced in comparison to other anthracycline-like drugs. Reduction of the side-chain carbonyl moiety by soluble aldo-keto reductases, which frequently gives rise to the major metabolite of anthracyclines containing that moiety, is not possible with menogaril. To date conjugates have not been identified, and reductive cleavage of methoxyl at C-7 does not appear to represent a major metabolic pathway, particularly in humans. A major limitation in metabolism studies with menogaril is the lack of availability of radiolabelled drug. It has not been possible to adequately characterize the distribution and fate of drug and metabolites with unlabelled drug. Despite relatively detailed metabolism studies, it is not clear whether or not unknown metabolites play a major role in the activity of menogaril, or even if metabolism plays a major role in the disposition of this interesting agent.

Teroxirone (NSC 296934)

Teroxirone (Figure 4) is a triepoxide triazine which has completed preclinical and Phase I evaluation under the auspices of NCI. Several features of the disposition and metabolism of this agent are of interest and serve as the basis for continuing investigations of teroxirone as an agent well suited for regional administration.

Teroxirone was one of several triepoxides prepared in West Germany for evaluation as potential alkylating anti-tumour agents (Budnowski, 1968). Teroxirone had activity against a variety of murine tumour models including L1210 and P388 leukaemias and B16 melanoma (Spreafico *et al.*, 1980). The mechanism of action of teroxirone has not been defined. However, protein–DNA and DNA–DNA inter-strand cross-links were detectable by DNA alkaline elution assay following incubation of teroxirone with murine and human tumour cells (Ames and Gretsch, 1985). Cross-links were not detected if teroxirone was first treated under conditions known to hydrolyse the epoxide moieties. The major toxicities identified in preclinical studies were haematopoietic, including leukopenia and neutropenia. In NCI-sponsored Phase I clinical trials, dose-limiting toxicities were thrombophlebitis at the site of drug administration and moderate myelosuppression (Rubin *et al.*, 1987).

The limited preclinical pharmacological studies conducted prior to Phase I studies suggested that teroxirone might be somewhat unique with regard to its metabolism and elimination. Following bolus intravenous infusion to rabbits, teroxirone plasma elimination was extremely rapid with an elimination $t_{1/2}$ of less than five minutes. Only trace amnounts of parent drug were recovered in 24 hour urine (Ames *et al.*, 1983, 1984). Despite the presence of epoxide moieties, teroxirone was relatively stable in aqueous solutions (including buffers at physiological pH). Complete hydrolysis of teroxirone required heating at 60–90°C in dilute acid (M. M. Ames, unpublished observations). While teroxirone was lesss stable in fresh rabbit plasma, human plasma or human whole blood, the rate of disappearance at 37°C ($t_{1/2}$ 20–40 min) did not account for the rapid plasma elimination.

Following bolus intravenous administration of teroxirone to Phase I

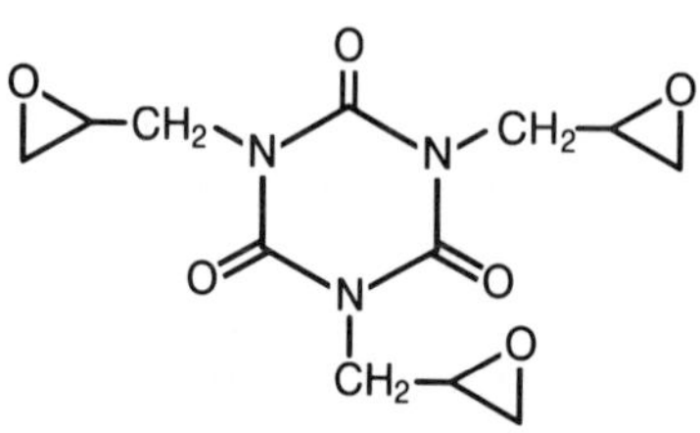

Figure 4. Structure of teroxirone.

patients at doses of 140–500 mg/m^2, teroxirone plasma elimination was extremely rapid (mean $t_{½}$ 1·4 min) and Cl_{TB} very high (mean value 5·7 l/min) (Ames *et al.*, 1984). When teroxirone was administered by constant intravenous infusion, steady-state concentrations were rapidly achieved, consistent with the rapid $t_{½}$ values observed in bolus studies. The clearance values were even greater as rates of infusion were reduced from 12·5 mg/min to 0·45 mg/min, suggesting that elimination may involve a saturable process (M. M. Ames, unpublished observations). Urinary recovery of parent drug (24 hours) was less than 1% in all patient studies.

Additional studies were carried out in an effort to characterize the mechanisms of plasma elimination and their possible roles in the activity of teroxirone. Teroxirone was avidly metabolized by rat and rabbit microsomal preparations in a non-NADPH-dependent reaction which was inhibited by cyclohexene oxide, a known inhibitor of microsomal epoxide hydrase (Ames *et al.*, 1984; Ames and Kovach, 1984). Teroxirone epoxide hydrolysis products were detected in incubation mixtures. The very large Cl_{TB} values obtained from patient studies implied extrahepatic sites of metabolism. In addition to blood (which did not avidly degrade teroxirone), the lung could provide the observed rapid clearance of parent drug. However, no evidence of metabolism was found when teroxirone was incubated with rabbit and rat lung homogenates and microsomal preparations. In another effort to determine the fate of teroxirone *in vivo*, rabbits were administered ^{14}C-ring-labelled teroxirone. The rapid plasma disappearance of parent drug ($t_{½} < 5$ min) was accompanied by a much slower (several hours) plasma disappearance of radioactivity (Ames *et al.*, 1984). The radioactivity passed freely through protein filter membranes, apparently ruling out rapid irreversible interaction of labelled teroxirone with proteins (Ames *et al.*, 1984). Thus, teroxirone appeared to be rapidly metabolized. While epoxide hydrolysis in the liver may account for a significant portion of teroxirone metabolism, it is likely that other sites are involved in the biotransformation of this drug *in vivo*. Metabolism appears to eliminate teroxirone cytotoxicity. Incubation of teroxirone with human tumour cells inhibits colony survival (Ames *et al.*, 1984), but inhibition was not observed when 9000 *g* rat hepatic preparations were co-incubated with cells and drug. When cyclohexene oxide was added to mixtures of drug, cells and hepatic supernatant preparation, cytotoxicity was partially restored.

Teroxirone clinical utility is limited by difficulties of parenteral administration, specifically significant thrombophlebitis at doses producing myelosuppression in Phase I trials (Rubin *et al.*, 1987). The extremely short plasma half-life and activity of parent compound (as opposed to hydrolysis metabolites) suggest that teroxirone might be a candidate for regional perfusion studies. Locally high concentrations of parent drug combined with the very rapid systemic clearance of teroxirone might provide a therapeutic advantage for the treatment of appropriate tumours. The NCI has recently reopened the investigational new drug (IND) status of teroxirone for regional therapy studies based on results of the pharmacokinetic and metabolism studies.

N^2-Methyl-9-hydroxy ellipticine (Elliptinium acetate, MHE, NSC 264137)

During the 1960s, several groups isolated natural products with anti-tumour activity from *Ochrosia elliptica* and related plants (Hayat *et al.*, 1974; Suffness and Douros, 1980; Svoboda *et al.*, 1968). The active compounds were pyridazo-carbazoles, specifically ellipticine and 9-methoxyellipticine (Figure 5), both of which had activity against L1210 leukaemia and a number of solid tumours (Hayat *et al.*, 1974; Suffness and Douros, 1980; Svoboda *et al.*, 1968). Development of the parent compound, ellipticine, was curtailed by cardiovascular toxicity problems and haemolysis of red blood cells observed during preclinical toxicology studies (Paoletti *et al.*, 1979). Interest subsequently shifted to development of 9-substituted compounds including 9-hydroxyellipticine, 9-methoxyellipticine and MHE (Figure 5). The naturally occurring analogue 9-methoxyellipticine was ultimately evaluated in clinical trials and shown to have limited activity against acute myeloblastic leukaemia (Mathe *et al.*, 1970). 9-Hydroxyellipticine, prepared synthetically and later found to be a metabolite of ellipticine (see below), was active against a number of model tumour systems (Hayat *et al.*, 1974; LePecq *et al.*, 1976). Only limited activity was seen in subsequent clinical trials (Juret *et al.*, 1978). MHE, the *N*-methyl quaternary nitrogen analogue of 9-hydroxyellipticine (Figure 5), was selected for further study based on reduced toxicity as compared to other

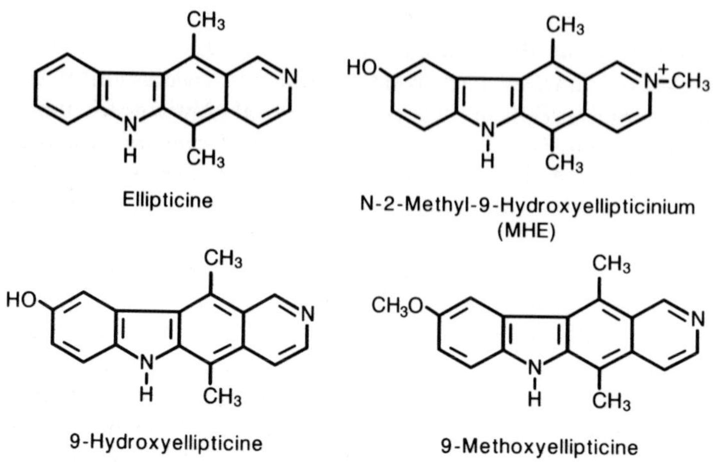

Figure 5. Structure of ellipticine, 9-hydroxyellipticine, 9-methoxyellipticine and MHE.

ellipticine analogues and evidence of increased binding to DNA (Elliptinium Investigator's Drug Brochure, 1982; Herman *et al.*, 1974). Among ellipticine analogues, MHE has received the most attention and study as an anti-tumour agent.

Toxicities observed during preclinical studies with MHE included moderate renal toxicity and reactions at the injection site, but only limited myelosuppression (Elliptinium Investigator's Drug Brochure, 1982). Phase I studies were first conducted in Europe. Toxicities included hypotension, haemolysis phlebitis, nausea and vomiting, dry mouth, neurotoxicity, renal toxicity, but only minimal myelosuppression (Brugarolas *et al.*, 1979; Dodion *et al.*, 1982; Juret *et al.*, 1978). Responses in Phase I and Phase II studies were observed primarily in breast cancers (Brugarolas *et al.*, 1979; Juret *et al.*, 1978, 1982). Several Phase I studies were conducted in the USA (Buzdar *et al.*, 1984; Einzig *et al.*, 1985). Toxicities were similar to those described in European reports. Dose-limiting toxicities were primarily nausea and vomiting and renal function impairment. Myelosuppression was either mild or not observed in these studies. Some time after initiation of Phase II trials in the USA, it was determined that, as formulated at that time, MHE could form short-chain polymers which may have been associated with some of the toxicities noted in Phase I and Phase II studies. Trials were halted at that time, and are due to begin again in the near future with a newly formulated product (Dr. A. Goodman, Ives Co., personal communication).

In preclinical pharmacology studies, the parent compound ellipticine was eliminated from mouse, rat and dog primarily via the bile (Chadwick *et al.*, 1978). Rat biliary metabolites included the sulphate and glucuronide of 9-hydroxyellipticine (Branfman *et al.*, 1978). NADPH-fortified rat liver microsomes converted ellitipticine to the 9-hydroxy metabolite in a cytochrome P-450 catalysed reaction (Lessa *et al.*, 1977). 9-Hydroxyellipticine was converted to the glucuronide conjugate by mice (Von-Bac *et al.*, 1980). Following intravenous administration of the quaternary analogue MHE to rats, drug was distributed to tissues including kidneys, liver, lung and thyroid glands (Von-Bac *et al.*, 1980). The $t_{1/2}$ of plasma elimination was 27 hours. Within three days, approximately 85% of the dose was excreted as unchanged MHE, primarily via the bile. No metabolites of MHE were reported in this study. Pharmacokinetics of MHE were reported as part of a Phase I trial in Europe (Gouyette *et al.*, 1982). Plasma elimination was best described by a three-compartment open model with a terminal phase $t_{1/2}$, Cl_{TB} and central compartment volume of distribution of 23·7 hour, 971 ml/min and 1·8 litres, respectively. Less than 20% of parent drug was recovered in the urine over a four-day period. Based on the above studies, it appeared that ellipticine was hydroxylated at the nine position and subsequently conjugated and eliminated in the bile. 9-Hydroxyellipticine was similarly conjugated, while MHE was eliminated primarily as unchanged drug, although it was appreciated that conjugation at the nine position was also likely for the quaternary compound.

The mechanism of action of ellipticines is thought to be related to interactions of these agents with DNA. Paoletti and his colleagues showed that most ellipticines bind strongly to DNA with binding constants between 10^5 and 10^7 M^{-1} (summarized in Paoletti *et al.*, 1980; LePecq *et al.*, 1974), The pyridocarbazole ring system approximates the geometry of a pyrimidine–purine base pair, and is ideally suited to position itself between DNA bases. Ellipticines are DNA intercalating agents. It was soon apparent however that DNA binding could not fully explain activity of ellipticines, since some analogues with very high binding constants possesed little or no cytotoxicity against cells in culture (Paoletti *et al.*, 1980).

It is possible that metabolism plays a role in the activity of ellipticine. Ellipticine analogues with a hydroxyl moiety at the nine position of the ring system, such as 9-hydroxyellipticine and MHE, have greater cytotoxic and anti-tumour properties than do their counterparts lacking the 9-hydroxyl moiety (LePecq *et al.*, 1974). It has been shown that ellipticine analogues bearing 9-hydroxyl moieties, and only those analogues, are converted to free radical and two-electron oxidation products by horseradish peroxidase and human myeloperoxidase in the presence of hydrogen peroxide (Auclair and Paoletti, 1981) (Figure 6). The two-electron oxidation products (e.g., quinone-imines, for MHE see Figure 6) will oxidize NADH, and the quinone-imine of MHE forms adducts with bovine serum albumin, presumably via nucleophilic attack of appropriate amino acid side-chains. At alkaline pH, and to a lesser extent at physiological pH, spontaneous oxidation of 9-hydroxyellipticine can also lead to formation of the free radical and the quinone-imine in aqueous

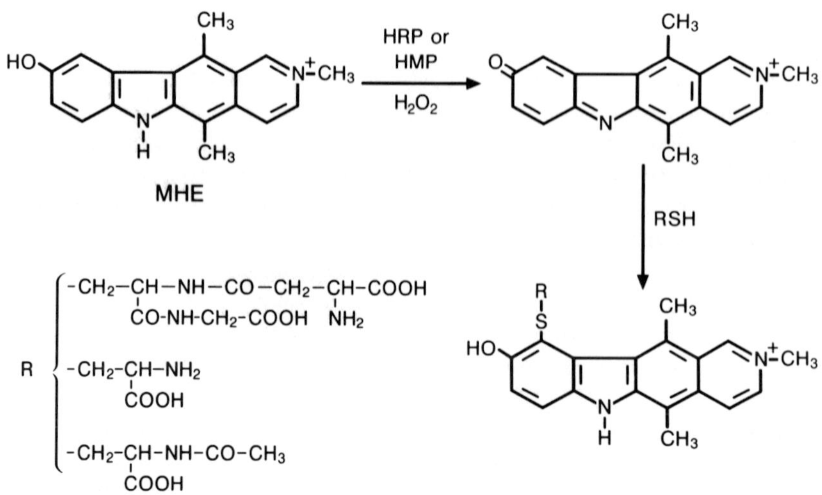

Figure 6. Oxidation of MHE by horseradish peroxidase or human myeloperoxidase and conjugation of the oxidation product with glutathione.

solutions (Auclair *et al.*, 1983). It has been suggested that the one-electron and/or the two-electron oxidation products of ellipticines might play a role in the cytotoxicity of these compounds via formation of toxic radical species and/or formation of alkylating species, respectively (Auclair and Paoletti, 1981; Auclair *et al.*, 1983). The quinone-imine product of MHE has been shown to react with nucleophiles including glutathione (Meunier *et al.*, 1983).

Evidence for formation of reactive electrophilic species *in vivo* has come from studies identifying urinary and biliary conjugates of MHE. A glutathione conjugate of MHE (Figure 6) was isolated and identified by nuclear magnetic resonance spectrometry and mass spectrometry as a rat biliary metabolite (Maftouh *et al.*, 1984). The *N*-acetylcysteine and cysteine conjugates of MHE (Figure 6) have recently been identified as urinary metabolites in rats and humans (Monsarrat *et al.*, 1983). The cysteine conjugate has also been identified as a human biliary metabolite of MHE (Bernadou *et al.*, 1985). The presence of glutathione and related conjugates is interpreted as strong evidence for oxidation of MHE followed by reaction of the electrophilic quinone-imine with nucleophilic sulphydryl of glutathione. This "reactive intermediate" or "oxidative bioactivation" pathway has been postulated to play a role in the anti-tumour activity of 9-hydroxyellipticine analogues including MHE (Bernadou *et al.*, 1985; Monsarrat *et al.*, 1983; Maftouh *et al.*, 1984). While there is strong evidence that ellipticines with 9-hydroxyl moieties are converted to species which covalently bind to macromolecules, the effects of such alkylation are more difficult to predict. The reactive species are monofunctional alkylating agents, and in that respect differ from most bifunctional alkylating agents with anti-tumour activity. Monofunctional alkylation could serve to anchor the intercalating agent in DNA, possibly exacerbating effects of such interactions. Most interesting are recent reports summarized by Pratviel *et al.* (1986) that the quinone-imine of MHE preferentially attacks the ribose moiety of nucleosides. The biological consequences of such ribose alkylations *in vivo* are not known.

There is a second type of DNA damage observed when ellipticines, including ellipticine, 9-hydroxyellipticine and MHE are incubated with murine or mammalian cells in culture. Exposure of cells to the ellipticines produces DNA single-strand and double-strand breaks (Ross and Bradley, 1981; Zwelling *et al.*, 1982). Protein is associated with the DNA strand breaks (Zwelling *et al.*, 1982). These specific DNA lesions are produced following incubation of cells with a variety of intercalating (adriamycin, 4-(acridinylamino)methansulphon-*m*-anisidide or *m*-AMSA) and non-intercalating drugs (etoposide or VP-16) (Ross and Bradley, 1981; Wozniak and Ross, 1983; Zwelling *et al.*, 1981). It is thought that the drugs stabilize a DNA–topoisomerase complex which prevents resealing of DNA following topoisomerase-catalysed cleavage of DNA, and that this stabilization leads to strand breaks. All of these agents, including the ellipticines, stimulate DNA cleavage when incubated with DNA and purified topoisomerase II (Chen *et al.*, 1984; Tewey *et al.*, 1984 a,b). In addition, precipitation studies show that the protein associated with the DNA strand breaks in whole cell studies is topoisomerase II (Chen *et al.*, 1984; Tewey *et al.*, 1984 a,b). It is widely speculated that these drug/DNA/topoisomerase interactions are related to the anti-tumour activity of this diverse group of molecules. The potential role of topoisomerases as targets of anti-cancer drugs has recently been reviewed (Ross, 1985). It is unlikely that the radical production associated with MHE (either by chemical or enzymatic means) is associated with the reported single-strand and double-strand DNA breaks produced by this agent, since equal or greater amounts of DNA damage occur after exposure of cells to ellipticine (Zwelling *et al.*, 1982). The oxidation pathways do not occur with ellipticine, which lacks the 9-hydroxyl moiety.

Summary

The conduct of detailed metabolic studies with new agents is a more difficult task than characterization of the parent compound. New analytical methods are required, radiolabelled drug may be needed, and isolation, purification and structure proof of metabolites is a time-consuming process requiring significant analytical resources. It is important to follow up the analytical studies with a variety of biochemical studies (cell culture, enzyme inhibition, interaction with macromolecules, etc.) to determine the role of metabolism in pharmacological activities associated with the parent drug. This chapter has included several examples for which appropriate analytical and biochemical studies provided information important in the understanding and use of new anti-tumour agents.

Acknowledgements

The author would like to thank Ms. Wanda Rhodes for her excellent preparation of the manuscript.

References

Allen, B. A., Newman, R. A., Griffin, J. P. and McCormack, J. J., 1981, Liquid chromatographic determination of an antineoplastic aziridinylbenzoquinone in human and murine serum. *J. Chromatogr.*, **222**, 146–151.

Ames, M. M. and Gretsch, S. K., 1985, DNA-DNA and protein-DNA crosslinking by the experimental anticancer agent Teroxirone (NSC 296934) in murine L1210 leukemia and human A204 rhabdomyosarcoma cell lines. *Fed. Proc.*, **44**, 1141.

Ames, M. M. and Kovach, J. S., 1984, Microsomal metabolism and in vitro cytotoxicity of the experimental triepoxide antitumor agent Teroxirone. 6th International Symposium on Microsome and Drug Oxidations, Brighton, England, August 5–10. Abstract P.3/50.

Ames, M. M., Kovach, J. S. and Rubin, J., 1983. Pharmacological characterization of Henkel compound (Teroxirone, NSC 296934) in animals and humans. *Proc. Am. Soc. Clin. Oncol.*, **2**, 29.

Ames, M. M., Kovach, J. S. and Rubin, J., 1984. Pharmacologic and characterization of Teroxirone, a triepoxide antitumor agent, in rats, rabbits, and humans. *Cancer Res.*, **44**, 4151–4156.

Auclair, C. and Paoletti, C., 1981, Bioactivation of the antitumor drugs 9-hydroxyellipticine and derivatives by a peroxidase-hydrogen peroxide system. *J. Med. Chem.*, **24**, 289–295.

Auclair, C., Hyland, K. and Paoletti, C., 1983, Autooxidation of the antitumor drug 9-hydroxyellipticine and its derivatives. *J. Med. Chem.*, **26**, 1438–1444.

Avramis, V. I. and Plunkett, W., 1983, Metabolism of 9-β-D-arabinosyl-2-fluoro-adenine-5′-phosphate by mice bearing P-388 leukemia. *Cancer Drug Delivery*, **1**, 1–10.

Bachur, N. R., Gordon, S. L. and Gee, M. V., 1978, A general mechanism for microsomal activation of quinone anticancer agents to free radicals. *Cancer Res.*, **38**, 1745–1750.

Bachur, N. R., Collins, J. M., Kelley, J. A., Van Echo, D. A., Kaplan, R. S. and Whitacre, M., 1982, Diaziquone, 2,5-diaziridinyl-3,6-biscarboethoxyamino-1, 4-benzoquinone, plasma and cerebrospinal fluid kinetics. *Clin. Pharmacol. Ther.*, **31**, 650–655.

Bender, J. F., Grillo-Lopez, A. J. and Posada, J. G., Jr., 1983, Diaziquone (AZQ). *Invest. New Drugs*, **1**, 71–84.

Bernadou, J., Monsarrat, B., Roche, H., Armand, J. P., Paoletti, C. and Meunier, B., 1985, Evidence for electrophilic properties of N^2-methyl-9-ellipticinium acetate [Celiptium] from human biliary metabolites. *Cancer Chemother. Pharmacol.*, **15**, 63–65.

Bhuyan, B. K., Blowers, B. L. and Shugars, K. D., 1980 a, Lethality of nogalomycin, nogalomycin analogs, and adriamycin to cells in different cell cycle phases. *Cancer Res.*, **40**, 3437–3442.

Bhuyan, B. K., Neil, G. L., Li, L. H., McGovern, J. P. and Wiley, P. F., 1980 b, Chemistry and biological activity of 7-con-O-methyl-nogarol [7-con-OMEN]. In *Anthracyclines: Current Status and New Developments*, edited by S. T. Crook and S. D. Reich (New York: Academic Press), pp. 365–395.

Branfman, A. R., Bruni, R. J., Reinhold, V. N., Silveira, D. M., Chadwick, M. and Yesair, D. W., 1978, Characterization of the metabolites of ellipticine in rat bile. *Drug Metab. Disp.*, **6**, 542–548.

Brink, J. J. and LePage, G. A., 1984, Metabolic effects of 9-β-D-arabinosyl-purines in ascites tumor cells. *Cancer Res.*, **24**, 312–318.

Brockman, R. W., Schabel, F. M., Jr. and Montgomery, J.A., 1977, Biological activity of 9-β-D-arabinofuranosyl-2-fluoroadenine, a metabolically stable analog of 9-β-D-arabinofuranosyladenine. *Biochem. Pharmacol.*, **26**, 2193–2196.

Brockman, R. W., Cheng, X. C., Schabel, F. M., Jr. and Montgomery, J. A., 1980, Metabolism and chemotherapeutic activity of 9-β-D-arabinofuranosyl-2-fluoro-adenine against murine leukemia L1210 and evidence for its phosphorylation by deoxycytidine kinase. *Cancer Res.*, **40**, 3610–3615.

Brown, T. D., Donehower, R. C., Grochow, L. B., Ettinger, D. S., Rice, A. P. and Waalkes, T. P., 1985, A Phase I study of menogaril (Men) in patients with advanced cancer. *Proc. Am. Soc. Clin. Oncol.*, **4**, 32.

Brugarolas, A., Gracia, M., DeJager, R., Mallarme, M. and Claryssse, A., 1979, 9-Hydroxymethylellipticinium [NNSC 264137]: Phase I clinical study. *Proc. Am. Ass. Cancer Res. Am. Soc. Clin. Oncol.*, **20**, 310.

Budnowski, M., 1968, Preparation and properties of the diastereo-isomers of 1,3,5-triglycidyl-s-triazine/triones. *Angew. Chemie*, Int. Edition English, **7**, 827–828.

Buzdar, A., Yap, H. Y., Goodman, A., Chou, C., Hortobagyi, G., Blumenschein, G., Benjamin, R. and Bodey, G., 1984, Phase I trial of elliptinium acetate in advanced cancer. *Proc. Am. Ass. Cancer Res.*, **25**, 182.

Chadwick, M., Silviera, D. M., Platz, B. B. and Hayes, D., 1978, Comparative physiological disposition of ellipticine in several animal species after intravenous administration. *Drug Metab. Disp.*, **6**, 528–541.

Chen, G. L., Yang, L., Rowe, T. C., Halligan, B. D., Tewey, K. M. and Liu, L. F., 1984, Nonintercalative drugs interfere with the breakage-reunion reaction of mammalian DNA topoisomerase II. *J. Biol. Chem.*, **259**, 13560–13566.

Chou, F., Khan, A. H. and Driscoll, J. S., 1976, Potential central nervous system antitumor agents. Aziridinylbenzoquinones. 2. *J. Med. Chem.*, **19**, 1302–1308.

Collins, J. M., Zaharko, D. S., Dedrick, R. L. and Chabner, B. A., 1986, Potential roles for preclinical pharmacology in Phase I clinical trials. *Cancer Treat. Rep.*, **70**, 73–80.

Curt, G. A., Kelley, J. A., Kufta, C. V., Smith, B. H., Kornblith, P. L., Young, R. C. and Collins, J. M., 1983, Phase II and pharmacokinetic study of Aziridinyl-benzoquinone [2,5-diaziridinyl-3,6-(carboethoxyamino)-1,4-benzoquinone, Diaziquone, NSC 182986] in high grade gliomas. *Cancer Res.*, **43**, 6102–6105.

Danhauser, L., Plunkett, W., Keating, M. and Cabanillas, F., 1986, 9-β-D-Arabinofuranosyl-2-fluoroadenine 5′-monophosphate pharmacokinetics in plasma and tumor cells of patients with relapsed leukemia and lymphoma. *Cancer Chemother. Pharmacol.*, **23**, 868–872.

DeSouza, J. J. V., Grever, M., Neidhart, J. A., Staubus, A. E. and Malspeis, L., 1984, Comparative pharmacokinetics and metabolism of fludarabine phosphate (NSC 312887) in man and dog. *Proc. Am. Ass. Cancer Res.*, **25**, 361.

DeSouza, J. J. V., Leiby, J. M., Staubus, A. E., Grever, M. R. and Malspeis, L., 1985, Altered pharmacokinetics of fludarabine phosphate (F) by 2′-deoxy-coformycin (DCF) in the dog and analysis of a route of fludarabine activation. *Proc. Am. Ass. Cancer Res.*, **26**, 358.

Diaziquone Clinical Brochure, 1979, National Cancer Institute, Bethesda, Maryland.

Dodion, P., Rosenczweig, M., Nicaise, C. *et al.*, 1982, Phase I clinical study of 9-hydroxy-2-N-methyl ellipticinium acetate (NSC 264137) administered on a five-day i.v. schedule. *Eur. J. Cancer Clin. Oncol.*, **18**, 519–522.

Dodion, P., Chang, B. K., Egorin, M. J., Olman, E. A., Englisch, K. L. and Bachur, N. R., 1984, The disposition of the new anthracycline antibiotic, menogaril, in mice. *Drug Metab. Disp.*, **12**, 365–370.

Dodion, P., Egorin, M. J., Englisch, K. L. and Bachur, N. R., 1985, Metabolism and disposition of menogaril (NSC 269148) in the rabbit. *Cancer Res.*, **45**, 5352–5357.

Dodion, P., Sessa, C., Joss, R., Crespeigne, N., Willems, Y., Kitt, M., Abrams, J., Finet, C., Brewer, J. E., Adams, W. J., Earhart, R. H., Rozenczweig, M., Kenis, Y. and Cavalli, F., 1986, Phase I study of intravenous menogaril administered intermittently *J. Clin. Oncol.*, **4**, 767–774.

Dorr, A., Von Hoff, D., Kuhn, J. and Kisner, D., 1985, Phase I clinical trial of menogaril. *Proc. Am. Soc. Clin. Oncol.*, **4**, 39.

Driscoll, J. S., Hazard, G. F., Jr., Wood, H. B. and Goldin, A. 1974, Structure-antitumor activity relationships among quinone derivatives. *Cancer Chemother. Rep.*, **4**, 1–363.

Driscoll, J. S., Dudeck, L., Congleton, G. and Geran, R. I., 1979, Potential CNS antitumor agents VI: Aziridinylbenzoquinones. III. *J. Pharm. Sci.*, **68**, 185–188.

Egorin, M. J., Van Echo, D. A., Whitacre, M. Y., Forrest, A., Sigman, L. M., English, K. L. and Aisner, J., 1986, Human pharmacokinetics, excretion, and metabolism of the anthracycline antibiotic menogaril (NSC 269148, 7-OMEN) and their correlation with clinical toxicities. *Cancer Res.*, **46**, 1513–1520.

El Dareer, S. M., Struck, R. F., Tillery, K. F., Rose, L. M., Brockman, R. W., Montgomery, J. A. and Hill, D. L., 1980, Disposition of 9-β-D-arabinosyl-2-fluoroadenine in mice, dogs and monkeys. *Drug Metab. Disp.*, **8**, 60–67.

Elliptinium Investigator's Drug Brochure, 1982, Ives Laboratories Inc., New York, pp. 4–29.

Einzig, A. L., Gralla, R. J. and Leyland-Jones, B. R., 1985, Phase I study of elliptinium (2-N-methyl-9-hydroxyellipticinium). *Cancer Res.*, **3**, 235–241.

Feun, L. G., Savaraj, N., Lu K, Guo Z, Raulston, L. G., Benjamin, R. S., Fields, W. S. and Loo, T. L., 1983, The pharmacologic fate of 2,5-diaziridinyl-3, 6-bis(carboethoxyamino)-1,4-benzoquinone (AZQ, NSC-182986) by intracarotid or intravenous administration in beagles. *J. Neuro-Oncol.*, **1**, 219–224.

Frytak, S., Eagan, R. T., Ames, M. M., Creagan, E. T. and Nichols, W. C., 1984, Phase I study of diaziquone. *Cancer Treat. Rep.*, **68**, 975–978.

Gormley, P. E., Wood, J. H. and Poplack, D. G., 1981, Ability of a new antitumor agent, AZQ, to penetrate into cerebrospinal fluid. *Pharmacology*, **22**, 196–198.

Gouyette, A., Huertas, D., Droz, J. P., Rouesse, J. and Amiel, J. L., 1982, Pharmacokinetics of 2-methyl-9-hydroxyellipticinium acetate (NSC 264137) in cancer patients (Phase I study). *Eur. J. Cancer Clin. Oncol.*, **18**, 1285–1292.

Grever, M. R., Malspeis, L., Kraut, E. H., Wilson, H. E., Staubus, A. E., Coleman, M. S. and Balcerzak, S. P., 1984, Combination of 2′-deoxy-coformycin and vidarabine in advanced malignancy: clinical and biochemical observations. *Cancer Treat. Symp.*, **2**, 97–104.

Grieshaber, C. K. and Marsoni, S., 1986, Relation of preclinical toxicology to findings in early clinical trials. *Cancer Treat. Rep.*, **70**, 65–72.

Griffin, J. P., Newman, R. A., McCormack, J. J. and Krakoff, I. H., 1982, Clinical and clinical pharmacological studies of Aziridinylbenzoquinone. *Cancer Treat. Rep.*, **66**, 1321–1325.

Grochow, L. B., Donehower, R. C., Ettinger, D. S., Cates A. E. and Rice, A., 1985, Pharmacokinetics of menogaril (MEN) *Proc. Am. Soc. Clin. Oncol.*, **4**, 32.

Gutierrez, P. L., Friedman, R. D. and Bachur, N. R., 1982, Biochemical activation of AZQ [3,6-diaziridinyl-2,5-bis(carboethoxyamino)-1,4-benzoquinone]. *Cancer Treat. Rep.*, **66**, 339–342.

Gutierrez, P. L., Fox, B. M., Mossoba, M. M. and Bachur, N. R., 1984, Free radicals in quinone-containing antitumor agents: Electrochemical reduction of diaziquone [2,5-diaziridine-3,6-bis(carboethoxyamino)-1,4-benzoquinone] and two analogues. *Mol. Pharmacol.*, **26**, 582–586.

Gutierrez, P. L., Egorin, M. J. and Fox, B. M., 1985, Cellular activation of Diaziquone [2,5-diaziridinyl-3,6-bis(carboethoxyamino)-1,4-benzoquinone] to its free radical species. *Biochem. Pharmacol.*, **34**, 1449–1455.

Hayat, M., Mathe, G., Janot, M. M., Potier, P., Dat-Xuong, N., Cave, A., Sevenet, T., Kan-Fau, C., Poisson, J., Miet, J., LeMen, J., LeGoffic, F., Gouyette, A., Ahond, A., Dalton, L. K. and Connors, T. A., 1974, Experimental screening of 3 forms and 19 derivatives of analogs of ellipticine: Oncostatic effect on L1210 leukaemia and immunosuppressive effect of 4 of them. *Biomedicine Express*, **21**, 101–106.

Herman, E. H., Chadwick, D. P. and Mhatre, R. M., 1974, Comparison of the acute hemolytic and cardiovascular actions of ellipticine and some ellipticine analogs. *Cancer Chemother. Rep.*, **58**, 637–643.

Hutton, J. J., Von Hoff, D. D., Kuhn, J., Phillips, J., Hersh, M. and Clark, G., 1984, Phase I clinical investigation of 9-β-D-arabinofuranosyl-2-fluoroadenine-5′-monophosphate (NSC 312887), a new purine. *Cancer Res.*, **44**, 4183–4186.

Juret, P., Tanguy, A., Girard, A., LeTalaer, J. Y., Abbatucci, J. S., Dat-Xuong, N., Lepecq, J. B. and Paoletti, C., 1978, Preliminary trial of 9-hydroxy-2-methyl-ellipticinium (NSC-264137) in advanced human cancer. *Eur. J. Cancer Clin. Oncol.*, **14**, 205–206.

Juret, P., Heron, J. F., Couette, J. E., Delozien, T. and LeTalser, J. Y., 1982, Hydroxy-9-methyl-2-ellipticinium for osseous metastases from breast cancer: A 5-year experience. *Cancer Treat. Rep.*, **66**, 1909–1916.

Kelley, J. A. and Siu Chong, E. D., 1981, Reverse phase hplc determination of AZQ in biological fluids. *J. Liquid Chromatogr.*, **4**, 1855–1867.

Khan, A. H. and Driscoll, J. S., 1976, Potential central nervous system antitumor agents. Aziridinylbenzoquinones. 1. *J. Med. Chem.*, **19**, 313–317.

King, C. L., Hittelman, W. N. and Loo, T. L., 1984 a, Induction of DNA strand breaks and cross-links by 2,5-diaziridinyl-3,6-bis [carboethoxyamino] -1,4-benzoquinone in Chinese hamster ovary cells. *Cancer Res.*, **44**, 5634–5637.

King, C. L., Savaraj, N., Yeung, K. L. and Loo, T. L., 1984 b, Mechanism of diaziquone (AZQ)-induced DNA cross-links and strand breaks. *Proc. Am. Ass. Cancer Res.*, **25**, 301.

Komiyama, T., Kikuchi, T. and Sugiura, Y., 1982, Generation of hydroxyl radical by anticancer quinone drugs, Carbazilquinone, Mitomycin C, Aclacinomycin A and Adriamycin, in the presence of NADPH-cytochrome P450 reductase. *Biochem. Pharmacol.*, **31**, 3651–3656.

Kovach, J. S., Beart, R. W., Svingen, P., Holley, K. E., Reiman, H. M., Buck, M. and Moertel, C. G., 1986, Concentration of 5-fluorouracil (FU) and metabolites in human colon carcinomas and normal tissues after i.v. FU. *Proc. Am. Soc. Clin. Oncol.*, **5**, 46.

Kufe, D. W., 1984, Clinical and cellular pharmacology of 2′-deoxycoformycin and vidarabine. *Cancer Treat. Symp.*, **2**, 85–95.

Kuhn, J., Kisner, D., Schwartz, R., Schick, M., Dorr, A., Clark, G., Von Hoff, D., Brewer, J. and Adams, W., 1985, Pharmacokinetics of the anthracycline analog menogaril (NSC 269148). *Proc. Am. Soc. Clin. Oncol.*, **4**, 46.

Le Page, G. A., Khaliq, A. and Gottlieb, J. A., 1973, Studies of 9-β-D-arabinosyladenine in man. *Drug Metab. Disp.*, **1**, 756–759.

Le Page, G. A., Worth, L. S. and Kimball, A. B., 1976, Enhancement of the antitumor activity of arabinofuranosyladenine by 2′-deoxycoformycin. *Cancer Res.*, **36**, 1481–1485.

LePecq, J. B., Dat-Xuong, N., Gosse, C. and Paoletti, C., 1974, A new antitumor agent: 9-hydroxy ellipticine. Possibility of a rational design of anticancerous drugs in the series of DNA intercalating drugs. *Proc. Natl Acad. Sci. USA*, **71**, 5078–5082.

LePecq, J. B., Gosse, C., Dat-Xuong, N., Cros, S. and Paoletti, C., 1976, Antitumor activity of 9-hydroxyellipticine (NSC 210717) on L1210 mouse leukemia and the effect of the route of injection. *Cancer Res.*, **36**, 3067–3076.

Lessa, P., Lecointe, P. and Paoletti, C., 1977, The hydroxylation of the antitumor agent, Ellipticine, by liver microsomes from differently treated rats. *Biochem. Pharmacol.*, **26**, 2169–2173.

Long, H. L., Powis, G., Schutt, A. J., Moertel, C. G. and Kovach, J. S., 1985, Menogaril by 72-hour continuous intravenous infusion: A phase I study with pharmacokinetics. *Proc. Am. Soc. Clin. Oncol.*, **26**, 9.

Maftouh, M., Monsarrat, B., Rao, R., Meunier, B. and Paoletti, C., 1984, Identification of the glucuronide and glutathione conjugates of the antitumor drug N^2-methyl-9-hydroxyellipticinium acetate [Celiptium]. *Drug Metab. Disp.*, **12**, 110–111.

Malspeis, L., DeSouza, J. J. V., Staubus, A. E., Neidhart, J. A. and Grever, M. R., 1984, Pharmacokinetics of 2-F-ara-AMP in man during a Phase I clinical trial. *Invest. New Drugs*, **2**, 116.

Mathe, G., Hayat, M., DeVassal, F., Schwarzenberg, L., Schneider, M., Schlumberger, J. P., Jasmin, C. and Rosenfeld, C., 1970, Methoxy-9-ellipticine lactate III. Clinical screening: its action in acute myeloblastic leukemia. *Rev. Eur. Etud. Clin. Biol.*, **15**, 541–545.

McGovern, J. P., 1980, Activity of the anthracycline agent, 7-con-*O*-methylnogarol [7-OMEN] administered orally to mice bearing P388 or L1210 leukemia. *Cancer Treat. Rep.*, **64**, 727–729.

McGovern, J. P., Neil, G. L., Denlinger, R. H., Hall, T. L., Crampton, S. L. and Swenberg, J. A., 1979, Chronic cardiotoxicity studies in rabbits with 7-con-*O*-methylnogarol, a new anthracycline antitumor agent. *Cancer Res.* **39**, 4849–4855.

Meunier, G., Meunier, B., Auclair, C., Bernadou, J. and Paoletti, C., 1983, Unexpected regiospecific alkylation of the antitumor agent N^2-methyl-9-hydroxy-ellipticinium acetate with N, O or S donors. *Tetrahedron Lett.*, **24**, 365–368.

Monsarrat, B., Maftouh, M., Meunier, G., Dugue, B., Bernadou, J., Armand, J. P., Picard-Fraire, C., Meunier, B. and Paoletti, C., 1983, Human and rat urinary metabolites of the antitumor drug Celiptium [N^2-methyl-9-hydroxyellipticinium acetate, NSC 264137]. *Biochem. Pharmacol.*, **32**, 3887–3890.

Montgomery, J. A. and Hewson, K., 1969, Nucleosides of 2-fluoroadenosine. *J. Med. Chem..*, **12**, 498–504.

Neil, G. L., Kuentzel, S. L. and McGovern, J. P., 1979, Treatment of mouse tumors with 7-con-*O*-methylnogarol and other analogs of the anthracycline antibiotic, nogalamycin. *Cancer Treat. Rep.*, **63**, 1971–1978.

Noker, P. E., Duncan, G. F., El Dareer, S. M. and Hill, D. L., 1983, Disposition of 9-β-D-arabinofuranosyl-2-fluoroadenine-5′-phosphate in mice and dogs. *Cancer Treat. Rep.*, **67**, 445–456.

Paoletti, C., Cros, S., Dat Xuong, N., Lecointe, P. and Moisand, A., 1979, Comparative cytotoxic and antitumoral effects of ellipticine derivatives on mouse L1210 leukemia. *Chem.-Biol. Interactions*, **25**, 45–48.

Paoletti, C., LePecq, J. B., Dat-Xuong, N., Juert, P., Garnier, H., Amiel, J. L. and Rousse, J., 1980, Antitumor activity, pharmacology, and toxicity of ellipticines, ellipticinium and 9-hydroxy derivatives: Preliminary clinical trials of 2-methyl-9-hydroxy ellipticinium [NSC 264137]. *Recent Results in Cancer Research*, **74**, 107—123.

Plunkett, W., Feun, L. G., Benjamin, R. S., Keating, M. and Freireich, E. J., 1984, Modulation of vidarabine metabolism by 2′-deoxy-coformycin for therapy of acute leukemia. *Cancer Treat. Symp.*, **2**, 23–27.

Plunkett, W., Iacoboni, S., Estey, E., Danhauser, L., Liliemark, J. O. and Keating, M. J., 1985, Pharmacologically directed ara-C therapy for refractory leukemia. *Seminars in Oncology*, **12**, 20–30.

Pratt, E. A. and Adams, W. J., 1983, Pharmacokinetics of intravenous menogaril (NSC 269148) in the beagle dog. *Proc. Am. Ass. Cancer Res.*, **24**, 259.

Pratt, E. A., McGovern, J. P., Adams, W. J. and Hamilton, R. D., 1982, Bioavailability and pharmacokinetics of orally administered 7-con-O-methyl-nogarol [7-OMEN, NSC 269148] in the mouse. *Proc. Ass. Cancer Res.*, **23**, 171.

Pratviel, G., Bernadeau, J., Ha, J., Meunier, G., Cros, S., Meunier, B., Gillet, B. and Guitte, E., 1986, Ribose as the preferential target for the oxidized form of elliptinium acetate in ribonucleos(t)ides. Biological activities of the resulting adducts. *J. Med. Chem.*, **29**, 1350–1355.

Preisler, H. D., Rustum, Y. and Priore, R. L., 1985, Relationship between leukemic cell retention of cytosine arabinofuranoside triphosphate and duration of remission in patients with acute nonlymphocytic leukemia. *Eur. J. Cancer Clin. Oncol.*, **21**, 23–30.

Richardson, C. L., Grant, A. D., Sehpok, S. L., Krueger, W. C. and Li, L. H., 1981,

Template specificity of DNA binding by nogalomycin and its analogs utilizing competitive fluorescence polarization. *Cancer Research*, **41**, 2235–2240.

Riggs, C. E., Jr. and Bachur, N. R., 1983, Clinical pharmacokinetics of anthracycline antibiotics. In *Pharmacokinetics of Anticancer Agents in Humans*, edited by M. M. Ames, G. Powis and J. S. Kovach (Amsterdam: Elsevier/North Holland), Chapter 10.

Ross, W. E., 1985, DNA topoisomerase as targets for cancer therapy. *Biochem. Pharmacol.*, **34**, 4191–4195.

Ross, W. E. and Bradley, M. O., 1981, DNA double strand breaks in mammalian cells after exposure to intercalating agents. *Biochem. Pharmacol.*, **654**, 129–134.

Rowland, M. and Tozer, T. N., 1980, Hepatic clearance and elimination. In *Clinical Pharmacokinetics, Concepts and Applications*, edited by M. Rowland and T. N. Tozer (Philadelphia: Lea & Febiger), 65–76.

Rubin, J., Kovach, J. S., Ames, M. M., Moertel, C. G., Creagan, E. T. and O'Connell, M. J., 1987, A Phase I study of two schedules of teroxirone. *Cancer Treat. Rep.* (in the press).

Sato, S. M., Iwaizumi, K. H. and Tamura, Y., 1977, Electron spin resonance study of the mode of generation of free radicals of daunomycin, adriamycin and carboquone in NADPH-microsome system. *Gann*, **68**, 603–608.

Schilsky, R. L., Kelley, J. A., Ihde, D. C., Howser, D. M., Cordes, R. S. and Young, R. C., 1982, Phase I trial and pharmacokinetics of Aziridinylbenzoquinones (NSC 182986) in humans. *Cancer Res.*, **42**, 1582–1586.

Spiegel, J. F., Egorin, M. J., Collins, J. M., Lerner, B. D. and Bachur, N. R., 1982, The murine disposition and pharmacokinetics of the antineoplastic agent, Diaziquone (NSC 182986). *Drug Metab. Disp.*, **11**, 41–46.

Spreafico, F., Atassi, G., Filippeschi, S., Malfiore, G., Noseda, S. and Boschetti, D., 1980, A characterization of the activity of α-1,3,5-triglycidyl-*s*-triazinetrione, a novel antineoplastic compound. *Cancer Chemother. Pharmacol.*, **5**, 103–108.

Struck, R. F., Shortnacy, A. T., Kirk, M. G., Thorpe, M. G., Brockman, R. W., Hill, D. L., El Dareer, S. M. and Montgomery, J. A., 1982, Identification of metabolites of 9-β-D-arabinofuranosyl-2-fluoroadenine, an antitumor and antiviral agent. *Biochem. Pharmacol.*, **32**, 1975–1978.

Suffness, M. and Douros, J., 1980, Miscellaneous natural products with antitumor activity. In *Anticancer Agents Based on Natural Product Models*, edited by J. M. Cassidy and J. Douros (New York: Academic Press), pp. 466–469.

Svingen, B. A., Appel, P. L., Lieber, M. M. and Powis, G., 1980, Radical formation during cellular and subcellular metabolism of the chemotherapeutic agent AZQ. *Pharmacologist*, **22**, 177.

Svoboda, G. H., Poore, G. A. and Montfort, M. L., 1968, Alkaloids of *Ochrosia maculata* Jacq. [*Ochrosia borbonica* Gmel.]. *J. Pharm. Sci.*, **57**, 1720–1725.

Szmigiero, L. and Kohn, K. W., 1984, Mechanisms of DNA strand breakage and interstrand crosslinking by diaziridinylbenzoquinone (Diaziquone) in isolated nuclei from human cells. *Cancer Res.*, **44**, 4453–4457.

Szmigiero, L., Erickson, L. C., Ewig, R. A. and Kohn, K. W., 1984, DNA strand scission and cross-linking by diaziridinylbenzoquinone (Diaziquone) in human cells and relation to cell killing. *Cancer Res.*, **44**, 4447–4452.

Tewey, K. M., Chen, G. L., Nelson, E. M. and Liu, L. F., 1984 a, Intercalative antitumor drugs interfere with the breakage reunion of mammalian DNA topoisomerase II. *J. Biol. Chem.*, **259**, 9182–9187.

Tewey, K. M., Rowe, T. C., Yang, L., Halligan, B. D. and Liu, L. F., 1984 b, Adriamycin-induced DNA damage mediated by mammalian DNA topoisomerase II. *Science*, **226**, 466–468.

Tseng, W. C., Derse, D., Cheng, Y. C., Brockman, R. W. and Bennett, L. L., Jr.,

1982, In vitro biological activity of 9-β-D-arabinofuranosyl-2-fluoroadenine and the biochemical actions of its triphosphate on DNA polymerases and ribonucleotide reductase from HeLa cells. *Mol. Pharmacol.*, **21**, 474–477.

Von-Bac, N., Moisand, C., Gouyette, A., Muzard, G., Dat-Xuong, N., Le Pecq, J. B. and Paoletti, C., 1980, Metabolic and disposition studies, of 9-hydroxyellipticine and 2-methyl-9-hydroxyellipticinium acetate in animal. *Cancer Treat. Rep.*, **64**, 879–882.

Wozniak, A. J. and Ross, W. E., 1983, DNA damage as a basis for 4′-demethyl-epipodophyllotoxin-9-[4,6-*O*-ethylidene-β-D-glucopyranoside] [Etoposide] cytotoxicity. *Cancer Res.*, **43**, 120–124.

Zimet, A. S., Ohnuma, T., Parlow, L., Coffey, V. A., Holland, J. F. and Goldsmith, M. A., 1985, A Phase I trial of menogaril [7-con-*O*-methylnogarol] in a daily × 3 schedule. *Proc. Am. Ass. Cancer Res.*, **26**, 167.

Zimm, S., Collins, J. M., Curt, G. A., O'Neill, D. and Poplack, D. G., 1984, Cerebrospinal fluid pharmacokinetics of intraventricular and intravenous aziridinylbenzoquinone. *Cancer Res.*, **44**, 1698–1701.

Zwelling, L. A., Micheals, S., Erickson, L. C., Ungerleider, R. S., Nichols, M. and Kohn, K. W., 1981, Protein associated deoxyribonucleic acid strand breaks in L1210 cells treated with the deoxyribonucleic acid intercalating agents 4′-[9-acridinylamino]methansulfon-*m*-anisidide and adriamycin. *Biochemistry*, **20**, 6553–6563.

Zwelling, L. A., Micheals, S., Kerrigan, D., Pommier, Y. and Kohn, K. W., 1982, Protein associated deoxyribonucleic acid strand breaks produced in mouse leukemia L1210 cells by ellipticine and 2-methyl-9-hydroxyellipticinium. *Biochem. Pharmacol.*, **31**, 3261–3267.

Index